GUIDE TO CLINICAL STUDIES AND DEVELOPING PROTOCOLS

Guide to Clinical Studies and Developing Protocols

Bert Spilker, Ph.D., M.D.

Head, Department of Project Coordination
Burroughs Wellcome Co.
Research Triangle Park, North Carolina; and
Clinical Assistant Professor of Medicine and
Adjunct Associate Professor of Pharmacology
University of North Carolina School of Medicine
Chapel Hill, North Carolina

Raven Press ■ New York

Raven Press, 1140 Avenue of the Americas, New York, New York 10036

Made in the United States of America

Library of Congress Cataloging in Publication Data

Spilker, Bert.
  Guide to clinical studies and developing protocols.

  Bibliography: p.
  Includes index.
  1. Drugs—Testing. 2. Medical research—Methodology.
3. Human experimentation in medicine. 4. Medical
protocols. I. Title. [DNLM: 1. Drug Evaluation—
methods. 2. Research Design.   QV 771 S756g]
RM301.S68   1984   615.5′8′0724   83-43220
ISBN 0-88167-018-9

*To my friends and colleagues at Burroughs
Wellcome, who instructed me in both the science
and the art of clinical research.*

Preface

This monograph focuses on the development of protocols and the conduct of clinical studies for the evaluation of drugs from a clinical and scientific perspective, although relevant statistical concepts are presented and discussed. With minor modification, the items presented can be applied to clinical protocols directed toward the evaluation of nondrug treatments, interventions, or methodologies.

A system of checklists, tables, and figures that detail practical information render this book a guide for either drug or nondrug clinical studies. The checklists enable the author of a protocol to ascertain whether he/she has forgotten any important detail in the planning, implementation, conduct, and/or analysis of a clinical study. The checklists also may be used as a peripheral memory by individuals planning and/or conducting several studies at the same time, as opposed to either the use of a large variety of different paper/forms or reliance on memory. These checklists may be modified easily for studies with special requirements.

Numerous tables and figures list and illustrate possible approaches for the investigator to use or consider in dealing with a wide variety of issues that arise during a clinical study, such as testing compliance or tapering the dose of a drug. In addition, many of the questions that arise regarding various aspects of the protocol are presented, and possible responses or solutions are discussed.

Section I of this book presents the steps involved in developing a study design by emphasizing the processes used in the conceptualization of a study. Section II describes and emphasizes the criteria and methodologies used to develop and write the study protocol. The study protocol is viewed as an expression of how the study design will be implemented. The order of chapters in Section II reflects the general order in which an individual develops and writes a protocol rather than the order in which the separate parts of the protocol appear in the finished version. Therefore, the chapter dealing with the Introduction appears near the end of Section II. The same concept motivates the ordering of the chapters in Section III, which traces the processes involved in planning, initiating, conducting, and analyzing results of a clinical study.

Brief examples are given to clarify many of the statements and points listed in the tables.

This book has five major objectives: (1) to help the neophyte in clinical study experience gain insight and knowledge about the complexities and procedures of planning, initiating, and conducting a successful clinical study, (2) to assist the experienced individual who either seeks a series of checklists to use or desires to evaluate new variations on familiar themes, primarily those listed in the tables and illustrated in the figures, (3) to guide the university student in a pharmacy, pharmacology, or medical curriculum in his/her coursework on clinical studies and to provide information that will prove helpful for making career decisions, (4) to orient marketing and sales personnel, journalists, and other nonscientists whose positions require the transfer of scientific and medical knowledge to other nonscientists, and (5) to serve as a reference source for any individual interested in clinical protocols and/or the conduct of clinical studies.

It is understood that a certain amount of overlap and repetition occurs between sections and chapters in this book. This is primarily because some aspects of a clinical study may be discussed in more than one of the categories described. An attempt has been made to minimize redundancy except where it is considered as useful emphasis and important to the discussion.

The volume intentionally avoids detailed discussions on the roles and applications of statistics and epidemiology in protocol development. Many protocols are designed with epidemiological research tools, and virtually all protocols utilize statistical techniques for development of study design and analysis of data. The importance of statistics in clinical research is acknowledged, and the importance of working with a statistician throughout a protocol's planning, conduct, and analysis phases is stressed. There are, however, numerous books that focus on these areas (e.g., Hill, 1971; Lancaster, 1974; and Friedman et al., 1981).

This book provides practical details beyond those found in previously published articles and books describing protocol development (Harris and Fitzgerald, 1970; Abrams, 1976; Chaput de Saintonge, 1977; Friedman et al., 1981; and Cato, 1982).

This book is directed to clinicians and scientists who will develop protocols and, possibly, conduct the clinical study as well. It is intended as a practical guide for professionals who are concerned with clinical studies, whether from the vantage of investigator, staff, sponsor, participant, or outsider, whether in an academic institution, private practice, sponsoring organization, regulatory agency, or organization approaching such studies from a different perspective.

Acknowledgments

It is my pleasure to acknowledge the help of many people who assisted me with this book. I am indebted to Dr. David Barry, Dr. John Rogers, and Dr. Hugh Tilson who reviewed the entire manuscript and made many valuable suggestions.

The author owes a special debt of gratitude to Dr. John Schoenfelder, who gave his time unstintedly to help improve the quality of this book and remove many ambiguities that were present.

Other individuals also contributed to this book in terms of valuable discussions and/or review of selected segments or chapters. The author appreciates their important input: Ms. Nancy A. Bauer, Drs. Larry Bell, M. Robert Blum, Gilles Cloutier, Ms. Kathryn Crean, Drs. Walter B. Cummings, Joanne Data, Ronald Deitch, Robert E. Desjardins, Richard J. Fleck, Michael F. Frosolono, Ms. Pamela Griffin-Lyon, Messrs. Dan W. Heatherington, Paul A. Holcomb, Jr., Dr. J. Heyward Hull III, Mr. M. James Louis, Drs. Loren Miller, Lawrence A. Nielsen, J. Greg Perkins, Warren C. Stern, Joel E. Sutton, Richard L. Tuttle, Ms. Judy Van Wyck Fleet, Drs. Tom Williams, and David Yeowell.

The author thanks Msses. Thomasine Cozart, Joyce B. Carpunky, and Rosemary K. Freeman for assistance in the preparation of this book and Messrs. David R. Price and Rolly Simpson for help with literature searches.

Contents

Section III: Planning and Conducting Clinical Studies

Terminology

A few comments should be made on some of the terms used throughout this work. Numerous words, including "patients," "volunteers," and "subjects," are used in the literature to denote participants in clinical studies. The term "patient" is used almost exclusively throughout this work but is intended to also cover those cases in which the term "volunteer" would be appropriate. The term "volunteer," when used, is defined as a normal individual who participates in a study for reasons other than medical need and who does not receive any direct medical benefit from the study. The term "disease" is used throughout this book in a broad sense, which includes reference to the patient's condition, problem, risk factors, or reason for treatment or evaluation. It is understood that some instances occur in which the use of this term is not entirely appropriate.

The phrase "adverse reactions" is used to denote physical and psychological symptoms and signs experienced by patients that may be related to the study drug. This term is also referred to as "side effects" by other authors. The term "adverse experience" is used to encompass adverse reactions plus any injury, toxicity, or hypersensitivity that may be drug related, as well as any medical events that are apparently unrelated to drugs that occur during the study (e.g., surgery, illness, and trauma). "Clinical studies" refers to the class of all scientific approaches to evaluate drugs. "Clinical trials" constitute a subset of drug studies that evaluate drug safety and efficacy according to official (or nonofficial) guidelines. Although drugs may be evaluated for their use in diagnosis, therapy, or prophylaxis, this distinction is not often made in this book, since the concepts discussed are generally germane for all types of drug studies.

List of Tables

Section I

Section II

Section III

List of Illustrations

Section I

Section II

Section III

Section I

Developing Study Designs

1 Establishing Study Objectives

Introduction • Types of Drug Studies • Study Objectives •
Phases of Clinical Testing

INTRODUCTION

Before a total commitment is made to initiate and conduct a study, careful consideration should be given to the question of why the study has been proposed. Is it based on someone's casual comment that such a study would be a "good idea" or an "important study to undertake"? Whatever the reason(s) for the study, they should be carefully evaluated from the point of view of whether that study is truly necessary to answer the question(s) posed.

The actual need for a study should always be addressed and demonstrated, since there are sometimes relatively simple alternatives to conducting a study. The questions that prompted the proposal to conduct a study may sometimes be answered through a literature search and evaluation, or possibly one or more "experts" or consultants could be asked for their views. A third possibility is that the study may have already been performed. This could be the case if a new question is raised on an established drug. One should inquire with the company that developed or markets the drug. If the potential author is in a pharmaceutical corporation, then older data in the files on the potential study drug should be reviewed.

A principle that many investigators consider fundamental is that one should seek the least complex approach to answering or addressing a clearly stated clinical problem, hypothesis, or question. In formulating an approach to the question to be addressed in the study and in establishing the study design to answer that question, it may be helpful to think of the approach as a balance between breadth and depth. For example, if the objective of a study were to examine the effect of a new drug for its general analgesic properties, it would not be as valuable in the initial study to evaluate a small group of patients intensively in great detail (in depth) as to study a larger group of patients more generally (in breadth). In-depth studies are usually directed towards determining the answers to, or information on, specific questions, such as bioavailability or mechanism of action. Studies that emphasize a broad approach (breadth) include many Phase III clinical studies, where the objective is to gain information on how a large population of patients will react to the study drug under usual (and unusual) conditions. (The four phases of drug studies in the United States are operationally defined later in this chapter.)

3

The study design is the framework by which the study objectives will be met. The design is generally established after the study objectives have been clearly elucidated. Otherwise, one may be in the position of attempting to fit the questions to be answered (i.e., study objectives) to an imposed or fixed study design. If it is not possible to implement a study design acceptable for addressing the objectives posed, then it may be necessary to refine or modify the study objectives.

There are several reasons why the specific study design required to address the study objectives may be either unsuitable or impossible to adopt. The design might require (1) methods that are beyond the state of the art in the particular field of medicine involved, (2) equipment that is too expensive or too difficult to obtain or operate, (3) too many patients, (4) efforts that are too arduous for patients to meet comfortably, (5) too long a period to conduct, (6) too much manpower to conduct, or any other numerous possibilities. Thus, it may be necessary to revise the study objectives to bring them within the limitations imposed on the study design by resources, state-of-the-art considerations, or other factors.

TYPES OF DRUG STUDIES

There are several basic classes of clinical drug studies that address different types of purposes (goals) for the study. Although the exact number and description of these classes are arbitrary, a brief synopsis of each category will provide a basis for orienting one's major and minor study objectives and for understanding the variety of different purposes for drug studies.

Safety Evaluation

Although a safety evaluation constitutes an important part of almost all clinical drug studies, some studies are designed with a safety evaluation as their primary purpose. These studies include most of those conducted in Phase I. Safety is a broad topic that encompasses dose tolerance (i.e., how high a dose patients can receive without having clinically significant adverse reactions, physical signs, and/ or laboratory abnormalities), dose frequency, and duration of exposure to a drug.

Pharmacokinetic Evaluation

Establishing the relevant pharmacokinetic parameters in humans is an important part of the development of all drugs. This type of study concentrates on investigating one or more of the following basic pharmacological concepts: absorption, distribution, metabolism, and excretion.

Efficacy Evaluation

Studies concentrating on efficacy are usually initiated in Phase II of clinical development, although important information can sometimes be gleaned from Phase I studies (e.g., when a drug is expected to cause a specific change in a laboratory parameter in normals as well as in patients).

Mechanism of Action Evaluation

Clinical studies may be designed to elucidate the mechanism of action of an investigational or marketed drug. This category would include evaluations of drug interactions.

General Population Evaluation

The therapeutic use of a new drug in a general patient population is primarily evaluated during Phase III and IV clinical studies.

Evaluation of Clinical Methodology

A drug may be used as a research tool in developing and/or testing new techniques for the evaluation and/or validation of a specific methodology.

Evaluation of Clinical Pharmacology

Although this group of studies overlaps to some degree with other types of studies, this category includes evaluation of new dosage formulations (e.g., tablets versus capsules), new routes of adminstration, new dosage regimens (e.g., b.i.d. versus t.i.d. dosing), and/or other characteristics of a drug's pharmacological profile.

Postmarketing Evaluation

This category consists of the varied types of Phase IV studies that are designed to identify rare or infrequent adverse reactions as well as beneficial effects not previously known or evaluated with a new (or established) drug. Specific types of epidemiological studies are described in Chapter 5.

After one of these broad types of studies has been identified as the major purpose or goal for the proposed study, study objectives must be established that are to be addressed within the framework of the above study type.

STUDY OBJECTIVES

Study objectives are concise statements of the major and minor questions that the study is designed to answer. The author should reflect on the objectives and confirm that they represent valid and proper questions, or series of questions, to propose. If an underlying question is the basis of the proposed objective, then it may be desirable to modify the objective to reflect the underlying consideration. If other individuals will assist in developing the protocol, one should obtain their agreement that the established objectives are appropriate, correctly stated, and will meet the goals or purposes of the study. The overall study goals (purposes) are differentiated from the objectives in that the former represent the type of study to be conducted (see previous section), whereas the objectives are the concise statements that will enable the goals to be achieved.

In all types of studies, the objective should be stated as specifically and succinctly as possible in the protocol. It is not suitable to write that the objective is "to determine the mechanism of action of drug X," since this objective is too general, vague, and merely restates the overall goal of the study. It is preferable to write that the study objective is to evaluate the effects of daily dose T of drug W in population X on parameters Y and Z by continuous or daily recording of results obtained in tests A and B during time period C, as compared with drug D at dose E, under the same experimental conditions.

Many methodological and statistical problems are created if too many questions are posed in one protocol. Posing many questions often creates an excessive number of subgroups of data, some of which may be insufficient in quantity to answer the questions posed. In addition, posing many questions often makes the study difficult to conduct and decreases the probability of having the study completed successfully. Nonetheless, one must be sensitive to the large number of potential questions from which the most optimal ones are chosen and be aware of the many potentially informative analyses that may provide valuable insights for future studies.

After the objective is agreed on, it must be determined whether it is feasible to address the objective with known clinical methodology. If the clinical methodology exists, then one must determine whether it is possible, in terms of time, money, manpower, and other practical concerns, to mount the effort necessary to complete the clinical study. It is understood that some practical considerations cannot be fully addressed until a general or detailed study design has been chosen, evaluated, and reviewed with statisticians. It is thus possible that in subsequent stages of developing the study design, the study objectives may have to be modified. These modifications will allow a protocol to be written that will address its goals within the framework of available methodologies and resources.

If the objectives of the study relate to the evaluation of drug safety, then the study design chosen will depend on which aspects of safety are of particular interest for evaluation. Safety considerations may focus on the doses used, laboratory results, physical examinations, adverse reactions, or other areas. If the purpose of the study is focused on determination of safe doses, then the study objective may relate to evaluating the safety of doses for (1) dose ascension (e.g., a rapid and/or slow rate of dose ascension may be evaluated), (2) "loading" the patient, (3) determining the maximally tolerated maintenance dose, or (4) defining a safe rate of dose taper. Numerous other questions related to "safe doses" may also be posed, such as the safety of a sudden withdrawal of the drug.

There are numerous other purposes for conducting a clinical study. Study goals and objectives may be developed that relate to comparative claims with other drugs, labeling of the drug, new dosage strengths or formulations, and establishment of various parameters related to pharmacokinetics. Although the study's primary objective(s) may be focused on efficacy or pharmacokinetics, an evaluation of safety or drug toxicity is virtually always performed at the same time, even if it is not a stated objective and is conducted in a nonrigorous manner.

Modifying or changing objectives after a study has been initiated will usually cause major problems in the analysis and interpretation of the data obtained and in the acceptance of that data by the medical community. An example of this problem arose in the Anturane Reinfarction Trial, but the details of that situation, which are not described here (see Anturane Reinfarction Trial Research Group, 1980; Temple and Pledger, 1980, for a description and discussion of the issues raised).

Thus, it is essential at the outset of a study to consider the evaluations and study objectives that may be important or useful to consider after the data have been collected. It is also well known that as the number of statistical tests performed increases, the chances of finding at least one result that is statistically significant by chance alone also increases. If 100 independent statistical comparisons are made, then on the average, five will be significant (if the level of statistical significance is $\alpha = 0.05$ and there are no differences between the comparison groups). Thus, the number of measurements made and analyses performed will have at least some bearing on the significance of the data obtained.

PHASES OF CLINICAL TESTING

The purpose and objectives of a study are usually related to some degree with the phase of clinical testing the study drug is in. In the United States, there are four phases of clinical testing, which are referred to frequently in this book. These phases may be defined in regulatory or operational terms. The following are operational definitions that are used throughout this book.

Phase I

Phase I consists of initial testing of a study drug in humans, usually in normal volunteers but occasionally in patients. Safety evaluations are the primary and almost always the sole objectives, and the attempt is made to establish the approximate levels of patient tolerance for acute and usually multiple dosing. Some preliminary efficacy data may be obtained in selected studies.

Phase II

Phase II studies are initial studies designed to evaluate efficacy in selected populations of patients for whom the drug is intended. The first part of Phase II often consists of pilot studies, which may be open label or single or double blind. The second part of Phase II consists of pivotal well-controlled studies that usually represent the most rigorous demonstration of a drug's efficacy. Relative safety information is also determined in Phase II studies.

Phase III

These studies are conducted in patient populations for which the drug is eventually intended. These studies generate additional data on both safety and efficacy in relatively large numbers of patients under normal use conditions in both controlled and uncontrolled studies. These studies provide much of the information that is needed for the package insert and labeling of the drug.

Phase IV

After a drug is marketed, studies are often conducted to provide additional details required to learn more about the drug's efficacy and/or safety profile. Different formulations, dosages, durations of treatment, drug interactions, and other drug comparisons may be evaluated. New age groups, races, and other types of patients can be studied. Detection and definition of previously unknown or inadequately quantified adverse reactions and related risk factors are an important aspect of many Phase IV studies. If a marketed drug is to be evaluated for another (i.e., new) indication, then those clinical studies are considered as Phase II studies. The term postmarketing surveillance is frequently used to describe those studies in Phase IV (i.e., following marketing), which are primarily observational or nonexperimental in nature, to distinguish them from Phase IV clinical studies.

2 Preliminary Considerations Relating to Study Design

Factors Involved • Role of the Statistician • Consideration of Study Bias • Prospective Versus Retrospective Approaches • Pilot Studies

FACTORS INVOLVED

It is important to consider several factors in creating a study design. A list of many of the factors that constitute a study design is presented in Table 2.1. Some of these are more important in certain protocols than in others. For example, the major objective of a clinical study might be to compare two routes of administration of a new drug, whereas in other studies the choice of the route of administration may be a relatively minor factor or not subject to choice (e.g., if the drug is only available in one form).

Establishing a rough hierarchy of the importance of the factors constituting the study design within a given study is sometimes helpful in deciding which of these factors to consider initially. Once this decision is made, a design can be chosen by evaluating the possible variations for each of the relevant factors. One must insure that the overall design created in this manner can be implemented within the resources available. If the design is complex and/or involves numerous options, it may be useful to construct algorithms or flow charts to help others to understand the study design more easily. The criteria for the choices to be made at each

TABLE 2.1. *Factors considered in constructing a basic study design*

1. Establishing study objectives
2. Preliminary considerations
    Role of the statistician
    Consideration of study bias
    Prospective versus retrospective approaches
    Pilot studies
3. Types of blinds
4. Controls used in clinical studies
5. Choice of overall study design
6. Sample size and number of parts of a study
7. Randomization procedures
8. Screening, baseline, treatment, and posttreatment periods
9. Patient population and methodological considerations
10. Dosing schedules
11. Considerations of pharmacokinetics and drug interactions
12. Forms of drugs
13. Routes of administration

decision point must be established in advance and clearly described in the protocol. Although algorithms may help to clarify complex study designs, it is the author's opinion that they are rarely necessary.

There may be constraints on choosing a study design imposed by the objectives of the study. One example is where investigational drugs are being evaluated in Phase I, II, or III. In such cases, the study design chosen must fit general Food and Drug Administration (FDA) guidelines for the specific phase of investigation. Also, if the data expected to be obtained from the study are to be combined with data from other studies, then the data collected should be able to be integrated with the other data. This may necessitate using a standard study design in multiple studies. This concern must also be reflected in the design of data collection forms in order to insure that data collected are in the desired format. Careful attention must be paid to using compatible, if not completely identical, systems of disease classification and terminology to describe the classification, especially if the data sets obtained in the various studies are to be merged.

ROLE OF THE STATISTICIAN

Before discussing each of the elements of a basic study design, it is important to review the role of the statistician in the following areas:

1. Study objectives. In most situations the statistician should review the objective(s).
2. Study design. This is discussed below in this chapter.
3. Interim analyses. If these are to be performed, then their influence on the study design must be determined.
4. Early termination of the study. Criteria must be established in advance for studies using a sequential design and are sometimes established in advance for fixed-sample-size studies in which interim analyses are contemplated.
5. Analysis of the data. The statistician should prepare his/her approach(es) to the data in advance. Prototype tables and figures may be prepared (see Section II and Appendix 2 for details).

Two statistical terms that should be familiar to investigators and clinical scientists are type I error (α) and type II error (β). The magnitudes of these errors are usually determined by the investigator before a study begins, often in collaboration with the statistician. These are important concepts, because they are used in the determination of sample size and also reflect how a study will be viewed by the medical community.

Type I error (α) is the probability of declaring a statistical difference when in fact there is none. It may be viewed as the significance level necessary for the statistical test to detect a difference between treatments that is clinically meaningful (e.g., $\alpha = 0.05$). This also means that the probability of a false–positive result is not greater than 0.05. Type II error (β) is the probability of not detecting the difference that is looked for if it is present (i.e., the chance of missing a real effect). Power (defined as $1 - \beta$) is the probability of detecting this difference. It is desirable to have a high power or probability of detecting a difference between treatments, and the goal of any study is to have small type I (α) and small type II (β) errors. If the study is limited by fixed resources, however, it will be difficult (or impossible) to achieve both goals. Since there is a trade off between the two types of errors, it will be necessary to decide which goal is more important.

CONSIDERATION OF STUDY BIAS

One of the main purposes in choosing and developing a clinical strategy to develop a new drug is to attempt to reduce known biases that may compromise the analysis and interpretation of the clinical data. Where biases cannot be eliminated, it is important to define them so that they may be considered when conclusions are drawn from a study.

In the early planning stages of a clinical study, one should be aware of biases that may either influence or become part of a study. Biases may be introduced into a clinical study at any stage in the planning, conduct, or analysis. Seven general stages or categories of bias were described by Sackett (1979). He indicated that the biases may occur in:

1. Examining the literature in the field.
2. Specifying and selecting the study sample.
3. Executing the experimental maneuver (or exposure).
4. Measuring exposures and outcome.
5. Analyzing the data.
6. Interpreting the analysis.
7. Publishing the results.

Sackett described 57 examples of biases in a "catalog" and gave a reference for many. This catalog (plus references) is presented in Appendix 1. Many biases may not be extirpated from a study if they are introduced as part of the study design, and these often represent the primary reason why otherwise well conducted and analyzed studies are not accorded credence by the medical community. Other types of pitfalls that may trap an unwary author are discussed in Chapter 26.

In trying to reduce bias, the author of a protocol should be familiar with the most common sources of bias and have a statistician evaluate the protocol, since many biases have a statistical basis. Randomized controlled studies have the greatest probability of reducing bias, and observational, cohort, case-controlled, or uncontrolled studies have the greatest propensity to include bias. Potential biases range from the more obvious to the arcane. Among obvious sources of bias, three can briefly be mentioned as illustrative examples:

1. Extrapolation of data from one group of individuals to the entire population often leads to substantial errors. This may occur in clinical studies if the initial choice of the population sampled is not a true cross section of the desired (reference) population.

2. Patients with a known disease may be questioned many times about factors possibily relating to etiologies, but a normal control group may be questioned less intensely and less frequently. This may lead to a "recall bias," especially if the questions are difficult to answer and/or sensitive.
3. Patients with a worse prognosis may be overwhelmingly assigned to receive one treatment rather than another. This will make it much more difficult for that treatment group to demonstrate the response that would have been noted if the two treatment groups were equal.

These and additional biases are described in more detail by Feinstein (1967) and Sackett (1979).

PROSPECTIVE VERSUS RETROSPECTIVE APPROACHES

It is widely accepted that well-designed prospective studies yield less biased, more scientifically acceptable data than do comparable retrospective studies. The retrospective (e.g., case-control survey) study is quite useful, however, under certain conditions. It is useful when the objective is to generate rather than to test hypotheses, and it is generally less expensive than a prospective study. The retrospective survey is subject to a great deal of bias, and thus results are often seriously questioned. For example, the criteria for patient inclusion and adequacy of documentation must be clearly established before a survey of patient records is initiated. The more precisely the patient entry criteria are defined, the better is the chance that a meaningful analysis and interpretation of the data will be obtained. A clinical survey may be either retrospective or prospective; in this book, however, a clinical study is defined as being prospective.

PILOT STUDIES

There are situations in which a pilot study is more appropriate to conduct than a full-scale or fully-controlled study. A pilot study is used to obtain information deemed necessary for further clinical studies. Although pilot studies are often unblind and use open-label drug, they may also be single or double blind and may include tight control on all appropriate variables. The term "pilot" refers to the purpose of the study. A number of common reasons that are advanced for conducting a pilot study are presented in Table 2.2.

Once a decision to conduct a pilot study is reached, a further decision must be made as to whether it should be conducted as a separate study or integrated into a controlled study. If the finalization of details in the study design of a controlled study would depend on data generated in an open-label pilot study, it is the author's view that the pilot and controlled study should be separate. If, however, the pilot study is intended to give the investigator experience with the drug and the controlled study has a finalized protocol and could be run independently, then combining these two parts may be beneficial from an administrative viewpoint.

TABLE 2.2. *Common reasons for conducting pilot studies*

1. Dose ranging with a new drug or with an old drug being evaluated in a new therapeutic area
2. Initial efficacy evaluation of a new drug
3. Initial efficacy evaluation of an established drug for a new indication
4. Determination or clarification of details requiring refinement prior to finalizing the protocol for a larger or similar clinical study (e.g., to estimate the degree of variation in the measurements obtained); this information can help estimate the required sample size more accurately
5. Determination of details required to finalize plans for the conduct of the study (e.g., to conduct "dry runs" through complex protocols; to determine the duration required to conduct a drug study)
6. Evaluation of the methodology to be used in another study
7. Evaluation of a variable related to the clinical pharmacology of a drug (e.g., b.i.d. versus t.i.d. dosing) in a rapid and noncontrolled manner
8. Development of clinical experience by research personnel with a drug under open-label conditions prior to initiation of a double-blind clinical study
9. Determination of the actual availability of patients for enrollment in a study as opposed to the expected availability
10. Exploration of ethical questions relating to whether a specific placebo-controlled double-blind study (or other study design) is ethically acceptable to conduct with the study drug

The concept of using pilot patients as a vanguard may be relevant in some studies to confirm that the study drug is safe or that the procedures are suitable, safe, and operational before exposing a larger number of patients. This is especially relevant in Phase I studies, where the safety of a new drug may be almost completely unknown. But the use of pilot patients is not advised in a well-controlled study.

The term "pilot study" sometimes has the connotation of being a "quick and dirty" evaluation. A sloppy approach, however, will not provide reliable information and may raise new questions (and problems) that have to be addressed. Therefore, a pilot study must be planned with as much care as a full-scale controlled study.

3 Types of Blinds

TYPES OF BLINDS

The term "blind" refers to a lack of knowledge of the identity of the study treatment. Patients, investigators, ancillary personnel, and monitors are the major groups of individuals who may be kept blind during a drug study. Blinding is used to decrease the biases that occur in a clinical study when patients are evaluated during treatment and to avoid a placebo effect that often occurs in open-label studies. The types of blind of patients and investigators in a clinical study are described below.

1. Open label. No blind is used. Both investigator and patient know the identity of the drug.
2. Single blind. The patient is unaware of which treatment is being received, but the investigator has this information. In unusual cases, the investigator and not the patient may be kept blind to the identity of the treatment.
3. Double blind. Neither the patient nor the investigator is aware of which treatment the patient is receiving. A double-blind design is generally considered to provide the "most" reliable data from a clinical study. This type of study, however, is usually more complicated to initiate and conduct than single-blind or open-label studies.
4. Combination of blinds. (a) In part 1 of a study, one type of blind may be used (e.g., single blind), and in part 2 of the same study, another blind (e.g., double blind) may be used. A third part of the same study may utilize the same blind as part 1 or use an entirely different type of blind. (b) Some patients may follow a protocol under one type of blind and others follow the same protocol under a different type of blind. (c) The blind used may be changed during the course of the study according to certain criteria (e.g., when inpatients are discharged, the double blind may be broken, and they may continue their treatment on open-label medication).

BLINDS IMPOSED ON INVESTIGATORS AND/OR PATIENTS

The use of a blind in a clinical study may adversely affect the physician–patient relationship, since in a double-blind study neither one will know what treatment is being given, and one (usually the patient) will not know the treatment in a single-blind study. This situation may create a strain on their relationship.

Maintaining an effective double blind is extremely challenging or even impossible in some studies. If certain data collected (e.g., blood levels of study or concomitant drugs, specific adverse reactions) would effectively destroy the blind, then a system may be constructed to keep this information from the investigator in order to preserve the blind. One imaginative technique that has been used to maintain the double blind in some studies may be referred to as the "two-physician method." Physician 1 speaks with and examines patients at each visit. Physician 1 also evaluates the therapeutic response and possible drug toxicity but does not receive any laboratory or other information that might unblind the study. Physician 2, who is unblinded, receives the report from Physician 1 as to possible drug toxicity on each patient as well as all laboratory data. Physician 2 is then able to adjust the dose of drug(s) the patient is receiving according to guidelines in the protocol.

In some studies it may be necessary to use a separate placebo tablet (or other drug form) for each study or active drug or for each size of two or more dose strengths of the study drug. In this "multiple-placebo" or "double-placebo" method, two (or more) separate containers are dispensed to each patient. Each bottle will contain either study drug or placebo and will provide the appropriate medication and dosage for patients when they take the required number of capsules or tablets from each bottle at each dosing time (i.e., group A receives drug A and placebo B; group B receives placebo A and drug B; and group C receives placebo A and placebo B). Two cases in which this technique is particularly useful are when two different routes of administration are being compared (e.g., a topical cream versus a tablet for treatment of a skin disorder) and when two different formulations are being compared (e.g., a long- and short-acting drug).

BLINDS IMPOSED ON THE MONITOR(S)

Monitors are individuals or groups who observe the conduct of a clinical study to confirm that it is adhering to its protocol and to assist with problems that may arise in the conduct of the study. These roles and other functions of the monitor are described in detail in Section III of this volume.

The decision of whether to impose a blind on the monitors should be made prior to initiation of a study. A number of possible approaches to imposing a blind on the clinical study monitors are listed below:

1. All monitors of a study are blind to patient treatment in order to avoid introducing bias.
2. Some but not all of the monitors are blind during the clinical study.
3. No blind is imposed on the monitors even though the clinical study itself may be double blind.

If a monitor remains blind to patient treatment, it must also be determined whether or not the monitor will be privy to interim summarizations and/or analyses generated during the study. If monitors are made cognizant of such data, then a bias could be introduced into their relationship with investigators, even though the blind in a study would literally remain intact.

BLINDS IMPOSED ON ANCILLARY PERSONNEL

In some double-blind studies, pharmacists or other personnel who package drugs must be unblinded. It is preferable that all individuals who normally interact with the investigator, patients, and others conducting the study remain blind. Some results (e.g., ECGs, X-rays) may be interpreted by a person blind to the identity of the patients' treatment even in an open-label study.

IMPORTANCE OF DOUBLE-BLIND STUDIES: TWO EXAMPLES

The importance of utilizing double-blind studies whenever possible and practical is illustrated by two actual examples. In the first, an antidepressant was evaluated for anti-Parkinson's Disease activity in two studies with identical study designs except that one was open-label and the other was double-blind (versus placebo). In the open-label study, eight of 12 (67%) patients significantly improved (by at least 30% in efficacy scores) on active drug treatment, but in the double-blind phase (conducted at the same time in different patients), only two of eight patients (25%) improved (C. G. Goetz, C. M. Tanner, and H. L. Klawans, *personal communication*). All patients received single-blind placebo for the first week of treatment in order both to identify and exclude early placebo responders from both the open-label and double-blind studies. These results are reminiscent of a report in the psychiatric literature that stated that 83% of uncontrolled studies reported positive results, but only 25% of controlled studies were positive (Foulds, 1958).

The second example is that of a single-blind study and a double-blind study conducted by the same group of scientists who evaluated the effect of zinc on hypogeusia (decreased taste acuity). In the single-blind study, patients who failed to respond to placebo significantly improved their hypogeusia with zinc therapy (Shechter et al., 1972). This led the same authors to perform a randomized, double-blind, crossover study in which no difference between zinc sulfate and placebo was observed (Henkin et al., 1976).

CHECKING THE VALIDITY OF A DOUBLE-BLIND STUDY

If a blind is to be incorporated into a study design, then it is important to check the validity of the blind prior to, during, and after the study is completed.

Prior to the beginning of the study, the blind is "validated" by considering how it will be implemented and maintained plus a review of ways in which it may be challenged or broken during the study. "What if" exercises may be useful in determining whether a sound system of blinding the study has been created.

During the study, the monitor or other appropriate individual(s) may evaluate how well the blind is being maintained. Discontinued patients may be closely questioned on this point. If it is apparent that the blind in a study is not effective, then measures may be taken to modify the protocol to strengthen the blind. Alternatively, nothing may be done, or the study may be changed to an open-label study. Other possibilities certainly exist for dealing with the situation in which the integrity of the blind has been compromised.

After the study has been completed, all patients and the investigator may be asked to guess which treatment each patient received. This technique is described in the section on "End of Study Questionnaire" in Chapter 37.

4 Controls Used in Clinical Studies

*Types of Controls in Clinical Studies ● Tightly Designed
Protocols ● Comments on Control Groups ● Number of Active Drug and
Placebo Control Treatment Groups*

TYPES OF CONTROLS IN CLINICAL STUDIES

There are several ways of defining "controls" in clinical studies. Two definitions are used in this book, one specific and one broad. In the specific definition, "control" refers to the existence of a group of patients who receive a treatment used for comparison with the study drug. Examples include placebo control, active drug control, and historical control groups.

The broad definition of control relates to the adherence of the study to a tightly designed protocol. The purpose of this control is to reduce the variability of many factors and biases that might influence the study. One of the factors that could be designed tightly would be the number of comparison groups of patients.

TIGHTLY DESIGNED PROTOCOLS

A controlled study using the broad context of the term is one in which at least some of the elements of the study design are relatively fixed and are not allowed to vary. The broad concept implies, however, that control is not all or none (i.e., a controlled or uncontrolled study) but rather involves a relative degree of control. The greater the number of factors of the study design that are specified and the more tightly they are delineated, the greater is the control that is built into the study. In a "well-controlled" Phase II study, there traditionally is tight control on most of the important factors that are expected to vary. Since almost all aspects of a study design may affect the degree to which a study is controlled, careful thought is required to evaluate which study design to choose and how tightly to control each aspect of that design. The final study design chosen is the basic framework or organization of the entire study, and it should be established only after comprehensive discussions with statisticians, experienced colleagues, and investigators.

Controlled drug studies do not always require the use of a placebo or active drug control group. For example, two groups of patients may be given the same fixed dose of a test drug with an additional factor (e.g., surgery, concomitant drug) that acts to help control the study design.

If patients cannot be taken off their present drugs, then the study may be designed as an "add-on" evaluation of the test drug. Under those circumstances, controlling the study requires that the name, dose, reason for use, and effectiveness of each concomitant drug be strictly documented and monitored. Another concern in the control of many studies relates to the presence of nondrug treatment modalities such as individual (or group) psychotherapy or other psychological therapies for testing many drugs that are acting on the central nervous system, or the heat, manipulation, braces, exercises, bed rest, and physiotherapy that are used concomitantly with medication to treat back pain. The presence of nondrug modalities may be ignored or either loosely or tightly controlled in the protocol of a drug study.

An example of a relatively minor factor that may be controlled is the number of physicians seen by a patient. In any clinical study in which more than one physician is involved, it is usually considered optimal to have each patient see the same physician at each visit. The same consideration applies to other study personnel. Evans (1979) has demonstrated, however, that this is not essential in all clinical situations.

COMMENTS ON CONTROL GROUPS

An important factor to control in any study is the makeup of the groups of patients being evaluated. The inclusion criteria are the major means by which these groups are made more (or less) homogeneous. The assumption is usually made that the greater the similarity between the groups, the more likely it will be that any differences found in the data from a well-controlled study are caused by the study drug and not by chance or other factors. In choosing the type(s) of individuals who will constitute the control group, it may be important to specify whether patients with the same (or related) disease, random volunteers, healthy medical students, blood donors, nearby laboratory technicians, professional personnel, or others are to be included in the study.

The use of multiple control groups (using the specific definition of control) may be the optimal means in some studies to solve the problem of establishing the most suitable control group. This solution may be especially relevant for clinical studies to which large amounts of resources are being devoted to achieve the study objectives. If, for example, a drug is being evaluated in patients with a given disease who undergo surgery, it may be necessary to have both a control group with the same disease who are not undergoing surgery and a control group without the disease who are undergoing the same surgery. The use of two (or more) control groups in a study should be considered if the additional groups will add valuable or essential information. There is a possibility, however, that adding unnecessary control groups in a study may yield equivocal data and raise additional questions. Another possible control group to include in a study could be a "no-treatment" observational group, although this approach is not commonly followed in Phase I, II, or III drug studies. The no-treatment control group fails to account for the pill-giving ritual and any effects that this event may have on efficacy. A group receiving a low dose of a study drug may act as a control group in a design where a dose-response relationship is being established (see Chapter 24). The principle to follow in establishing a control group is that the control patient population should be as identical to the study population as possible.

NUMBER OF ACTIVE DRUG AND PLACEBO CONTROL TREATMENT GROUPS

When a new drug is being evaluated, it is often important to incorporate an active drug and/or a placebo medication as controls into the study design. A well-established standard drug (active drug) may be used as a control in addition to, or in place of, a placebo control group. Active drug controls such as the use of aspirin in evaluating new analgesics and antiinflammatory agents are an accepted tradition in some areas of drug development. Before an active control may be incorporated into a pivotal study design, however, it must be unequivocally demonstrated that the active drug actually does work (i.e., is active) and is generally accepted to work. This latter point is especially relevant when pivotal studies on investigational drugs are submitted to regulatory bodies, and these agencies must be willing to accept an active drug's inclusion into the study. As a general principle, placebo-controlled drug studies are preferable to active drug-controlled studies. If both an active drug and placebo may be incorporated into a study design, then this design is preferable in almost all cases to either the inclusion of an active or placebo control alone. The case against using an active drug as a control without a separate placebo group was presented by Temple (1982).

In nonpivotal drug studies, the investigator or clinical scientist need not have the same constraints about including an active drug without placebo. The same comments, however, apply to how the results of the study will be viewed in the medical community. That reception will depend on the quality and nature of the results obtained as well as on the disease being studied. It is not considered ethical to compare a new investigational study drug as monotherapy with placebo in certain diseases (e.g., epilepsy). In the case of evaluating a new antiepileptic drug, add-on studies are often performed with a study drug versus placebo. After a new drug has demonstrated efficacy, then future studies may be designed in which concomitant drugs are removed one at a time (perhaps at 2- to 4-month intervals) to arrive at the point where the new drug is evaluated as monotherapy.

5 Classification of Study Designs

INTRODUCTION

It must be stressed that the present system of classification of study designs is somewhat arbitrary and is not necessarily considered to represent the most ideal manner of describing study designs. There are various other systems or means of classifying study designs that might be more appropriate for some individuals to use. One of the reasons this situation exists is that there is some degree of overlap between various study designs.

SINGLE GROUP OF PATIENTS

In some open-label or single-blind studies, all patients are treated with the same drug throughout the study. Criteria may be established to change patients from one drug to another or to allow for dosage reductions (e.g., for adverse reactions) or dosage increases (e.g., for lack of toxicity and/or lack of optimal improvement). Thus, a single homogeneous group of patients at the start of a clinical study may complete the study as a heterogeneous group of patients because each was treated with a different dosing regimen.

Study designs utilizing historical controls could be considered as either a single group of patients or two groups of patients. In this book, studies using historical controls are discussed as designs with two groups of patients.

TWO GROUPS OF PATIENTS

Parallel and Crossover Designs

The two most common designs utilizing two groups of patients are the parallel (noncrossover) and crossover designs. The parallel design is applicable to most experimental situations. It is "robust" (i.e., tolerant) to many kinds of problems that can occur in clinical studies (e.g., missed visits, missing data). In the parallel design, patients are randomized to one of two treatment groups and usually receive the assigned treatment during the entire study. The treatments assigned to the two groups differ. Each group generally receives either study drug or placebo, one of two different study drugs, or one of two doses of the same study drug. Two placebo medications could also be evaluated. One variation of the parallel design is for each group to receive alternating (and escalating) doses of the same drug. Some of the possible variations of a parallel design are shown in Fig. 5.1.

In the crossover design, each patient receives both treatments being compared in the study. If one of the treatments is placebo, then the effect of the study drug may be expressed as the difference between responses to the two treatments. The variability of data obtained with this design is less than that associated with those obtained with the parallel design (i.e., within-patient differences are used to assess treatment differences in a crossover study, whereas between-patient differences are used to assess treatment differences in a parallel design). Because of its increased sensitivity and smaller variability, the crossover design requires fewer patients than does the parallel design to detect the same effect. For the same sample size, the parallel design is less sensitive in detecting differences between two treatment groups than is the crossover design.

In order to use a crossover design, the patient must have a stable (usually chronic) disease during both treatment periods, and a similar baseline condition must be present at the start of each of the two treatment periods. It is obvious that if the patient's baseline differs markedly at the start of each treatment, then it is impossible to compare the two treatment effects accurately. Not only must the baselines be similar, there must not be any carryover (i.e., residual) effects (even psychological ones) after either treatment. This means that the disease manifestations should revert to the same baseline and that the effect of the treatment should disappear when either treatment is stopped. One of the major reasons that this design is not used more frequently is that a carryover effect is noted after many drugs are stopped. The test for carryover effects may not be adequately sensitive to confirm the absence of this phenomenon. Thus, the data obtained with a crossover design may be challenged even when no carryover is observed. An additional reason why this design is not used more often is that many chronic diseases vary in their intensity or in frequency and number of episodes; thus, similar baselines are not likely to occur. The crossover design is also well suited to bioavailability studies. A period of at least 10 half-lives is usually allowed between the two periods of the crossover.

The order of the two treatments in a crossover design is usually randomized so that half the patients receive treatment A in period 1 and treatment B in period 2, whereas the other half receive treatment B and then treatment A. It is possible in an open-label crossover design for one treatment to be an "observation" and not a

---

FIG. 5.1. Selected schemata for treatment periods of parallel studies. Baselines are not illustrated, and time is along the *abscissa*. Unless indicated, each part may be conducted in either a single-blind or double-blind manner. In **schemata 1 to 4**, each treatment group may constitute a different dose or drug. In **schema 3**, the placebo trial may be conducted at the end of the study. In **schema 4**, the placebo trial may be conducted at an announced or unannounced time during the treatment and for a specified or unspecified duration. In **schema 5**, each dose is of a fixed or variable length, and doses may be given in an ascending or random order. One or more of the doses in each treatment group may be a placebo, or each of the two treatment groups could be subdivided into two or more subgroups (e.g., drug and placebo) at each dose period.

I. COMMON PARALLEL DESIGNS

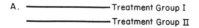

A. ─────────── Treatment Group I
    ─────────── Treatment Group II

B. ─────────── Treatment Group I
    ─────────── Treatment Group II
    ─────────── Treatment Group III

2. TWO PART PARALLEL STUDY

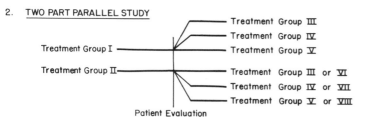

Treatment Group I ────────── Treatment Group III
                             Treatment Group IV
                             Treatment Group V

Treatment Group II────────── Treatment Group III or VI
                             Treatment Group IV or VII
                             Treatment Group V or VIII

Patient Evaluation

3. PARALLEL DESIGN WITH PLACEBO INITIATION

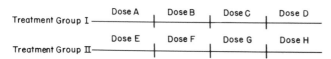

Placebo ────────── Treatment Group I   (ex: Test Drug)
                   Treatment Group II (ex: Different Dose of Test Drug,
                                             or Active Control)
                   Treatment Group III (ex: Placebo)

Patient Evaluation

4. INTRODUCTION OF PLACEBO DURING TREATMENT

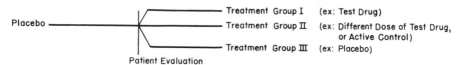

Treatment Group I	Placebo	Treatment Group I
Treatment Group II	Placebo	Treatment Group II
Treatment Group III	Placebo	Treatment Group III

5. MULTIPLE DOSES WITHIN EACH TREATMENT GROUP

Treatment Group I ── Dose A │ Dose B │ Dose C │ Dose D

Treatment Group II── Dose E │ Dose F │ Dose G │ Dose H

6. PARALLEL EVALUATION OF A COMBINATION DRUG

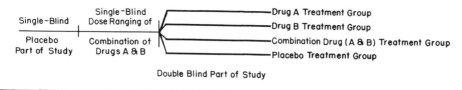

Single-Blind Placebo Part of Study	Single-Blind Dose Ranging of Combination of Drugs A & B	Drug A Treatment Group
		Drug B Treatment Group
		Combination Drug (A & B) Treatment Group
		Placebo Treatment Group

Double Blind Part of Study

◄───►
TIME

drug or placebo. The analysis of data obtained with a crossover design is adversely affected by patient dropouts and missing data (i.e., the analysis is not as "robust" as with a parallel design).

In designing a crossover study, it must be determined whether the change from one treatment period to another will be time dependent (e.g., after 10 weeks on treatment A all patients will be switched to the second treatment), or whether it will depend on the condition of the patient's disease state. The former practice is usually preferable. Another issue is whether or not to inform the patient at the time when their treatments are switched. It is not necessary to do this if the patient has been generally apprised of this event in the informed consent.

A "double-crossover" design refers to a study in which each group of patients receives each treatment twice during the study. Three or more crossovers are also possible in a study. Figure 5.2 illustrates a number of variations of the crossover design. The extra-period design attempts to avoid one of the major problems of the crossover design, i.e., the presence of residual effects.

If the data are examined at the end of the first treatment period, and the difference between treatment groups is highly significant, then it may not be ethically permissible to continue the study (see section on early study discontinuation).

Matched-Pair Designs and Historical Controls

Two other study designs using two groups of patients are matched pairs and historical controls. Neither of these designs is as scientifically and statistically reliable as the parallel and crossover designs, although there can be certain exceptions. Both matched pairs and historical controls were used more frequently in the past.

The matched-pairs design is a type of parallel design in which pairs of patients who are "identical" in respect to all relevant factors are identified. One patient is randomized to receive treatment A and the other to receive treatment B. This method is more applicable to acute drug studies than to chronic ones. Because of the difficulty of identifying well-matched pairs, this technique is difficult to use if recruitment proceeds slowly, but if all patients begin a drug study at approximately the same time, this technique becomes easier to implement. The matched-pairs design can also be implemented within one individual; in this case, one arm, eye, or foot receives one treatment, and the other arm, eye, or foot receives the other treatment. One major problem with this design, however, is that all relevant factors may not be known.

With the historical control design, all patients receive the same study drug treatment. The control group is composed of similar patients who were previously treated, sometimes by different investigators. The weakness of this method is that it is almost impossible to have an adequately controlled historical group and to have known all the relevant information required. Even if the historical study included the same patients as in the active treatment part of the study, major differences might still be present. Using the same patients, however, would add a

I. SINGLE CROSSOVER WITH NO INTERVENING BASELINE

(i.e., No drug-free interval)

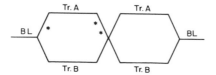

2. SINGLE CROSSOVER WITH INTERVENING BASELINE

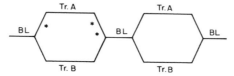

3. DOUBLE CROSSOVER WITHOUT INTERVENING BASELINES

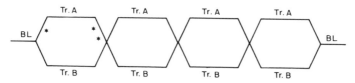

4. DOUBLE CROSSOVER WITH INTERVENING BASELINES

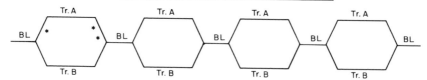

5. EXTRA PERIOD CROSSOVER

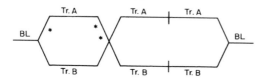

6. OPEN-LABEL CROSSOVER WITHOUT RANDOMIZATION

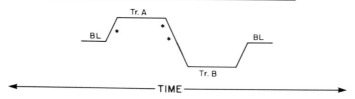

← TIME →

FIG. 5.2. Selected schemata for crossover studies. **Schemata 1 to 5** may be open label, single blind, or double blind. BL, baseline; Tr.A, treatment A; Tr.B, treatment B. *, Dose ascension part of each period. **, Dose taper part of each period. All baselines that occur after treatment has been initiated include washout of drug. In **schema 1**, there is usually a brief washout period between treatments A and B. Although the change from one treatment to another in all schemata is shown as being time dependent, it is possible that this change may be dependent on the condition of the patient's disease state.

degree of credibility to the study, but no randomization would have been performed, and significant investigator and/or patient bias could easily have entered the study (e.g., differences may have arisen through changes in diagnostic criteria, personnel treating the patient, or concomitant therapy).

Historical control data may be derived from the literature, from patients' medical charts, or from a centralized and possibly computerized data bank within a large institution. This latter technique for obtaining patient information is one means of improving the quality of historical controls. If adequate data are retained from completed clinical studies, they will help to surmount one of the major problems of this type of study, i.e., lack of sufficient information to confirm that patients in the two groups are comparable.

Another method of improving the validity for the use of historical controls is to include two control patients for each test patient and to analyze for differences between patients. It is preferable to use unpublished data for historical controls, since there is a well-known bias towards publishing positive data. The case for using historical controls in certain situations was recently presented by Lasagna (1982). The inclusion of historical controls (i.e., clinical experience) is frowned on in current medical research, and data obtained are seldom accepted as definitive. The degree to which historical controls in a study design are accepted depends in large measure on their objectivity.

Sequential Designs

A novel study design that has not been widely used to date is called sequential design and analysis. Sequential designs are variations of parallel studies in which patients are assigned to receive one of two treatments. Figure 5.3 shows the results of a hypothetical double-blind study to illustrate the use of sequential analysis. Each patient in this study would have received simultaneous treatment with a new

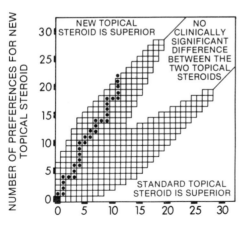

FIG. 5.3. Illustration of sequential design procedure. (Reprinted by permission of Futura Publishing Co. from Rodda, 1974.)

and standard topical steroid on different lesions (e.g., drug A on one limb and drug B on the contralateral limb) for a period of time. After each patient completes the protocol, a choice is made by the investigator (based on various criteria) as to which of the two steroids was preferable or whether it was impossible to discern a distinction in efficacy. For every preference for the new steroid, one mark in a vertical direction is made in the figure, and for each preference for the standard steroid, one mark in the horizontal direction is made. No marks are placed on the figure when a choice cannot be made between the two treatments. Patients are entered into the study until one of the three boundaries illustrated in the figure is reached. In the case illustrated, 33 preferences were made before a decision was reached (i.e., that the new topical steroid was superior to the standard drug). The graph does not indicate the number of patients in whom no distinction between the two treatments was made. The major emphasis of sequential design and analysis is focused on the time at which sampling in a study should be stopped.

Another type of sequential design is the group sequential approach. In this design, a number of patients are entered and studied. An interim analysis of the data is then conducted, and if the results are significant or if the treatment groups are totally alike, then the study is stopped. If there is a difference between the two groups that is nonsignificant (statistically), then a second group of patients is enrolled, and the same type of randomization is used as was employed for the original group.

A third type of sequential study design is the "play-the-winner" design. If patients are entered into a study in specific blocks (e.g., 20 patients at a time), then patients in the second and subsequent blocks are assigned to treatment groups as data are generated in the study. In this "play-the-winner" design, there may be 20 patients in the first group studied, 10 on placebo and 10 on active drug. If positive data (preferably, "all-or-none" responses are determined) are found in eight of 10 on active drug and in four of 10 on placebo, the assignment of treatments to the second group of 20 patients will overplay the winner and put 15 patients on active drug and only five patients on placebo. Because of the relatively recent introduction and unproven validity and acceptance of this method, this approach should be reviewed thoroughly with a statistician before it is adopted as a study design. This design provides several potential advantages: (1) fewer patients are needed to complete a study with a highly effective drug than for a study with a fixed sample size, (2) if only a few patients with a particular disease or problem are available, then this design may offer a significant advantage over more traditional study designs, (3) there is a savings in the cost of the study, and (4) a more rapid answer may be reached about a supposedly superior therapy.

The negative aspect of this methodology is that it is not suitable for most clinical studies, since a study must have a number of characteristics for this design to be appropriate, including simple study design, limited scope of hypotheses, and rapid evaluability of effects (i.e., the results of the study must be able to be determined in a short time interval). Planning budgets, packaging drugs, and other practical aspects of the study are more difficult administratively with this design, and data for different sites cannot be pooled even if the same protocol is followed at all sites. An additional negative aspect is that if the two therapies being evaluated are comparable in their efficacy, this technique may require more patients than would be required in a conventional drug study design. The reader is referred to Rodda (1974) and Thompson (1980) for more details on this technique.

MULTIPLE GROUPS OF PATIENTS

Although many variations of study design are possible using multiple groups (i.e., more than two), the vast majority are based on the two main concepts described above, parallel and crossover designs.

A well-known type of crossover design involves the use of the Latin square. In this "complete-crossover" design, each group of patients receives each treatment, but in a random order. In addition, the design is balanced in that each treatment is given first to one group, second to one group, third to one group, etc. for the number of groups included in the design. An example of this is shown below. This permits each patient to serve as his/her own control. A period of time usually elapses between successive parts of the study to allow for any carryover effects from prior treatment to disappear and to establish a new baseline.

| | Treatment | | |
	Period 1	Period 2	Period 3
Group I	A	B	C
Group II	B	C	A
Group III	C	A	B

When a decision is made to select the number of groups of patients in a study design, the opportunity also exists to form a number of subgroups. For example, two doses of a study drug plus placebo may be evaluated in a parallel study. Each of the three groups may be subdivided on the basis of gender or disease severity or other characteristics. Many imaginative and useful variations are possible in the formation of subgroups. One potential "trap" is to establish a large number of subgroups with too few patients in each to yield meaningful statistical analyses.

If the results of a study are difficult to anticipate, and one does not wish to expose a substantial number of patients to the risks of toxicity from a particular drug or dose, it may then be appropriate to use a pilot group of patients. The pilot group would consist of a small number of patients who are given the drug (or dose) before the larger group is exposed. The pilot group could remain in the vanguard and test each higher dose of a new drug, with the larger group(s) following after initial assurance of relative safety has been obtained.

TYPES OF EPIDEMIOLOGICAL STUDIES

Studies of drugs may be performed using the techniques of epidemiological research. These may be either experimental or nonexperimental in design. Some of these study designs are similar to those previously discussed but are presented here specifically as they relate to their epidemiological application.

Experimental Study Designs

The epidemiologic designation for experimental studies is appropriate when those studies involve large populations and/or address public health rates and issues. In general, experimental epidemiologic studies utilize prospective designed protocols and are of three basic types.

Clinical Studies

These are the traditional prospective Phase III type disease treatment studies described in detail in this book, but in the present context, they address "epidemiological" questions or issues such as the ability to reduce transmission rates of infectious disease through treatment of a segment of the community. In such studies, outcomes are often measured at the population level (in terms of attack rates) as well as at the individual level. An interesting variation of this approach is the so-called risk factor reduction study in which the study measures nontraditional outcomes rather than the disease parameters usually monitored in clinical studies.

Field Trials

These studies involve the evaluation of large-scale field studies of drugs, vaccines, or other biologicals for the prevention or management of disease. These studies usually require more patients than clinical studies and are conducted at the patients' homes, schools, workplaces, or central locations. They often use observational approaches but are considered experimental designs inasmuch as they actively select persons who will or will not be exposed to treatment.

Community Intervention Studies

These studies are essentially field studies in which one or more entire communities may be involved (Morgenstern and Bursic, 1982). In a strict sense, the community intervention study requires that the entire community be exposed, since results are compared to control communities in which the treatment was not implemented. Examples of community intervention studies include analysis of the effects of water fluoridation and evaluation of the presence of paramedical rescue teams in a given community.

Nonexperimental (Observational) Study Designs

Drug development and evaluation do not always require, nor is it always appropriate to conduct, randomized clinical studies. There are clinical situations in which it is either unethical, undesirable, or unnecessary to conduct double-blind, randomized, controlled studies. In these situations, it is often possible to conduct observational studies to determine the outcome of drug treatment. Observational studies record specific events that are occurring in a defined population without any intervention with the population studied.

Nonexperimental studies include most of the studies performed in pharmaco-epidemiology and usually measure drug safety in routine use. Attempting to utilize experimental studies to address many specific epidemiological issues would incur enormous expenses. Another reason for using nonexperimental methods to answer epidemiological questions is that it is ethically unacceptable to expose people to toxic drugs or other conditions that may have been encountered as a result of industrial, natural, or man-made disasters or situations (e.g., radiation exposure resulting from a nuclear weapons explosion). Nonexperimental epidemiological studies differ from usual clinical studies in that the former (1) generally observe medical or health outcomes without actually intervening in patient encounters, (2) usually involve more patients (often over 1,000), (3) study situations in which patients receive drugs through normal prescribing practices, and (4) follow patients who are treated according to routine clinical practice, often over long periods of time. Approval of the study protocol by an ethics committee and the obtaining of patient informed consents are not always required and may be inappropriate in some cases, since it would compromise the basis and assumptions of the observational approach.

There are two major types of nonexperimental (observational) studies, (1) passive monitoring of events and reports and (2) active surveillance that includes cohort and case-control studies.

Passive Monitoring of Events and Reports

The primary use of passive observational monitoring studies is for assurance of safety and/or early detection of relatively uncommon but clinically important adverse reactions.

Although not "technically" a form of study at all, relatively unstructured monitoring for signals in medicine represents the backbone of epidemiology, including pharmacoepidemiology. Known as "epidemiologic intelligence," this approach deploys a wide spectrum of "sentinel" devices in an attempt to elicit from the background incidence of disease (1) unusual clusters, (2) increases in incidence, or (3) unexpected or (4) inexplicable phenomena. For adverse reactions attributable to medications, such monitoring consists of ongoing solicitation of "news" about problem cases in medical practices in which practitioners suspect that a drug may have caused a problem—solicitation by pharmaceutical sales representatives on their "detailing" visits, solicitation by the Food and Drug Administration (FDA) through its *FDA Drug Bulletin*, requests for examples of unexpected drug-associated events by specialty groups (e.g., the drug-induced ocular side-effects registry), and, of course, spontaneously discovered associations by concerned practitioners reported voluntarily to the manufacturer, the FDA or United States Pharmacopeia (USP), or, if unusual enough, through the published literature as an article, case report, or letter to the editor.

Active Surveillance

On the basis of extensive public debate and detailed evaluations of the limitations of the "epidemiologic intelligence" approach, the Joint Commission on Prescription Drug Use (Melmon, 1980) recommended that more active postmarketing surveillance (observational cohort or case-control) studies should be instituted (perhaps even mandated) for all major new drugs. The Commission also emphasized the usefulness of large-population observational studies for the possibility of developing new hypotheses and uncovering serendipitous discoveries about drugs. These are two important areas that (like detecting adverse reactions) are not expected to be compromised by the biases of nonblinded techniques. Nonetheless, numerous other biases would be present (e.g., biases of patient selection, different treatment regimens, lack of standardized evaluation criteria) when nonblinded techniques are used.

Observational studies to explore efficacy have the greatest potential to provide useful clinical data when the desired effects of the drug are opposite to the inherent tendencies and trends within the study. Examples of this would occur when a drug (1) saves patient lives that would be lost if no treatment were provided, (2) arouses a patient from a coma, (3) provides immunological protection against a common disease such as measles, or (4) provides prophylactic protection in well-characterized medical situations. Observational studies are most often used in Phase IV postmarketing surveillance studies to evaluate drug safety. Observational Phase IV studies to further explore drug efficacy are described by Strom et al. (1983).

Despite the recommendations of the Joint Commission on Prescription Drug Use, experience with large observational studies monitoring for drug safety has not been entirely satisfactory. An FDA review of three major postmarketing studies (cimetidine, cyclobenzaprine, and prazocin), which included from 7,607 to 22,653 people, concluded that the studies did not reveal any adverse reactions to these drugs that were not previously known. But physician case reports that were spontaneously submitted ("epidemiologic intelligence") provided information on new adverse drug reactions for two of these three drugs (Rossi et al., 1983). Lasagna (1983) commented on this report with sobering statistics indicating that rare adverse reactions (one event in 10,000 or more patients) will almost never be observed with formal Phase IV studies, which for logistic and/or financial reasons rarely involve even 10,000 patients. Lasagna concluded that spontaneous physician reports will remain an important source of new information about previously unknown benefits and risks of marketed drugs. It is clear that new approaches and methodologies are required to improve the usefulness of postmarketing surveillance studies.

The basis for choosing either the cohort or case-control study methodology is dependent on the amount of drug use and whether the suspected events being studied occur frequently or rarely. For rare (but identifiable) events of a frequently used drug, the case-control methodology is superior, whereas for more frequent events of a less frequently or rarely used drug, the cohort methodology is better. If both drug use and the event studied are frequent, then either method will be adequate to use, but if both drug use and the event studied are rare, then neither method will work well.

If the cost, logistics, and feasibility of case-control and cohort designs are comparable, the cohort method is preferable because of the inherent biases of the case-control methodology. When use of a newly approved drug is to be monitored for early detection of adverse reactions, only the prospective cohort method is applicable.

Cohort Studies

A cohort is a population or group that is followed forward in time. The cohort study is similar to clinical studies except that patients are not randomly assigned to a specific treatment or group prior to the study. One type of cohort study is the situation in which two or more groups of people (with one major difference between them) who do not have a disease are followed forward in time, and the incidence of the disease is periodically measured in each group. The Framingham, Massachusetts cardiovascular disease study is an example of a public health cohort study. Cohort studies may be either prospective, retrospective (historical), or a combination of both. The control group (i.e., control cohort) may be defined to be similar to the study cohort, or data obtained in the general population may be used.

The application of this methodology in the pharmaceutical area involves assembly of a population exposed to a drug or class of drugs and a comparable population that has not been exposed. The study may be designed to generate or test a hypothesis. Outcomes are compiled in both populations, and the rates compared. Unusual or unexpected results may be evaluated in additional studies.

Case-Control Studies

In this type of study, a group of cases and a group of controls are chosen, or a matched patient is located for each "case" patient; they are equivalent in all relevant factors except for the disease that only the case patient has. The investigator then looks back in time to learn what important differences existed between the two patients or the two groups, especially in terms of exposure. Such historical investigation may provide valuable information as to why the case patient developed this particular disease.

For this method to be most effective, all cases with the disease in a defined population must be included in the study. The controls would be chosen from the same defined population such that they would qualify as case patients if they had the disease. Two examples of defined population are (1) all persons seen at a given clinic or clinics and (2) all persons within a given geographical area. The case group may represent the entire population of patients who have the disease, or they may be a subset of the entire population.

There are several rules that apply to the proper choice of a control, but these are not described in detail here. Suffice it to say that a process that requires recall is highly sensitive to problems of scientifically unacceptable bias, both subtle and obvious. The interested reader is referred to the epidemiological literature for additional methodological details. It is recommended that expert counsel be obtained before case-control studies are initiated.

6 Sample Size and Number of Parts of a Study

Sample Size • Number of Parts of a Study

SAMPLE SIZE

The number of patients required for a clinical study (sample size) refers to the number of patients who finish a study rather than the number who enter. Thus, in planning a study the definition of a "completed" patient is important to establish, as is the expected rate of patient dropouts. An important result may fail to be detected if too few patients complete a study. Another problem that may occur if too few patients complete a clinical study is that a false–positive result may occur. Although a false–positive result may occur in all studies, the chances of its happening are higher with fewer patients. It follows that "guesstimates" of sample size are not scientifically acceptable for controlled studies even if made by experienced individuals. For all studies, the required sample size is usually determined by statisticians on the basis of (1) the magnitude of the effect expected (and/or desired), (2) the variability (often estimated) of the variables being analyzed, and (3) the desired probability (power) of observing that effect with a defined significance level. A power of 80% (0.8) is usually chosen as adequate for most controlled studies.

There are two main types of sample size to consider: fixed and sequential. When a fixed sample size is used in a study, the number of patients in each group may be fixed (1) at a defined number, (2) within a narrow or broad range, (3) by a minimum number, or (4) by a maximum number. In a sequential study design, the final number of patients enrolled will depend on analyses performed throughout the study. In this design, a significant result can be obtained more rapidly and probably with fewer patients than with a fixed sample, provided that there is a real difference to be detected.

If multiple objectives (e.g., both safety and efficacy) are included in a study, then each will probably require a different sample size. The larger the expected difference in magnitude of the effect between drug and placebo or between two drugs, the smaller is the sample size that will be required to detect this difference. Thus, a study generally requires larger sample sizes to demonstrate the smaller differences expected in safety parameters between a drug and placebo and smaller sample sizes to demonstrate the larger differences expected in efficacy parameters. On the other hand, the smaller variability in data obtained (e.g., with vital signs) may mitigate against the requirement for larger sample sizes to show smaller differences. When multiple sample sizes are computed, the most reasonable one should be utilized. This often requires compromises and an ordering of the most important objectives to be addressed.

In determining sample size, one must address the consideration of establishing a suitable ratio of patients between the two (or among three or more) treatment groups. There are basically two choices: either using equal-size samples in all treatment groups or using unequal- but proportional-size groups (e.g., using a 2:1 ratio that assigns 12 patients to receive drug X and six to receive placebo). The general rule to follow is that groups of equal size are preferable from a statistical perspective for clinical studies, although not all statisticians would require equal-size groups in all situations. An advantage of using equal-size treatment groups is that the study gains in power. Losses of power are not great, however, and may be acceptable if the ratios are no more than 2 or 3 to 1. A disadvantage of using equal-size groups is that more information may be gained on patient responses to a new drug if unequal-size groups are used and more patients receive the study drug.

Some statisticians advocate that all patients should have an equal chance of receiving a study drug and thus would assign patients in a study with a high- and low-dose group and placebo group in the ratio of 1:1:2 (i.e., twice the number on placebo as in either of the other groups). From a practical and often ethical point of view, patients are usually more willing to enroll in a drug study when the chance of their receiving active drug is greatest. Thus, this particular apportionment of patients would make the study more difficult to initiate than an equal distribution of patients among groups, or an apportionment in favor of the drug group. The relative importance of the patient's feelings in determining the ratio of group size in a study relates to a large degree on the particular disease studied and the severity of its symptomatology. A patient with severe chronic pain will be less willing to enter a study in which the chances of getting placebo are 50% than one in which the chances are about 10%.

NUMBER OF PARTS OF A STUDY

If two or more study designs are included within one protocol, then the study may be said to have two (or more) parts. Even with only one study design, there may be two (or more) parts if different patient populations are treated in each part. There are a number of possibilities to consider in determining the number of parts to incorporate into a study. These parts may be essentially independent, or they may be dependent on each other. A protocol with dependent parts means that a decision must be reached or an evaluation made after the first part has been completed (or has reached a certain point in the protocol) about whether to proceed, or on what basis to proceed, with the next part. It is also possible that specific aspects of the study design in the second part cannot be finalized until data from the first part are available and analyzed [e.g., an ED_{50} (dose that elicits 50% of the total response) may have to be calculated after part 1 of a study is completed so that this dose may be given to patients in part 2].

When planning the protocol design, one must decide if significant decisions are to be incorporated into a protocol. If they are, it must be clearly defined who will be making each decision, that is, whether it will be the sponsor, the investigator, or both. It should also be specified if decisions will be made on the basis of blinded or unblinded data and what criteria will be used in reaching the decision.

There are two opposite positions that are often taken in incorporating major decisions affecting study design into a protocol. Most investigators and individuals who design studies prefer that a protocol have a clearly defined problem that can be addressed in a clearly defined manner and limit the protocol to that evaluation. According to this viewpoint, any decision that must be made during a study to define or modify the design requires a new protocol.

The opposite position allows for decisions to be incorporated at specific points in the protocol, which will then permit continuation of the study with a modification not fully defined at the outset of the study. The logical extension of this latter approach, however, is a protocol that allows more and more decisions and modifications of design during the study and becomes progressively more vague at the outset as to exactly what will be done at each step of the study. One variation of this approach is to define the criteria for all modifications to the protocol in advance. Obviously, the Institutional Review Board, regulatory bodies, and other groups that must approve the study will act to prevent extreme examples of allowing unspecified changes in a protocol to occur during a study.

The number of distinct parts of a study must be determined in advance even if progression between subsequent parts of the study is "automatic" and does not require any decisions to be made. For example, if a given drug is evaluated in patients with two different diseases using the same protocol design, the drug may be studied in patients with disease A in part A and disease B in part B. Another example occurs when a pilot and well-controlled study are both incorporated into one protocol rather than separated into two distinct protocols. Since there are many possibilities of which types of studies may be combined into a single protocol, practical and realistic guidelines, as well as the established guidelines of a sponsoring institution (for sponsored studies), must be followed in determining the number and types of parts of a study.

7   Randomization Procedures

Background • Simple Randomization • Block Randomization • Systematic
Randomization • Stratification • Minimization • Other Variations of
Randomization Procedures • Obtaining and Using Randomization Codes

BACKGROUND

Randomization is the process by which patients in a clinical study are "randomly" assigned to receive one of the treatments being evaluated. Randomization is used to reduce bias in assigning patients to treatment and is usually implemented through a randomization code that assigns patients to different treatments. In a two-period crossover study, a randomization code usually determines the order by which patients receive treatments. In a Latin-square design (usually with three or more periods), a randomization code is also used to determine the order in which patients receive treatments. Patients may be randomized to different treatment groups in open-label, single-blind, or double-blind studies, but its use is most important in double-blind studies. It is in double-blind studies that a suitable process of randomization is essential to determine how well the blind will be maintained and, in part, how the results of the study will be viewed and judged.

Simply using an alternating ABABAB order for assigning patients to one of two treatment groups (coded A and B) is not acceptable for double-blind clinical studies. The investigator will tend to develop biases that one treatment is preferable, and patients may be purposely placed in one group or the other by the investigator. Also, if the study code is broken for one patient, then it is effectively broken for all patients.

Advantages of using randomization in a controlled study include the following:

1. Randomization procedures attempt to decrease the effect of interjecting one's own biases (either known or unknown) in assigning patients to treatment groups. They should minimize the differences in relevant characteristics of the groups receiving treatment in a parallel design.
2. Randomization permits certain statistical methods to be used with the resulting data.
3. Randomization allows for blinding of the patient and/or the investigator in the sense that if the blind is broken for one patient, it is not broken for all.
4. Randomization procedures are the current norm for demonstrating efficacy and safety of investigational drugs.

Two limitations of using randomization in a clinical study are these:

1. The randomization procedure alone often will not adequately eliminate the differences between the treatment groups. If baseline values were widely

divergent between the two treatment groups, it could create a major problem for the interpretation of the results. If there was a characteristic known to have a bearing on the outcome of the study that was not found to be equal in the two groups studied, then an interpretation of the results obtained might be seriously challenged. For example, if a drug is being evaluated for prevention of myocardial infarction in patients with heart disease and the risk factors for having a myocardial infarction were not evenly divided between the two groups chosen by randomization procedures, then an interpretation of the results might be seriously questioned. Randomization will not insure an equal distribution of risk factors or other relevant patient characteristics to each treatment group. There is a technique called stratification that can minimize the probability of obtaining an unequal distribution of important patient or disease characteristics between groups. The pros and cons of stratification are discussed later in this chapter.

2. Incorporating an appropriate randomization process into a clinical study may be complex and/or difficult to administer and thus pose practical problems that will have to be considered and solved in advance.

There are many methods used to randomize patients. The basic types of randomization are (1) simple randomization, (2) block randomization, (3) systematic randomization, (4) stratification, and (5) minimization.

SIMPLE RANDOMIZATION

Simple randomization is a procedure that uses a code to assign all patients to receive one of two (or more) different drug treatments at the start of the study (i.e., prior to treatment). This code is usually generated prior to the initiation of the study and usually assigns treatments based on the order of patients admitted to the study.

In studies in which the same patients receive progressively higher doses of a study drug at each visit, as in some Phase I single-dose studies, it may be advantageous to carry out a new randomization at each clinic visit (dosing period) for patients to receive either the study drug or placebo. Alternatively, the original randomization of patients to treatment groups could be maintained throughout the study. One advantage of conducting a new randomization of patients prior to each dosing is that it may minimize the psychological apprehension of volunteers who had experienced adverse reactions and believe that they have received the active study drug. Another advantage is that a larger number of patients will be exposed to the test drug. One disadvantage, however, is that the pharmacokinetic data obtained will not be as complete, since each patient may receive different doses of a drug or different numbers of doses. Another disadvantage will be that interpretation of dose–response data will be more difficult.

BLOCK RANDOMIZATION

In the block randomization method, a block size (e.g., four, eight, or 20 patients) is chosen, and the number of patients assigned to each treatment is proportional (1:1, 2:1, 3:1) within the block size chosen. For example, if a block size of eight is chosen and there are two treatments, then for every block of eight patients entered, if a balanced block (equal numbers of patients are assigned to each treatment) is used, four will receive one treatment and four will receive the other. It follows that the block size chosen should be divisible by the total number of treatments (e.g., for three treatments, block sizes of six, nine, and 18 are possible). The main advantage of using a block randomization is that if the study does not enroll the full number of patients expected, there will still be an equal or approximately equal number of patients in each treatment group for a balanced block and proportional numbers of patients in each group for a proportional block randomization.

A variation on the block randomization is to use blocks of variable size, although there are not many instances when this precaution would be necessary. The first block is sometimes larger than subsequent blocks, especially if it is believed that the investigator will attempt to "second guess" the assignment of patients to treatment. A block size of two is not used (except for matched pairs), since only two possibilities exist for randomizing patients to treatment A or B (i.e., AB and BA). If a block size of four is chosen, then there are six possible choices for randomizing patients in balanced blocks of four patients: ABAB, AABB, ABBA, BABA, BBAA, and BAAB. As the block size increases, the number of possible combinations of creating a balanced or proportional block increases.

SYSTEMATIC RANDOMIZATION

In systematic randomization, patients are assigned to receive treatment based on (1) a random order in the first block, which is then repeated in all subsequent blocks, or by (2) a sequential assignment to treatment. Two examples are when alternate treatments are assigned to patients as they are enrolled in a study and when every nth patient receives a different treatment.

STRATIFICATION

It is quite common to assign patients to treatment groups, based on their sex, age, weight, race, intensity of disease, disease risks, or any other relevant factor that is expected to have an important influence on the outcome of the study. Assignment of patients to groups based on a relevant factor is termed stratification. Although patients may be stratified on the basis of several factors, the resulting increase in the number of strata obtained and decrease in stratum size limit the number of factors that may be used with this method. Thus, patients are stratified based on the smallest number of characteristics possible. Within each stratum, patients are randomized to receive one of the study treatments.

Stratification is more important with small sample sizes since the need for this technique usually decreases to a degree in studies with an extremely large sample size. One problem of stratification is that it creates additional administration to deal with, beyond that imposed by other types of randomization. It may also divide a study of two groups into a study of several smaller groups if the outcome of the data is not consistent in the subgroups and cannot be combined. Stratification may be performed either prospectively or retrospectively in regard to the time of conducting the clinical study. If it is performed prospectively, then one usually cannot also use stratification at the end of the study (using subgroup analyses) to balance treatment groups. If stratification is only performed retrospectively, then it involves subgroup analysis, which is a topic that has strong proponents and critics.

MINIMIZATION

An interesting variation of the randomization process is a technique termed minimization (Taves, 1974). Minimization is a sophisticated form of stratification. In stratification, only one or a few factors believed to have a significant impact on the results are used to construct similar groups, whereas in minimization all known factors that might possibly have an important effect on treatment outcome are generally included. The goal of this technique (as well as stratification) is to minimize the differences in makeup of the two (or more) treatment groups at the outset of the study. Parameters may be weighted differently to give selected ones more importance. This process can be most effectively utilized if patients are entered slowly or in groups. Clinical examples of the use of minimization are illustrated in two studies by Weintraub et al. (1980, 1983).

OTHER VARIATIONS OF RANDOMIZATION PROCEDURES

There are instances in which one does not wish to have a particular patient group overrepresented in the study. Instead of stratifying patients to balance the treatment groups, it may be a useful ploy to introduce a quota system. In this method, a specific group (e.g., patients over a specified age) is restricted to a specific percentage of the total study sample. Thus, one subgroup cannot be overrepresented in the total sample beyond the desires of the protocol's authors.

Other variations of the traditional randomized clinical studies are occasionally proposed (e.g., Zelen, 1979). Zelen proposed a means to compare new and standard treatments whereby one-half of the patients choose between the new treatment and the standard treatment. The other half of the patients receive the standard treatment. It usually takes a number of years before the medical community evaluates and accepts the merits of new approaches. The trend in clinical study methodology over the last 25 years has been towards including more appropriate control groups and objective approaches to developing study designs.

Another variation on the theme of randomization concerns the nature and size of the unit that is being randomized. Although this unit is the individual patient in most studies, there are occasions where it may be more practical to randomize treatments by hospital, investigators, communities, large geographical areas, or other factors. This approach may be considered for studies conducted in developing countries with limited resources. In such cases, entire geographical areas may be randomized. This approach, however, may severely confound treatment with centers (geographical areas) and hamper the interpretation of statistical tests. Another approach has entire treatment centers arbitrarily assigned to one group, especially when one treatment requires the use of expensive or rare equipment that is not widely distributed. There are obvious disadvantages to this technique, but this method may allow useful studies to be conducted when more traditional randomization schemes are not practical.

OBTAINING AND USING RANDOMIZATION CODES

The process that is usually followed to obtain and use a randomization code is shown in Fig. 20.20. The randomization procedures should be developed and the codes generated by individuals trained in statistics who have adequate resources for obtaining the necessary codes. Numerous questions relating to group size and stratification should be discussed with statisticians, and all elements in the study design clarified prior to the request for a randomization code(s). The method by which the investigator assigns patients to treatment (i.e., does he call the monitor or a central office, or does giving the appropriate bottle with the patient's number assign the proper treatment, etc.) must be determined and clearly specified prior to initiation of the study. If the monitor(s) is to remain blind to patient randomization, then the code that is generated must be delivered to other study personnel or to individuals who will package the drug, whether at the investigator's site or at the sponsoring institution.

8

Screening, Baseline, Treatment, and Posttreatment Periods

Screening Period • Baseline Period(s) • Treatment Period(s)
• Posttreatment Period

SCREENING PERIOD

The time period during which a screening examination may be conducted is usually indicated in the protocol (e.g., 2 to 6 days prior to initiation of baseline). An initial screen is often conducted by telephone or medical record review prior to the first clinic visit. This may be performed with a prepared form that addresses the most salient points of inclusion and exclusion, which helps to "screen" many patients who do not meet the inclusion criteria. Pharmacy records may also be "screened" in some instances (e.g., in nursing homes) to find suitable patients. A relatively straightforward approach of conducting this initial screen is to list all inclusion (and exclusion) criteria that can be requested by telephone or evaluated in medical records as a series of questions on a preprinted form.

When the number of patients "screened" is described, it must be clarified whether this number refers to the patients "interviewed" or to the number tested and examined to determine their suitability for the study. In some studies, additional numbers are presented, such as the number of patients who constituted the total pool of potential patients and the number of those who were eligible for the study but did not consent to take part.

The time that may elapse between the completion of screen and onset of baseline (or treatment period) is usually specified in the protocol. If an "excessive" time elapses between screen and baseline, and certain entry criteria (primarily clinical signs and symptoms) have changed, it is possible to allow a modified screen to be used for reevaluating potential patients who had already been screened. The specific tests that may be conducted during the screening period are usually listed in a time and events schedule. This schedule is described in detail in Chapter 19 of this book.

Results of all relevant screening tests should be obtained and reviewed (if at all possible) prior to formally initiating the baseline or treatment period. Patients have been admitted to the treatment (or baseline) period in many studies while the results of some of their screening (or baseline) tests were still pending. If important abnormal results (e.g., laboratory data) are noted after the patient has already entered the study, and the patient is allowed to continue with treatment, the entry criteria will probably be breached. In addition to this "technical" problem, a serious medical and ethical problem may develop if a patient was already treated with the study drug and developed a severe adverse reaction that could have been prevented.

BASELINE PERIOD(S)

The baseline period is used to obtain measurements that will determine whether the study groups are comparable at the start of treatment and also to provide values (in some studies) against which treatment values may be compared. Baseline periods are not required in all protocols, and the screening period may function as a baseline in some studies; that is, the data obtained during screening may serve as baseline values for comparison with treatment values.

Baselines may be active, historical, or both. Active baselines refer to a time period when data are collected after the protocol has been initiated, whereas historical baselines utilize data (often collected during screen) that were generated, though not necessarily recorded, before the patient entered the protocol.

The baseline period does not always follow the screening period. If an active baseline is incorporated into the study design, then it usually follows the screening period and formal admission of the patient into the study. When historical baselines are to be obtained, then this baseline period may actually precede or overlap the screening period. The protocol should clearly define the time limits of each of these periods and their relationship to each other.

Baselines are not restricted to pretreatment assessments. Baselines may be interspersed during a study, such as between different doses of the same drug, between the two periods of a two-period crossover, or between successive periods of a Latin-square design study. Utilizing multiple baselines in a study has the advantage that carryover (residual) effects may be more easily investigated.

Numerous factors must be considered in determining the length of a baseline period. These factors relate to the nature of the disease, characteristics of the patients and drug(s), location and setting of the study, and available resources. One must determine whether any time may elapse between termination of baseline and start of the treatment period. It is the author's view that this would be a poor practice in most studies.

At least two sets of measurements should be obtained during baseline (whenever possible) to optimize the validity of the data and calculate its variability for comparing baseline data with those obtained during treatment within a group or for comparing baseline values between groups. If more than one baseline value is obtained in a specific test, there is the question of whether all values should be averaged or whether only specific values (e.g., the last two or three) should be averaged, or possibly only the most recent (last) value should be used. These are all relevant concerns to address prior to initiating a study, although it may be necessary to conduct or utilize data from a pilot study in order to obtain a sound basis for reaching a decision on this issue.

It may be impossible to obtain all necessary information on a patient during baseline (e.g., if the treatment must start before it is possible to obtain either important laboratory data or various measures of a disease needed to assess the patient's suitability for enrollment based on the inclusion criteria). This situation often occurs when one wants to initiate treatment rapidly in patients with an acute disease. Patients are therefore sometimes entered before their eligibility is fully assessed. Various alternatives for dealing with this potential problem should be addressed in the protocol or by providing verbal and/or written instructions to the investigator. For example, the entry criteria could be adjusted prior to the study to allow for this possibility. Alternatively, patients who are later found not to fit the protocol's entry criteria could be dropped or possibly enter an open-label or single-blind study that is conducted simultaneously.

Patients are usually randomized to one of the treatment groups at the end of the screening period or baseline.

TREATMENT PERIOD(S)

Establishing the length of the treatment period requires careful consideration of many factors. The primary factors relate to the objective(s) of the study. Other important factors include previous drug experience with the study drug, toxicological data, stability and variability of the disease, phase of drug evaluation, and the intended duration of drug use in the general patient population that may be given the drug.

The frequency of outpatient visits (or inpatient evaluations) during the treatment period is usually an issue that is evaluated in planning a clinical study. Many factors will influence the decision of when patient visits (evaluations) are scheduled and whether the visits are to be equally or unequally spaced throughout the treatment period. In general, visits are often scheduled more frequently at the start of a study and less often as the study progresses. Each study will have different factors to consider in determining the appropriate number of patient visits, but the additional time, cost, and energy that each visit entails must be considered for patient, staff, and investigator in addition to consideration of the value of the additional data that will be generated. It is often convenient to schedule patient visits in even multiples of days, weeks, or months (e.g., every two weeks for four visits, then every four weeks for the remaining visits).

An important aspect of treatment that is related to study design concerns the endpoint chosen for use in a study or treatment. The endpoint is usually merely alluded to in the study objectives in terms of assessing the efficacy and/or safety of the treatment even when specific tests are identified.

If drug effects on safety parameters are the major objectives of the study, then a decision should be reached in the planning stage as to whether the endpoint or termination of the study is defined as (1) the point at which adverse reactions begin to appear or (2) the point at which adverse reactions become more marked and drug intolerance appears. Another alternative is to test the safety of doses that have been, or are expected to be, tested for efficacy in other studies. A pharmacological, laboratory, or clinical endpoint or a combination of these may be used in a study.

Other aspects related to drug treatment, including dosage and adverse reactions, are dealt with in other chapters of this section.

POSTTREATMENT PERIOD

Posttreatment refers to the time after the study drug has been discontinued. The major purposes of a posttreatment period are to check for any withdrawal effects and to insure the patient's safety. The posttreatment period may also be useful to study residual effects of treatment. In evaluating the need for a posttreatment period in a drug study (as well as its duration), one may consider (1) previous experience with the drug in similar patient populations, (2) whether the drug dosage is being tapered slowly or abruptly stopped, (3) the clinical status of the patients, (4) whether patients are in a secure and/or controlled environment, and (5) the pharmacokinetic characteristics of the drug.

The posttreatment period may last for a fixed number of days (or weeks or months) after treatment is completed, or it may last until a predetermined date is reached. In the latter case, each patient may have a different length of posttreatment evaluation. Either one or several posttreatment clinic visits may be scheduled for all patients, and the return of specified (or all) parameters to their original baselines may be required. It is important to schedule a clinic visit at a time when virtually all of the drug has been eliminated from the patient's body (five or more half-lives) and any expected withdrawal reactions will have had a chance to occur. The posttreatment evaluation and/or data collection may be conducted by telephone in appropriate studies or under selected conditions (e.g., if the patient has moved).

The term "follow-up" is used in different ways depending on the type of clinical study described. If the study evaluated a surgical procedure rather than a drug, then the postsurgical period is usually described as follow-up. In the case of therapeutic or Phase I drug studies, as described in this book, follow-up is used synonymously with posttreatment. In studies where a drug (or vaccine) is given for prophylactic protection, follow-up is the period of time after the drug (or vaccine) is given, during which contact is maintained with the patient. This definition is also used in many cases where diet, exercise, or some other factor is altered in an attempt to reduce a known risk factor for a given disease. The distinction among the above usages of the term "follow-up" is that in a therapeutic drug study it is usually a short period of minor importance to the study objectives, whereas in many surgical, prophylaxis, and risk-factor reduction studies it is usually an extremely important part of the study, in which critical data is obtained that addresses the study objectives.

9 Patient Population, Methodologies, and Measurements

Choosing a Patient Population • Choosing Variables and a Methodology for Measuring Them • Choosing the Patients' Environment • Defining Drug Activity • Placebo Effect • Interim Analysis • Duration of Study

CHOOSING A PATIENT POPULATION

General Considerations

Numerous questions must be addressed in determining the general makeup of patients who will enter a clinical study. Some of these are:

1. Will normal volunteers or patients with a specific disease be most suitable?
2. What total number of patients should be enrolled to adequately address the study objectives? Is it likely that the required number of patients can be enrolled at one site, or will a multicenter study (two or more sites) be required? Those questions are generally discussed with statisticians, and the power of detecting clinically meaningful treatment differences should be evaluated.
3. Should some patients be enrolled as alternates at the start of a drug study? "Alternate" patients are defined as those patients who complete the screen and usually the baseline periods and are ready to be enrolled in the treatment period. Alternate patients may enter the study without delay if they are housed nearby in the event one or more of the enrolled patients does not arrive at the study site at the scheduled time, does not pass the screen (or baseline) examination, or must be discontinued for any reason once the study has begun. "Replacement" patients refers to patients who have not completed the screen or baseline even though they might have been recruited prior to the dropout of the patient they have replaced.
4. Should the study be conducted with inpatients (patients kept in a hospital or clinic setting), outpatients, or both? In some studies, patients are entered and studied as inpatients and then continue the study on an outpatient basis. In other studies, outpatients enter the hospital (or clinic) one or more times for various periods and, after discharge, return to their outpatient status. Another alternative is to enroll both inpatients and outpatients in a study, although this approach may have significant drawbacks for interpreting the data obtained.

It may be relevant to measure or assess the expectations of patients entering a drug study. It has been shown in a double-blind study of two antiinflammatory drugs plus placebo that treatment outcomes were related in part to patient expectations (Berry et al., 1980).

Phase I Studies

Numerous Phase I drug studies were often conducted on prisoners, prior to 1970, but this practice is infrequently followed in the United States today. The major reason that prisoners are no longer allowed to participate in clinical studies is that it is believed that they are not able to provide a freely given informed consent. There are individuals who believe that the "loss" of this population for drug studies represented both a gain and loss for these prisoners and our society because of benefits that this population gained from participation in these studies (Lasagna, 1977; Shubin, 1981). In addition, the relative safety of virtually all drugs tested meant that few individuals experienced long-term adverse reactions to the studies.

Most Phase I studies are currently performed with normal volunteers. There is, however, a growing belief that patients may sometimes be appropriate to use in Phase I studies to test new drugs for safety (Weissman, 1981). This may be especially useful if patients metabolize drugs differently than do normal volunteers. For example, epileptic patients who are currently receiving microsomal enzyme-inducing drugs may metabolize a new drug differently than will a normal volunteer. Another example in which patients may be used for Phase I studies relates to the use of drugs with expected toxicity, such as evaluating the safety of new anticancer drugs that are potentially toxic. In this situation it is usually not ethically acceptable to enroll normal volunteers in a Phase I study.

Factors to consider in determining whether to use patients or volunteers depend on whether the investigator will be able to complete the study more rapidly, efficiently, safely, ethically, and cost-effectively and also obtain more reliable information with patients or volunteers.

It may be preferable in some Phase I studies to expose a larger number of patients to a maximally tolerated dose than to lower doses. This has the advantage that more information may be obtained on the specific dose or doses that are of greatest interest. If a study has two treatment periods, then a smaller group of patients may be enrolled in the first period, in which a maximally tolerated dose is determined. A larger number of patients are then enrolled in the second treatment period, where they receive a dose based on the results obtained in the first period.

A Phase I rising single-dose study may expose one group of patients (or volunteers) to each dose evaluated, or a new group of patients may be enrolled to receive each dose. There are numerous advantages and disadvantages of each approach, but these are not enumerated here.

CHOOSING VARIABLES AND A METHODOLOGY
FOR MEASURING THEM

In evaluating the efficacy (or safety) of a new or established drug, the precise target(s) for evaluation should be identified. Possible types of targets for evaluation of efficacy include the following:

1. Clinical parameters. These include symptoms and signs of the primary or coexisting disease.
2. Clinical tests. Abnormalities present are determined by tests used to measure or study the disease or from a manifestation of the disease.
3. Disease abnormality. This may include a biochemical defect attributable to the primary or coexisting disease, an anatomical lesion attributable to the primary or coexisting disease, or any other abnormality attributable to the primary or coexisting disease.

The term "coexisting disease" is used to include risk factors.

The study may evaluate treatment of an active disease or risk factor, diagnosis of the disease state, or prophylactic treatment to prevent a disease from occurring. In discussing the nature of measurements as part of the study design, measurements that relate to meeting the study's objective will be emphasized. For example, the exact time of day that a drug (given once daily) is administered is usually not specified in the design section of most protocols; however, that time could be critical if the study is primarily concerned with diurnal rhythms and is designed to evaluate the effects of a drug given at 8 P.M. versus those effects measured when it is given at 8 A.M.

The major variables chosen to evaluate efficacy or safety are often indicated in the design section of a protocol. Parameters that provide objective measurements of drug efficacy are almost always preferable to subjective measures of response, although it is often reasonable to include both types of measurements. When no objective or even semiobjective measurements are available, then subjective measurements must be used. A double-blind controlled design will provide some degree of control and assurance that results obtained with subjective data will be reproducible and interpretations will be meaningful.

As a general principle, one should not employ any methodology that is not well documented and/or widely accepted as providing valid data. In particular, measurement of the major indicator of efficacy should utilize validated procedures. It may be relevant to determine the scientific basis for the proposed methods, since many widely used tests have never been adequately validated.

In choosing the correct tests to include in a clinical protocol, both the specificity and sensitivity of the tests should be evaluated. A specific methodology detects a signal for the desired event and does not detect signals for other events. Specificity refers to the probability of correctly diagnosing a negative case as negative. Specificity in a test is lacking if a positive result occurs when it should be negative. This is a false–positive result. Sensitivity refers to the probability of correctly diagnosing a positive case as positive. Sensitivity in tests is lacking if a negative result occurs when it should be positive. This is a false–negative result. A methodology with high sensitivity, therefore, has the ability to detect a small change in the magnitude of the signal measured.

It may be important to specifically indicate details in the protocol that are related to tests used. The details may be given in either the protocol or an appendix and may vary from model numbers of specific equipment used to paper speed of the recording paper [e.g., for electrocardiogram (ECG) recordings]. The amount of relevant detail to include for each test must be determined. If multiple tests are included in a study, their order of use may be controlled or scheduled in a fixed (or random) order, and the time allowed between the tests specified. The number of repeat measurements should be determined and indicated for each test (at least on the data collection forms). It may be important to document whether responses to a test remain constant in the absence of any drug, since a major error would be introduced if normal changes in a test score were inappropriately ascribed to a drug.

If pertinent efficacy measurements may be obtained in outpatient studies while the patient is at home (e.g., blood pressure measurements, number of bowel movements and consistency of stool), then more choices of suitable study designs will be available. Many factors (e.g., patient reliability, adequate measuring devices) have to be considered before this type of data collection is endorsed.

CHOOSING THE PATIENTS' ENVIRONMENT

If patients have to be hospitalized to test a new agent, this may have a moderate or strong influence on the characteristics and nature of the patients' disease. Many (if not most) diseases treated in outpatients will appear to change in nature or severity when outpatients are hospitalized. This has been demonstrated for patients with various forms of epilepsy (Riley et al., 1981). In addition, responses to pain and pain thresholds appear to differ between clinical and laboratory settings (American Medical Association, 1983). Data obtained at an early stage of a drug's development in a setting where the disease process is altered from the patient's usual environment may not yield a valid impression of the study drug's true potential efficacy.

DEFINING DRUG ACTIVITY

In establishing the standard(s) for defining drug activity, the differences between statistical and clinical significance must be considered. Statistical significance may be precisely defined. Clinical significance is a subjective parameter that indicates the minimal difference between two treatments that would affect a clinician's judgment of how to treat patients with the same or similar problem. Although the difference between two treatments that is considered clinically significant will differ among physicians, these differences generally tend to cluster around a specific figure or range.

The degree or magnitude of change in efficacy parameters that will be considered to represent a true clinical improvement should be established in the planning phase of a study. An efficacy test that demonstrates a 10% change after drug treatment may be statistically significant, but a change of 50% may be required for the results to be clinically significant (clinically meaningful). Statistically significant changes in many parameters used to evaluate safety are not always clinically significant. For example, a statistically significant change in heart rate of four beats per minute, either within or outside the normal range, will almost never be clinically significant. In some cases, however, such minor changes may indicate an effect that should be evaluated in greater detail or closely monitored in future studies.

PLACEBO EFFECT

The term placebo is generally used to refer to (1) medication taken, (2) effect observed, or (3) control group of patients. As medication, it is "blank" (i.e., without any active drug) and is given to some or all patients one or more times during a study. The term placebo is also used to describe the "placebo effect" that is elicited by the placebo drug or is caused by the influence of nonstudy drug or nontreatment factors, usually on efficacy measures. The "placebo group" refers to a control (comparison) group in a study made up of those patients who were given a placebo medication. Placebos are used in drug studies to control for major sources of misleading data: (1) prejudice on the part of the investigator and/or (2) patient and (3) spontaneous alterations and variations that occur during treatment and are related to the disease studied or to other factors. Prejudices may be based on psychological and emotional factors that enter a study plus physical effects that are related to receiving medication.

Several types of placebo responses are observed in clinical studies, based primarily on the number of placebo responders and the magnitude of their response. The placebo effect may be observed in all patients, or it may only be present in a subset of the total number studied. The magnitude of the placebo response may be either 0 or 100% in a specific parameter (e.g., where a placebo drug affords either no pain relief or complete pain relief), but usually the placebo effect is noted as a relative change between 0 and 100% (e.g., 20% decrease in the number of anginal attacks). The placebo response is a major factor that must be considered when evaluating analgesics, antidepressants, and many other types of drugs. Substantial clinical data have been obtained in recent years that indicate that most disease states may be significantly affected by placebo medication. It is important to note that the placebo response may increase or decrease over time.

It is commonly accepted that a small or moderate placebo effect will be present in most drug studies conducted in conscious individuals. Although a variety of approaches exist to control or diminish the placebo effect, in some cases the placebo effect is ignored in developing a study design. Either a separate placebo group or a placebo treatment period for all patients may be incorporated into the study design to evaluate and/or control for the placebo effect.

Certain techniques may be used to exclude those patients from a study in whom a large placebo response is anticipated. For example, all patients could be given a placebo medication (single or double blind) for a fixed period, after which they would be tested; any patients who improved by more than a specified amount would be excluded from further participation in the study. This technique may not only eliminate placebo responders from a study but, if a pill count is also performed during this period, may sometimes eliminate noncompliant patients as well. Any procedure for excluding placebo responders from a study introduces a bias that would generally make this practice inappropriate during Phase III. In Phase III studies, a drug is evaluated in a general population with a given disease, and "all" types of responders and patients that satisfy entry criteria should receive the drug to develop more clearly the full spectrum of the drug's safety and efficacy profile. The bias that is introduced by excluding placebo responders, however, may be acceptable in an early Phase II study, where the primary objective is to determine if the drug possesses the desired activity. Minimizing the placebo effect in Phase II is desirable, since it allows the drug's efficacy to be more clearly assessed.

The magnitude of the placebo response may be determined by evaluating the response of patients in a double-blind study to placebo and an active study drug. Another approach to evaluating the magnitude of the placebo response is to compare the results of an active study drug in an open-label study with results obtained in a double-blind study utilizing the same design. The assumption made in this comparison is that if more individuals respond to a drug (or respond better) in an open-label study than in a double-blind study, then at least part of the difference is attributable to a placebo effect, which in turn may reflect greater expectations of patients who enter the open-label study.

Other approaches for evaluating or controlling placebo responses are to interject a placebo treatment at an unannounced time(s) in the protocol. This could occur at the start or termination of the study or at intermittent points during the study, depending on the nature of the drug and study design. In this situation, both patients and investigator are informed that each patient will receive active drug and placebo, but they are not told when each will be administered or if several placebo periods will be introduced. Information on the length of each placebo period could also be withheld from the investigator and patient if this were considered ethical by the relevant ethics review board(s). A discussion of placebo control groups may be found in Chapter 4.

INTERIM ANALYSIS

If data are to be examined during the course of a study, the evaluation is referred to as an interim analysis. An interim analysis may be performed to follow the progress of a study and/or to further develop the clinical program of the study drug by using the results of the interim analysis to help plan additional studies. The results of the analysis may also be used to adjust the protocol during the conduct of the study, or a decision may be made prior to performing the interim analysis that the results will not be used to alter the conduct of the study being analyzed.

The statistical evaluation performed may involve a formal analysis of all available data with criteria established for the various possible consequences (e.g., stop the study prematurely, increase the sample size). The analysis could also consist of an informal evaluation of limited data by a person blinded to patient randomization to obtain a perspective of one or more specific points that will not be used to affect the study. In between these two types of evaluations, many other possible analyses may be performed. It is usually possible to decide prior to performing an interim analysis whether the results will be used to modify the study in any way.

One of the "dangers" in performing interim analyses is that many statistical tests assume that the data are only being analyzed once, and multiple analyses of the data using these tests violate this assumption. This implies that, if interim data analyses are planned, they (1) should be discussed with statisticians prior to the study, preferably while it is being designed, (2) the statisticians should perform the analyses under defined conditions, and (3) the potential ramifications of performing the interim analyses should be considered in advance.

DURATION OF STUDY

The duration of each patient's treatment in a study may be (1) fixed (e.g., 2 hr, days, weeks, or years), (2) variable (e.g., the study lasts until a specified measure of efficacy returns to normal, 12 to 18 weeks), (3) indefinite (e.g., ongoing treatment of chronic disease), or (4) unspecified. The type and length of duration chosen for the study should almost always be indicated in the protocol.

The duration that is established for treating patients in a study is often dependent on the expected or established therapeutic use of the drug as well as the extent of toxicological data. Many studies have a duration that parallels the duration of the disease or exposure to an external factor (e.g., prophylactic study of an antimalarial in people visiting a specific country for a defined period of time). The terms acute, subacute, subchronic, and chronic are often used to describe the duration of drug therapy as well as the duration of diseases. Their definitions vary to some degree among diseases and among clinicians. Therefore, these terms should be clearly defined in any protocols in which they are used.

Acute studies are often used for acute diseases or for chronic diseases with acute episodes, and chronic studies are often used to study chronic diseases. Nonetheless, even in testing drugs for a chronic disease, there are occasions when an acute study design is preferable. Some common reasons are:

1. To evaluate bioavailability and the pharmacokinetics in patients with the disease who may be expected to absorb, distribute, metabolize, or excrete the drug differently than the normal population (e.g., in epileptic patients receiving drugs that induce hepatic microsomal enzymes) or in a subset of patients with a "specific" problem (e.g., patients with renal impairment).
2. To evaluate the acute effect of a drug on a specific test in patients, such as studying acute electroencephalographic (EEG) effects caused by a new antiepileptic drug.
3. To avoid a placebo effect that is observed in chronic studies. For example, the relatively marked placebo effect observed in chronic drug studies in

patients with angina is primarily absent in acute drug studies (Redwood et al., 1971).

In addition to establishing the duration of a patient's treatment, it may also be important to establish the duration of the entire study. An important consideration relating to a study's total duration is the pattern in which patients are entered into a study. Examples of enrollment patterns include those in which (1) all patients start a study at the same time, (2) defined groups of patients start a study at fixed times, (3) different numbers of patients start a study at fixed times, (4) variable dates are used for patient entry and study initiation, (5) no specific dates are used, and patients enter the study as they are enrolled, or (6) another pattern of patient enrollment is established.

A target date for completion of a study is usually established at the outset. There are a wide variety of reasons, however, why this date is commonly not achieved, and it requires a great deal of planning, effort, and even luck in most cases to achieve the goals that are established.

10   Dosing Schedule

Choosing a Starting Dose of a New Drug • Choosing Dose
Increments • Factors Involved in Developing Dosage Schedules

CHOOSING A STARTING DOSE OF A NEW DRUG

The choice of a starting dose for the initial study of a new drug in man is based on several factors. These include the ED_{50} (the effective dose that elicits 50% of the total response) of the most sensitive animal species, a comparison of the drug's potency and activity with the potency and activity of known standards that have a similar mechanism of action, LD_{50} (the dose that kills 50% of the test animals; median lethal dose) values in various species, available pharmacokinetic data of blood levels obtained in animals, and information on the drug's expected absorption, distribution, metabolism, and excretion. After a conservative dose is found that is expected to represent the threshold of the dose–response relationship in humans, a fraction of that dose is chosen as the starting dose. The fractions used by most investigators generally range between one-half and 1/10 of the expected threshold dose for human efficacy. Some investigators choose a starting dose based solely on the use of a fraction of the threshold dose that caused an adverse reaction or positive effect in the most sensitive animal model tested.

In cancer research it had been customary to initiate Phase I human clinical studies of anticancer drugs at one-third of the lowest dose (per square meter) that caused reversible toxicity in the most sensitive large animal species (dog or monkey) (Penta et al., 1979), although some authors believe that toxicology data in normal and tumor-bearing mice should also have been considered (Goldsmith et al., 1975). Retrospective analysis of preclinical and clinical data for a large number of compounds indicates that 1/10 mouse LD_{10} (on a body surface basis) should provide a safe starting dose for Phase I studies. This starting dose is both safe and efficient in that the minimal number of Fibonacci escalation steps (see next section for details) is required to achieve the maximally tolerated dose (Rozencweig et al., 1981). Current accepted practice at the National Cancer Institute is to utilize rodent lethality studies to derive the human starting dose and large animal toxicology results to predict those toxicities that may be encountered in initial clinical studies.

The methods described above attempt to provide a margin of safety in case a hypersensitive reaction or unexpected effect is manifested by a patient. A survey of scientists in academic and industrial institutions was conducted to compare their views on the conduct of initial drug studies in man (Blackwell, 1972a). It would be interesting to determine how these views have changed (if at all) over the intervening years.

TABLE 10.3. *Various options to consider in developing a dosing schedule for the different periods of a study protocol*

A. Frequency of dosing
   1. Fixed intervals (e.g., q.i.d., t.i.d., b.i.d., q.d., q.o.d.)
   2. Variable intervals (e.g., p.r.n., titrating to a given effect or blood level)
   3. Combination of above
B. Drugs allowed between screen and dose ascension[a]
   1. Take patients off all drugs
   2. Take patients off specifically designated drugs or classes of drugs
   3. Allow specific drugs or a specific number of drugs to be taken
   4. Switch all patients to a standard drug
   5. Allow patients to continue taking any or all drugs they were previously taking
C. Dose ascension[b]
   1. None, start the study drug at a maintenance dose
   2. Use a loading dose, then decrease dose to maintenance level
   3. Use a fixed dosage ascension for all patients
   4. Use a variable dosage ascension based on established criteria. Either the amount of the dosage, the time of administration, or both may be varied
   5. Taper a concomitant drug during dose ascension of the study drug
D. Dose maintenance[c]
   1. A fixed number of doses or dose ranges allowed. Doses may not be changed during the maintenance period of the study
   2. Doses may be raised during this period for lack of an adequate therapeutic effect or for other reasons
   3. Doses may be lowered for adverse reactions, laboratory abnormalities, or other reasons
   4. Doses may be subsequently raised or lowered after an initial dosage change
E. Dose taper and discontinuation
   1. Dosage stopped without taper
   2. Fixed dosage taper schedule used for all patients
   3. Variable dosage taper schedule is based on established criteria or clinical judgment
   4. Study drug is tapered as another drug is added
   5. Study drug is tapered after another drug is added

[a]The doses and durations associated with each step must be specified.
[b]In several of these procedures, dose ascension may be performed in a fixed number of steps, or the number of possible steps may vary between patients. See Fig. 12.7 for an illustration of alternative methods for dose ascension.
[c]The frequency of allowable dose changes must be specified for any of these four choices (e.g., one change may be made per week or per study or without limit).

CHOOSING DOSE INCREMENTS

The increments between increasing doses of the same drug should reflect a consistent pattern in terms of absolute or percentage increments. If doses of 50, 100, 200, 400, and 800 mg are tested in a study, then the next dose to be given should not be 900 mg but either 1,200 or 1,600 mg. If the adverse reactions observed at the 800-mg dose warrant, then the next dose may be adjusted downward to 1,000 mg. Dose increments in animals and in *in vitro* studies tend to increase in a logarithmic manner (e.g., x, $10x$, $100x$, $1,000x$ or x, $3.3x$, $10x$, $33x$, $100x$), but doses in humans usually increase arithmetically by (1) equal amounts (e.g., x, $2x$, $3x$, $4x$, $5x$), (2) approximately equal percentages (e.g., x, $2x$, $4x$, $8x$, $16x$), or (3) according to a specific formula (e.g., the modified Fibonacci dose escalation

1. RAPID (R) GRADUAL (G) OR SLOW (S) DOSE ASCENSION

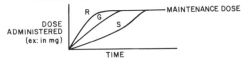

2. LOADING DOSE(S) FOLLOWED BY MAINTENANCE DOSES

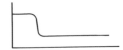

3. NO DOSE ASCENSION

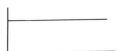

4. STEPWISE ASCENSION

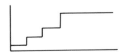

5. ASCENSION OF STUDY DRUG AS ANOTHER DRUG IS TAPERED

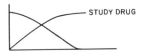

6. ASCENSION OF STUDY DRUG FOLLOWED BY TAPER OF ANOTHER DRUG

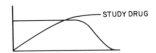

7. COMBINATION OF ABOVE METHODS

8. TEMPORARY OR PERMANENT DECREASES IN DOSES DURING ASCENSION

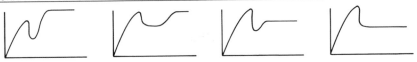

FIG. 10.4. Options available for dose ascension with a new or established drug. Dose taper may follow the same schemata as those presented for dose ascension. Each **graph** is intended to have the same *ordinate* (dose administered) and *abscissa* (time). In the example of stepwise ascension, the number of steps may be optional or fixed, and the time between steps may be variable or fixed. In options 5 and 6, the dose ascension of the new drug may follow any of the dose ascensions shown in options 1 to 4.

TABLE 10.4. *Options for choosing fixed and/or flexible dosages[a]*

---

1. Fixed/unchanging

   Dosage held constant at a fixed level (e.g., 100 mg/day for 5 days) or within a specified range (e.g., 10–20 mg/day for 5 days) for entire study

2. Fixed/changing

   Dosage held constant at a fixed level (e.g., 5 mg/day for the first week, 10 mg/day for the second week, and 30 mg/day for the third and fourth weeks) or within a specified range (e.g., 5 to 10 mg/day for the first week, 20 to 40 mg/day for the second week) with increasing and/or decreasing levels

3. Flexible

   Dosage changes according to the patient's needs; e.g., dose may be titrated to achieve and maintain a given clinical endpoint or laboratory effect such as blood level. An upper and lower dose limit are usually provided

4. Fixed/flexible[b]

   Dosage fixed for initial and/or earlier administrations, but with an option for the investigator to individualize dosage according to patient needs after a certain point is reached in the protocol. Dosage changes may be based on time, number of doses given, amount of drug given, toxicity, or therapeutic effect. The optional (i.e., flexible) dosages may be (1) limited to one or a set number or range of doses chosen according to specified criteria or (2) limited to a set amount or range (or other measure), (3) limited or specified by other criteria, or (4) not specifically limited at all

5. Flexible/fixed[b]

   Dosages are flexible in the initial phases of the protocol, often until a specific effect or blood level is achieved, and then the dosage is fixed for the remainder of the study

---

[a]These options refer to one group being treated with a study drug. Different groups may be treated in the same manner with different doses or dose ranges of the study drug to create a dose-response relationship.

[b]Variations of these options are possible using a third part (e.g., a fixed/flexible/fixed schedule or other criteria in choosing study doses).

scheme of x, $2x$, $3.3x$, $5x$, $7x$, $9x$, $12x$, and $16x$; Penta et al., 1979). There are numerous options to consider in planning dose ascension, maintenance, and withdrawal as well as the frequency of dosing. Some of these are shown in Table 10.3, and alternatives to use in dose ascension are shown in Fig. 10.4.

FACTORS INVOLVED IN DEVELOPING DOSAGE SCHEDULES

The dosage form and route of administration to be used (see Tables 12.10 and 13.11) have a major impact on the dosage schedule developed. The choice of these variables is generally determined at an early phase of the study's conceptualization and is sometimes related to the study's objectives (e.g., comparing effects of an i.v. and oral form of a drug). The topics of dosage form and route of administration are presented in Chapters 12 and 13, respectively.

It is pertinent to determine whether to study a fixed or variable dose(s) of the study drug. If a substantial amount of information is available about the study drug, then using fixed doses rather than a dose range(s) offers a number of advantages. If, however, a new drug is being initially evaluated for efficacy, then it may be preferable to use variable doses. This is because insufficient data exist on a new drug that could be used to choose the most appropriate fixed doses to study, and using dose ranges allows for flexibility in evaluating more doses.

TABLE 10.5. *Sample tables of dosage regimens for acute single dose drug studies*

Study day	Patient group code[a]	Dosing period no.[b]	Medication capsules		Total active dose (mg)
			Active group (N = 12)	Placebo (P) group (N = 6)	
1	A	1	1 × 200 mg + 5 P	6 P	200
4	B	2	2 × 200 mg + 4 P	6 P	400
8	A	3	3 × 200 mg + 3 P	6 P	600
11	B	4	4 × 200 mg + 2 P	6 P	800
15	A	5	5 × 200 mg + 1 P	6 P	1000
18	B	6	6 × 200 mg + 0 P	6 P	1200

Dose period	Placebo group (N = 6) no. of placebo capsules	Active drug group (N = 12)				Placebo capsules (no.)	Total dose (mg)
		No. of study drug capsules					
		0.5 mg	1.0 mg	4.0 mg	8.0 mg		
1	4	1	0	0	0	3	0.5
2	4	0	1	0	0	3	1.0
3	4	0	2	0	0	2	2.0
4	4	0	0	1	0	3	4.0
5	4	0	0	2	0	2	8.0
6	4	0	0	0	2	2	16.0

[a]A and B are two separate groups of patients.
[b]The time between dosing periods may be specified in terms of a fixed time, the minimum or maximum time allowed, or a range of times.

Dosages may be specified on the basis of a patient's (1) weight (e.g., mg/kg), (2) size (e.g., mg/m^2 of body surface area), (3) result of a laboratory test (e.g., creatinine clearance), or (4) other characteristics of the patient. Doses are often given in milligrams per kilogram instead of a total number of milligrams (1) for newly tested drugs with steep dose–response curves, (2) when safety and/or efficacy are not well defined, or (3) if toxicity (or efficacy) has been found to be directly proportional to the dose per body weight. The general options of utilizing fixed and/or flexible dosages are shown in Table 10.4. Dosage regimens (schedules) are based on both the quantity of the dose and the intervals chosen for drug administration; i.e., a dosing regimen includes a measure of both quantity and time.

For most studies a plan for frequency of dosing, dose ascension, taper, and withdrawal must be based on previous clinical experience, pharmacokinetics, and relevant preclinical data. In a safety study, patients may be dosed either to intolerance or to a dose expected to yield a therapeutic effect or prespecified blood level. It is usually valuable in at least one Phase I study to increase the dose of a new drug to the point at which clinically significant adverse reactions appear. This provides information on the upper limits of safety and indicates a dose range in which efficacy studies may be conducted. A list of many of the parameters used in selecting drug dosages is given in Table 11.7.

TABLE 10.6. Sample tables of dosage regimens for multidose drug studies

Day of study	Placebo group (tablets)	Low-dose group					High-dose group				
		75-mg tablets	150-mg tablets	P[a]	Total (mg/dose)	Total (mg/day)	75-mg tablets	150-mg tablets	P	Total (mg/dose)	Total (mg/day)
1	3	1	0	2	75	300	0	1	2	150	600
2–5	3	0	1	2	150	600	0	2	1	300	1200
6–10	3	1	1	1	225	900	0	3	0	450	1800

Daily time of dosing (days 1–21)

			No. of capsules to be taken		Total (mg/day)	
				Active drug		
Elapsed time (hr)	Actual time (hr)	Placebo (P) group (N = 6)	Low dose (N = 12)	High dose (N = 12)	Low dose	High dose
0	8–10 A.M.	2 P	1–5 mg + 1 P	2–5 mg	20	40
4	12–2 P.M.	2 P	1–5 mg + 1 P	2–5 mg		
8	4–6 P.M.	2 P	1–5 mg + 1 P	2–5 mg		
12	8–10 P.M.	2 P	1–5 mg + 1 P	2–5 mg		

Total dose of study drug (mg) for three groups of patients in each of the 9 weeks of study[b]

Weight of patient (kg)	1	2	3	4	5	6	7	8	9
10–19.9	50 (50)	100 (100)	100 (100)	150 (50, 100)	150 (50, 100)	200 (200)	200 (200)	100 (100)	0
20–39.9	100 (100)	150 (50, 100)	150 (50, 100)	200 (200)	200 (200)	300 (100, 200)	300 (100, 200)	150 (50, 100)	0
40–60	150 (50, 100)	200 (100, 100)	200 (100, 100)	300 (100, 200)	300 (100, 200)	400 (200, 200)	400 (200, 200)	200 (100, 100)	0

[a]P, placebo.
[b]The tablet sizes required for each dose are in parentheses (tablets are assumed to be available in 50, 100, and 200 mg). Placebos are used to make up two tablets per dose.

The particular study being designed may be part of a larger plan to develop a new drug or to explore a specific clinical area through a number of studies. If this is so, then the goals of the clinical program as they relate to dosage (e.g., b.i.d. or q.d. dosing; narrow or broad dose ranges) must be kept in mind as one proceeds from study to study, developing clinical data that one hopes will support the established goals. For example, in order to maximize the chances of demonstrating efficacy, it may be prudent to dose patients four times a day initially even though the goal of the clinical program may be eventually to dose patients twice a day.

It may be relevant to note in a protocol whether the dosages of the study drug are given in terms of salt or free base and also whether the drug(s) should be ingested in a fixed relationship to meals or with a certain amount of fluids. Phase I studies often specify the amount of water to be used for ingesting each oral dose (often 200 to 400 ml) and the relationship of drug dosing to meals. These factors are not generally indicated in Phase II and III protocols unless the drug is (1) known or believed to cause local irritation, (2) not adequately dissolved without ingestion of an appropriate volume of fluid, or (3) affected by some or all foods (e.g., tetracyclines are bound by dairy products).

After the dosage schedule has been determined, it must be clearly presented in the protocol. A few sample table headings that could be adapted or modified are shown for single-dose clinical studies in Table 10.5 and for multiple-dose studies in Table 10.6.

11

Considerations of Pharmacokinetics and Drug Interactions

Introduction • Pharmacokinetic Parameters • Selected Mathematical Models Using Pharmacokinetic Data • Drug Interactions

INTRODUCTION

Pharmacokinetics concentrates on describing the absorption, distribution, metabolism, and excretion of a drug. This chapter is not intended as a review of pharmacokinetics but rather is a brief nonmathematical synopsis of some pharmacokinetic parameters that an investigator would consider in developing a study design. An attempt is made to emphasize practical considerations.

The pharmacokinetic behavior of a new drug is usually determined in animals before the drug is tested in humans. Additional tests in animals usually progress at the same time that a clinical program evaluating the drug is developing. There are often important differences between pharmacokinetic results obtained in humans and laboratory animals, which emphasizes the relevance of pharmacokinetic studies performed in humans.

PHARMACOKINETIC PARAMETERS

A number of pharmacokinetic parameters evaluated in humans are discussed, and a few examples of cases in which these parameters have had a significant outcome on the results of clinical studies are provided. The parameters to be described include those used to choose a drug-dosing regimen (Table 11.7). These parameters are often evaluated in clinical studies designed specifically to characterize and understand the pharmacokinetic profile of a drug. It should be stressed that at least several of the parameters listed in Table 11.7 must be considered in selecting a drug dosage or dosing regimen. A number of the most important pharmacokinetic parameters described below are illustrated in Fig. 11.5.

Bioavailability

Bioavailability of an orally administered drug describes the net result of all processes from oral ingestion of the drug to the appearance of the drug in the systemic circulation. The term is sometimes used to describe both the amount and rate of drug present in the systemic circulation, but the amount of drug present is the more commonly described parameter. Bioavailability is usually expressed as a

TABLE 11.7. *Selected parameters used to choose drug dosages and regimens*

Parameters related to the drug's pharmacokinetics and pharmacological characteristics	Parameters related to the patient's characteristics
1. Peak blood[a] levels	1. Age
2. Time to peak concentration	2. Sex
3. Duration of blood[a] concentration	3. Weight
4. Duration of biological effects	4. Race or ethnic background
5. Drug half-life	5. Geographical location
6. Bioavailability	6. Severity of disease
7. Accumulation	7. Concomitant drugs
8. Microsomal enzyme induction	8. Concurrent diseases
9. Distribution characteristics	9. Other inclusion criteria
10. Plasma protein binding	
11. Metabolism	
12. Excretion	
13. Synergism	
14. Drug interactions	
15. Tachyphylaxis	
16. Tolerance	

[a]Usually determined in plasma or serum.

percent of the drug administered that is available within the body intact (unmetabolized) compared to an appropriate reference.

The bioavailability data of an oral dosage form may be compared to the same drug administered i.v. (absolute bioavailability) or compared to a standard oral dosage form or solution (relative bioavailability). Many factors (e.g., food, disease, age, other drugs) can enhance or diminish the degree of a drug's bioavailability, and these factors must be controlled in a study in which bioavailability is measured (Table 11.8). The three main factors to evaluate in a bioavailability study are (1) peak plasma concentration, (2) time to peak plasma concentration, and (3) area under the plasma concentration-versus-time curve (see Fig. 11.6). The means by which a different formulation of the same drug can affect these parameters is shown in Fig. 11.6. In this example, the rate of absorption for formulation B is slower, as reflected by the greater time required to reach the peak plasma concentration. Nonetheless, the extent of the two dosage forms absorbed is the same, as reflected by equivalent areas under the curve. The biological advantage of formulation B is that the maximum blood level remains below that which causes toxicity.

Peak Blood Levels

If a peak blood level above a certain value is associated with a high incidence of drug toxicity (e.g., phenytoin levels above 20 μg/ml), then this level should be avoided through periodic monitoring. There are numerous other reasons why it is desirable to monitor study drug levels in plasma and/or other physiological fluids.

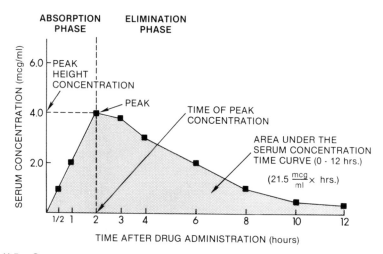

FIG. 11.5. Serum concentration–time curve following a single dose of a drug, illustrating a number of basic pharmacokinetic concepts. (Reprinted by permission of American Pharmaceutical Association from the *Journal of the American Pharmaceutical Association*, from Dittert and DiSanto, 1973.)

TABLE 11.8. *Factors influencing absorption of oral drugs into the systemic circulation*

---

1. Physical–chemical properties of the drug (e.g., solubility in stomach and small intestine, molecular size, type of molecule, crystal form)
2. Formulation used (e.g., characteristics of excipients, amount of pressure under which a tablet is compressed, range of particle sizes, enteric or other coating of tablet)
3. Gastrointestinal contents (e.g., presence of food or other drugs)
4. Gastrointestinal characteristics (e.g., gastric pH and emptying time, metabolic activity of the intestinal surface, intestinal emptying time, gastrointestinal secretions, disease)
5. Gastrointestinal flora (e.g., bacteria in the gut)
6. Hormonal secretions into the gastrointestinal system
7. Activity of the autonomic nervous system
8. Metabolic state of the patient (e.g., malnourishment)
9. Pathological diseases (e.g., malabsorption diseases)
10. First-pass phenomenon in the liver
11. Biliary flow
12. Other factors

Some of the reasons are listed in Table 11.9. Simulations of expected peak plasma levels based on relevant pharmacokinetic models made prior to the study are useful in selecting an appropriate dosage regimen to avoid undesirable plasma levels. It is difficult to include consideration of all potentially important factors in developing this mathematical model, since many of the factors that can influence blood levels are difficult to quantitate (e.g., drug interactions, elevated or decreased liver microsomal enzymes).

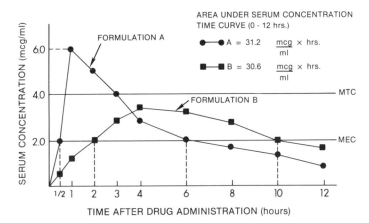

FIG. 11.6. Serum concentration–time curves for two different formulations of the same drug given at the same dose. The relationship of the curves to the minimum toxic concentration (MTC) and the minimum effective concentration (MEC) is shown. (Reprinted by permission of American Pharmaceutical Association from the *Journal of the American Pharmaceutical Association*; from Dittert and DiSanto, 1973.)

TABLE 11.9. *Reasons for measuring study drug concentration in plasma and/or other biological fluids*

1. Evaluate drug bioavailability and kinetics under different conditions
2. Measure patient compliance
3. Determine presence and degree of tolerance
4. Evaluate and quantify a clinical impression of underdosage or overdosage
5. Help to differentiate between the causes of an adverse reaction that could be caused by the patient's disease or the study drug
6. Establish suitable dosage schedules
7. Provide a guideline for when multiple drugs will be given and when drug interactions are probable
8. Provide a baseline when long-term treatment in a chronic disease is initiated
9. Evaluate errors in dosing
10. Evaluate different responses due to genetic factors
11. Evaluate whether the drug has a plasma range at which beneficial clinical effects are observed
12. Monitor the course of patients who are experiencing adverse reactions and/or an overdose
13. Other reasons

Time to Steady-State Concentration

The time to reach steady-state concentration is solely influenced by the drug's half-life. For example, 50% of the steady state is reached in one half-life, whereas 90% of the steady state is reached in 3.3 half-lives. If the time to reach steady-state concentration is relatively long (e.g., several days or longer), then a loading dose of a drug may be useful. If the time to steady-state concentration is quite short (because of a short half-life) and the drug is rapidly eliminated, then a controlled-release (long-acting) formulation may be useful to develop.

Duration of Blood Concentration

The duration of an adequate (above a minimum therapeutic concentration) blood concentration of a drug is an important factor in determining the frequency at which to administer the doses (see Fig. 11.6).

Duration of Biological Effects

For some drugs there is no direct correlation between drug plasma concentration and biological response to the drug. The duration of a drug's presence in the plasma may be relatively short, but the biological effect elicited may be prolonged. In this situation, less frequent drug administration can be utilized.

Drug Half-Life

This parameter is the time for half of the drug to have disappeared from the blood serum or plasma (see Fig. 11.5). The half-life of a drug is the sole determinant of the time necessary for steady-state concentrations to be reached on chronic dosing. Dosage interval considerations are most often based on drug half-life values, although they may be based on the duration of the biological half-life.

Accumulation

This refers to the build-up or increased levels of a drug in the body on multiple drug administrations. The potential for accumulation must be carefully considered in drugs with long half-lives or whenever the second dose is given while a significant fraction of the first dose is still present in the body.

Microsomal Enzyme Induction

When certain study or concomitant drugs are given chronically (e.g., phenobarbital, phenytoin), there is usually an increased level of microsomal enzymes in the liver. These enzymes metabolize a number of other drugs and thus increase their rate of elimination from the body. Therefore, a given dose of a drug that is metabolized by the induced microsomal enzymes may exert less of an effect than anticipated. This issue is especially important in testing new antiepileptic drugs, since most patients will be taking drugs that have caused enzyme induction. It must also be remembered that a drug that induces microsomal enzymes may also increase its own rate of metabolism, thus reducing its own pharmacological (i.e., therapeutic) effect. This generally occurs, however, only after a period of about 3 to 10 days, when the microsomal enzymes have been induced.

Distribution Characteristics

The rate and pattern of drug uptake into various body tissues can affect the selectivity and duration of drug action. For example, barbiturates are rapidly removed from the blood and enter fat tissues, from which they are slowly released. Different barbiturates have different affinities for fat tissues and differ in their distribution characteristics. These characteristics affect the size and frequency of doses to use in clinical studies.

Plasma Protein Binding

Many drugs interact reversibly with plasma proteins such as albumin. Because the unbound or "free" concentration of a drug generally correlates with pharmacological responses, any alteration in binding (especially for highly bound drugs) can affect therapeutic and/or toxic effects of a drug. Hypoalbuminemia or concomitant administration of other drugs that are highly protein bound (which would compete for binding sites) could elevate the "free" concentrations of the drug of interest. It may be necessary to consider these factors in protocol design and in establishing patient inclusion criteria.

Metabolism and Excretion

These topics are too enormous in scope to be summarized in a short space. Readers are referred to standard pharmacology and pharmacokinetic textbooks and references for information on these topics and for the myriad of ways in which they may influence drug study design. Major routes of excretion for drugs involve the kidneys and biliary system. The following routes are usually of minor significance: lungs, skin, saliva, hair, intestines, gastric secretions, and milk. Patients with altered liver function can be expected to metabolize drugs normally metabolized by liver differently than individuals with normal livers. This difference may have significant clinical consequences. Likewise, patients with altered renal function will excrete drugs (normally excreted in urine) differently than normals. The altered blood levels of a drug or duration of tissue levels in patients with abnormal renal function may yield significantly different clinical effects than those observed in a population of patients with normal renal function. Pathological conditions such as hypo- and hyperthyroidism or malnutrition states also affect metabolism of many drugs, as do environmental chemicals and diet (Conney et al., 1977).

Tolerance

Individuals may show tolerance to a drug (i.e., a decreased response or pharmacologic effect of a drug resulting from previous exposure to that drug) and may require a greater dose to yield an equivalent effect. Tolerance may be viewed as developing through either of two mechanisms. In one mechanism, the drug's concentration at the receptors will have decreased as a result of diminished drug absorption, increased drug elimination, altered binding of a drug, or other factors.

The other mechanism involves a diminution of the drug's effects once it has reached the target tissue.

Acute tolerance, in which a progressively decreased effect is observed on repeated dosing, is known as tachyphylaxis. This is an example of tolerance occurring at the cellular site of a drug's effect. This effect may be easily demonstrated with repeated i.v. doses of many sympathomimetic drugs.

If a drug is known to cause tolerance, then this factor must be considered in developing the study design, particularly with regard to frequency of dosing, amount of drug per dose, duration of the study, concomitant drugs, frequency of patient evaluation, and other factors.

SELECTED MATHEMATICAL MODELS USING PHARMACOKINETIC DATA

After limited pharmacokinetic data are available (e.g., rate of absorption and elimination and a constant for the volume of distribution) on a new drug, it is usually possible to simulate expected steady-state plasma concentrations under other conditions (e.g., using multiple doses). It may be possible to simulate certain pharmacological responses after information on blood levels and pharmacological responses is available (e.g., one may simulate the time necessary for 90% recovery from neuromuscular paralysis induced by a neuromuscular blocking drug).

Models have been developed that consider the body as consisting of one, two, or more compartments for understanding how a drug is distributed. A two-compartment model of rapidly equilibrating tissues (generally plasma and highly perfused organs such as the liver or kidney) or of more slowly equilibrating tissues is often used to study the effects of many drugs, although a single homogeneous compartment (one-compartment model) is used for some drugs.

Models are also used to determine the type of kinetics involved in excretion of a drug. Commonly used models allow mathematical description of the time course of drug levels under various dosing conditions. This description permits one to make predictions about both optimal amount and rate of drug dosing.

DRUG INTERACTIONS

Two or more drugs may interact in a myriad of ways and at various stages of drug administration, action, metabolism, and excretion. The effects of the interaction may lead to (1) a synergism of beneficial effects, (2) decreased therapeutic effects, (3) toxic adverse reactions, (4) unusual or complex effects that defy easy categorization, or (5) any other net result. A few common mechanisms that are involved in drug interactions include (1) drug incompatibility on administration, (2) induction of hepatic microsomal enzymes by one drug that affects the metabolism of another, and (3) renal effects of one drug that alter the elimination of another.

If drug interactions in a study are anticipated, then there are measures that can be followed either to prevent or minimize their impact. If the interactions are expected to occur during the absorption stages, then the times of administration of the two (or more) drugs may be staggered. The same approach may be followed for preventing problems of incompatible solutions of i.v. or other parenteral liquids. Two drugs should never be placed together in the same syringe or physiological solution unless well-documented compatibility tests have been performed. If the anticipated drug interactions are expected to occur after the absorption phase and to arise from physiological effects that will cause adverse reactions, then an alternative drug(s), dose, or dosage regimen should be sought whenever possible to avoid or minimize the problem. If these procedures are not possible, then appropriate laboratory and/or clinical monitoring of the patient should be considered.

12 Forms of Drugs

Drug Formulations • Forms of Drugs that May Be Taken Orally • Forms of Drugs that May Be Used Topically or Placed in Natural Orifices • Other Forms of Drugs • Long-Acting Dosage Forms

DRUG FORMULATIONS

In the majority of clinical studies, both the form of the drug to be studied and route of administration are known prior to development of the study design, and these factors are not raised as issues to be evaluated. Nonetheless, there are instances when either the forms of the drugs and/or routes of administration are the major focus of the study (e.g., comparison of two different forms or two different routes of administration). It is also possible that the pros and cons of each form (or route) that could be used must be considered prior to a determination of the most appropriate choice. A description of possible forms of drugs and routes of administration is presented in this and the following chapter.

The different forms of a drug shown in Table 12.10 are briefly described below, and a few considerations relating to their use in clinical studies are presented. Most of these drug forms contain a wide variety of additives or vehicles (e.g., lubricants, disintegrants, antioxidants, binders, diluents, buffers, surfactants, antibacterials, bulking agents, chelating agents, solubilizing agents, and tonicity-adjusting agents). Some of these additives may cause allergic responses in some individuals, and this factor must be considered in the clinical testing of the drug. Formulating a placebo for controlled studies may pose pharmaceutical problems for some of these drug forms. (Table 20.31 lists many factors in a placebo that must be matched to the study drug.) The preparation of a placebo should be initiated early in the process of drug development.

The comments below are generally brief and limited in scope. Additional information is presented in *Remington's Pharmaceutical Sciences* (Osol, 1980), *Modern Pharmaceutics* (Banker and Rhodes, 1979), *The Theory and Practice of Industrial Pharmacy* (Lachman et al., 1976), and in numerous other sources.

FORMS OF DRUGS THAT MAY BE TAKEN ORALLY

Tablets

Tablets are solid forms of a drug that are usually prepared by compression and are the most common form of drugs sold. Tablets may be coated or uncoated. If coated, they may be film coated to aid in swallowing, give a cosmetically acceptable appearance, and also to protect the drug from rapid dissolution. Enteric coating is one type of film coating that prevents a tablet from dissolving in the acid medium

TABLE 12.10. *Forms of drugs*

A. Forms of drugs that may be administered via the mouth
  1. Tablet
  2. Capsule
  3. Solution
  4. Suspension
  5. Emulsion
  6. Aerosol
  7. Gas
B. Other forms of drugs that may be used topically or placed in natural orifices in the body
  1. Powder
  2. Ointment
  3. Cream
  4. Gel
  5. Lotion
  6. Paste
  7. Suppository
  8. Transdermal patch
  9. Sponge
C. Long-acting dosage forms
  1. Sustained action
  2. Prolonged release
  3. Repeat action
  4. Depot

of the stomach. The tablet is thus absorbed in the intestines and not in the stomach. Tablets may also be sugar coated, which masks objectionable odors or tastes and protects the drug from many interactions (e.g., the sugar coating serves as an antioxidant). Sugar coating is a more time consuming process than is film coating. Layered tablets contain two or three different layers in each tablet. Press-coated tablets have a core tablet that is surrounded by a different material (i.e., it is a tablet within a tablet).

Active ingredients released from tablets may be absorbed under the tongue (e.g., sublingual nitroglycerin) or in the buccal cavity. These two routes of administration are useful for drugs that would otherwise be extensively metabolized in the liver in a "first-pass effect," and the sublingual route can achieve rapid absorption of a drug (e.g., nitroglycerin). Tablets may be chewable (e.g., aspirin has been sold in a gum form) or effervescent (e.g., Alka Seltzer™ contains sodium bicarbonate and citric acid and releases CO_2 when placed in water) or prepared as lozenges (candy-like forms of a drug) that dissolve slowly and maintain contact with the oral cavity and are especially useful in treating pediatric patients. Some examples of drug classes put into lozenges (also called pastilles or troches) are antibiotics, local anesthetics, antitussives, analgesics, and decongestants.

Disadvantages of tablets are that they require more excipients than do capsules or other dry forms of drugs. The types of excipients that may be required in tablets include lubricants (e.g., magnesium oxide) to keep the drug powder from sticking to the manufacturing punches, binding agents or gums (e.g., sucrose, gum acacia) to hold the tablet together, and disintegrants (e.g., starch, cellulose) to facilitate disintegration of the tablet in the gastrointestinal tract. Each excipient placed in a tablet may influence the bioavailability of a drug.

Capsules

Capsules may be composed of hard or soft gelatin, although hard gelatin capsules are more common. Soft gelatin capsules are generally used to contain a drug in the liquid form. Capsules may be enteric coated for the same reasons as tablets. Capsules are filled with loose powders, granules, beads, lightly compressed plugs, or even tablets. The outside covering may be clear, semiclear, or opaque. One of their advantages is that many patients find them easier to swallow than tablets.

Disadvantages of capsules are that they (1) are often more expensive than tablets to produce, (2) may require too large an empty capsule shell to include all drug required, and (3) are slower to manufacture than are tablets.

Drugs in Phase I studies are usually prepared in capsules since less pharmaceutical development work and less expense are required to produce capsules rather than tablets.

Solutions

Solutions are mixtures that are formed by dissolving a solid, liquid, or gas homogeneously in a liquid. Solutions are especially useful for pediatric and some geriatric oral drugs and are the most common form of all parenteral drugs. Potential problems must be considered in relation to solubility, stability, irritation to tissues, compatibility with preservatives, and other factors. Freeze drying is a process used for solutions and colloidal solutions. Freeze-dried forms of drugs are generally reconstituted shortly prior to use.

Suspensions

Suspensions are usually formed when the preparation of a solution is not possible. Suspensions are finely divided solids mixed or dispersed in a solid, liquid, or gas; the term is mainly applied to solids dispersed in liquids. A stable suspension that does not have to be shaken has advantages over suspensions in which settling occurs. Potential problems must be considered in relation to taste, odor, aftertaste, color, stability, compatibility with preservatives, and other factors.

Emulsions

Emulsions are mixtures of two immiscible liquids, one of which is uniformly dispersed throughout the other. Emulsions are usually oil in water or water in oil. They may be applied topically, or given orally or parenterally. There are extremely few emulsions used parenterally. A 10% intravenous (i.v.) fat emulsion (Intralipid 10%) is an example of one such product and is used for parenteral nutrition.

Aerosols

Aerosols are pressurized containers with a valve and have been used to administer drugs both orally (into the mouth and lungs) and topically. Many drugs have been placed in aerosol containers for treating numerous cutaneous or systemic diseases (e.g., asthma). They contain two major ingredients, the drug (with excipients) and the propellant, which forces the drug out of the container when the valve is pressed open.

The advantages of aerosols include ease and rapidity of use, protection of the contents from contamination by air, moisture, and light, and the ability to deliver "precisely" measured doses with metered valves. Disadvantages include the presence of fluorocarbon propellants (in some aerosols), which may cause environmental problems related to their effects on ozone, possible allergic and toxic reactions to some propellants, and generally high cost.

The types of aerosol products available may be described as (1) fine space sprays of small particles of the active drug, (2) surface-coating sprays, which use larger particle sizes to cover the surface with a film, and (3) aerated sprays, which dispense various foams and creams, although this latter type is not used orally. Aerosols may be used to deliver either liquids or small particles of solids. Pump sprays and the intermittent positive-pressure breathing apparatus are other methods of delivering inhalationally applied drugs.

Gases

Gases are usually given by mouth but may also be administered via the nasal cavity. General anesthetics are the most common type of drug given in this form and are supplied as gases (e.g., nitrous oxide) or as liquids that volatilize (e.g., halothane).

FORMS OF DRUGS THAT MAY BE USED TOPICALLY OR PLACED IN NATURAL ORIFICES

Powders

Powders are most often packaged in sprinkling cans, aerosols, and jars. Powders and crushed tablets may be mixed with foods (e.g., applesauce) for administration to children. Advantages of powders include flexibility in preparation (compounding with excipients) and generally good chemical stability.

Powders are useful in certain applications, including foot powders, powders for decubitous ulcers, dental powders, douche powders, dusting powders (applied to the skin for various hygienic purposes), and insufflation. Insufflation describes the delivery of powder directly into the lungs (e.g., the Spinhaler™ turbo-inhaler is used to deliver micronized cromolyn sodium powder to lungs). The drawbacks of powders often include (1) poor adhesiveness to the skin, (2) that they are time consuming to prepare and package, (3) difficulty of patients obtaining equal doses, especially if the powder is affected by humidity, is hygroscopic, or is fluffy, and (4) unsuitability to drugs that have an unpleasant odor or taste.

Ointments, Creams, and Gels

Ointments, creams, and gels are semisolid formulations. Ointments are generally translucent, creams are usually opaque white, and gels have a clarity that ranges from clear to a translucence similar to that of petrolatum. The term "cream" has been used both for oil-in-water emulsions and for water-in-oil emulsions, although the former are more prevalent. Ointments are high-viscosity suspensions of the active drug(s) in a vehicle.

One limitation of these formulations is the difficulty encountered in delivering a precise dose with commercially available products. There are a number of techniques used to measure the dose of drug delivered from a jar or tube containing ointment, cream, or gel. Probably the best method is to weigh the tube or other container before and after either one or several applications. It is understood, however, that not all of the drug expressed from the tube or removed from the jar or other container will have been applied to the target lesion. Another system to calculate the dose is to measure the length of the ribbon squeezed from a tube (e.g., this system is used with nitroglycerin 2% ointment). A third approach is to measure the area covered with the medication and to express the dose as the amount of drug required to cover a defined area, but this latter method is the least reliable of the three described to define dosage. It is often preferable to prepare unit-of-use foil packs or other units that contain precise amounts of drug. This presupposes, however, that the contents of one (or more packs) will contain the appropriate quantity of drug for all patients and for all lesions.

Lotions

Lotions are usually liquid suspensions that are used externally on the body. The decision to develop a lotion usually depends on the intended use (e.g., shampoo, special skin treatment). In preparing drug dosages for clinical studies, it may be useful to consider unit-dose containers, each having a fixed amount of lotion to apply. An alternative means of measuring the dose is to weigh containers before and after treatment(s).

Pastes

Pastes are stiff semisolid mxitures of powders (e.g., starch, zinc oxide, talc) dispersed in petrolatum as a base (i.e., an ointment) intended for use on the skin. Pastes are often used to treat oozing and moist lesions such as burns and open wounds, where pastes absorb serous fluids and secretions. They adhere well to the skin and form an opaque layer. Pastes may be removed with a vegetable or mineral oil. Examples of pastes are zinc oxide paste and those used by outdoor athletes on their face to prevent windburn.

Suppositories

These solid forms are usually placed in the rectum, where they melt and deliver drug that is absorbed through mucus membranes. Suppositories are also placed in the vagina and, albeit rarely, in the urethra. Local effects occur within 30 min and usually last for at least 4 hr. This form is also used to elicit systemic effects. In the formulation of suppositories, special attention is concentrated on achieving the optimum size, shape, hardness, melting characteristics, and bioavailability. Under situations in which an individual has difficulty swallowing, suppositories may be given orally for patients to suck in order to deliver a drug.

This form was used by ancient Egyptians, Greeks, and Romans, and today suppositories are more widely used in some countries than others. In the United States, this form is most widely used for pediatric and geriatric patients. In pediatrics, suppositories are used to treat emesis and other conditions. The adult population mainly uses this form to treat hemorrhoids and constipation, but suppositories are suitable as a carrier for many classes of drugs.

Transdermal Patches

Transdermal patches have recently been introduced for the gradual absorption of nitrates in patients with angina and for scopolamine to prevent motion sickness. The use of this drug form will probably expand in the future as a means of obtaining constant but low level of drug delivery over a prolonged period.

Sponges

Sponges impregnated with drugs are currently being used for contraception. A disposable vaginal polyurethane sponge with nonoxynol-9 is now sold over the counter in the United States.

OTHER FORMS OF DRUGS

Depot

Depot drugs are placed inside body tissues or cavities for prolonged periods. The depot acts as a reservoir from which the drug is slowly leeched over an extended period at a relatively constant rate. There are a variety of physical–chemical means whereby release of the drug from the depot may be delayed and controlled. Examples of depots include depot injections given i.m. (e.g., procaine penicillin G, medroxyprogesterone acetate suspension) and s.q. (e.g., protamine zinc insulin), and implants that are professionally placed (e.g., Progestosert®). Silicon rubber (Silastic) inserts that contain drugs have been more widely used in recent years. Drugs are either sealed inside an inner cavity or may be made as part of the inert Silastic matrix itself, from which it diffuses. Silastic has been formed into many shapes, including tubes, membranous sacs, rings, and other shapes. There

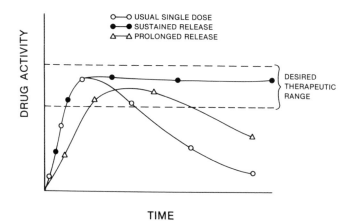

FIG. 12.7. Two types of hypothetical long-acting formulations of a single drug (sustained release and prolonged release) compared to activity over time of a single dose of the same drug. (Reprinted by permission of Philadelphia College of Pharmacy and Science from Osol, 1980.)

is wide speculation that implants will be used more widely in the future to provide drug release close to the target organ.

LONG-ACTING DOSAGE FORMS

Long-acting dosage forms have been referred to by many names, including controlled release, timed release, delayed action, and extended release, plus the three names used in this section to describe long-acting dosage forms: sustained action, prolonged action, and repeat action. There are occasions when it is desirable to release the drug from the formulation over an extended period to provide an adequate drug level during the entire sleep or waking period (e.g., to maintain sleep, an antibacterial effect, or many other effects) or at other times when the drug used does not have the desired duration of effect. There are various types of long-acting dosage forms and various techniques of formulating these products. Three types of long-acting dosage forms are:

1. Sustained action. The drug is absorbed and acts the same pharmacologically as the usual single dose, but its effect continues for a longer period, and constant drug levels in blood are maintained (see Fig. 12.7).
2. Prolonged action. The drug is absorbed somewhat less rapidly and for a longer period than the usual single dose, and its total duration of effect is greater than that provided by the single dose, although constant drug levels in blood are not necessarily maintained (see Fig. 12.7).
3. Repeat action. The drug is manufactured to have a usual dose absorbed at two different times (e.g., by placing an enteric coated tablet inside a regular tablet).

The most difficult form of the above three types to prepare is the true sustained-action dosage form, and this is rarely achieved. Several different manufacturing methods are used to prepare sustained- and prolonged-action dosage forms. These include the use of (1) tablets with slow-release cores, (2) capsules containing coated slow-release beads, (3) multilayered tablets, (4) porous inert carriers or (5) ion-exchange resins to complex drugs, and (6) tablets compressed from different types of granules (e.g., coated and uncoated) that provide release at different times.

Sustained release of parenteral drugs may be attained through the use of relatively insoluble salts or esters of the active parent molecule. Vehicles may be chosen for use from which the active drug is slowly absorbed. Newer techniques for creating long-acting liquids have begun to provide new drugs with this property, and there are many novel ideas being evaluated for new forms of drug delivery (Merz et al., 1983).

13 Routes of Administration

Introduction ● Routes of Administration in Which Drugs Are Placed into a Natural Orifice in the Body, Including Oral Routes of Administration ● Routes of Administration in Which Drugs Are Injected into the Body or Placed Under the Skin ● Topical Routes of Administration

INTRODUCTION

Routes of drug administration may be considered as being of two types—enteral and parenteral. The enteral routes place the drug directly into the gastrointestinal tract by oral, sublingual, buccal, or rectal administration. All other routes, including topical routes, may be defined as parenteral, although topical routes are not commonly described as a parenteral route of applying drugs.

Routes of drug administration may also be divided into one of four general categories: (1) oral, (2) topical, (3) injected into the body or placed under the skin, or (4) placed into a natural orifice in the body other than the mouth. Examples of routes that are included in these four broad categories are presented in Table 13.11. The choice of a particular route to use in most studies is usually evident to the author of a protocol, but there are occasions when a choice among several routes is possible. Each route of administration has a number of potential and actual advantages and disadvantages. There are also considerations that should be familiar to individuals using these routes. A number of these factors are described in the sections that follow.

ROUTES OF ADMINISTRATION IN WHICH DRUGS ARE PLACED INTO A NATURAL ORIFICE IN THE BODY, INCLUDING ORAL ROUTES OF ADMINISTRATION

Drugs placed into a natural orifice exert local effects and in many instances systemic effects as well. The possibility of systemic effects occurring when local effects are desired or of local effects occurring when systemic effects are desired should be considered.

For routes of administration in which the drug is taken orally or placed into an orifice other than the mouth, clear instructions about the correct application of the drug must be provided. Many cases are known of oral pediatric drops for ear infections being placed into the ear, and vice versa (ear drops being swallowed). Errors in drug utilization are especially prevalent when a drug form is being used in a nontraditional manner (e.g., suppositories that are taken by the buccal route).

Many patients are not familiar with terms such as sublingual (under the tongue), buccal (between the cheek and gingiva), otic, and numerous others. A clear de-

TABLE 13.11. *Routes of administration*

A. Oral routes
1. Oral
2. Inhalational[a]
3. Sublingual
4. Buccal
B. Placed into a natural orifice in the body other than the mouth
1. Intranasal
2. Intraauricular
3. Rectal
4. Intravaginal
5. Intrauterine
6. Intraurethral
C. Injected into the body or placed under the skin
1. Intravenous
2. Subcutaneous
3. Intramuscular
4. Intraarterial
5. Intradermal
6. Intralesional
7. Epidural[b]
8. Intrathecal[c]
9. Intracisternal
10. Intracardiac
11. Intraventricular
12. Intraocular
13. Intraperitoneal
D. Topical routes
1. Cutaneous
2. Transdermal[d]
3. Ophthalmic

[a]This route is usually via the mouth, although the nose may be used.
[b]This route is also referred to as peridural and extradural.
[c]This route is also referred to as subarachnoid.
[d]This route is also referred to as transcutaneous and percutaneous.

scription of each of these nontraditional (i.e., nonoral) uses should be discussed with patients, and instructions may also be written and given to patients. Demonstrations are often useful to illustrate selected techniques of drug use (e.g., how to use an inhaler or aerosol for asthma). Some drugs must be placed by physicians into body orifices (e.g., medicated intrauterine devices such as Progestasert™).

The inhalational route via mouth or nose is used for drugs that are in a gaseous state (e.g., anesthetic gases) and for liquids and solids (via aerosols). Both the liquid and solid particles are so small that they remain suspended in air as they are inhaled into the lungs. In general, the smaller the particle size, the further the particles travel before depositing along the tracheopulmonary tree. There is less of a tendency for smaller particles to sediment at the upper end of the pulmonary system, where they are inhaled. When patients inspire a large volume of air, the velocity of the air moving into the respiratory tract is greater, forcing all particles to go further into the tracheopulmonary tree before they are deposited. Thus, aerosols of mixed particle size will cause less consistent pharmacological responses than will those of a more uniform size. Also, smaller-size particles are generally deposited closest to the alveolar membranes, from which they will be absorbed more rapidly into the circulation. Finally, patients should be instructed to inhale with a strong effort when they use an aerosol to deliver a drug.

Significant systemic absorption occurs with many drugs given by inhalational techniques, which use small particles. Although pressurized and nonpressurized aerosols have been used to deliver numerous drugs into the systemic circulation, this approach has not been widely used.

ROUTES OF ADMINISTRATION IN WHICH DRUGS ARE INJECTED INTO THE BODY OR PLACED UNDER THE SKIN

General Considerations

Most injected routes of administration place the drug directly or indirectly into the systemic circulation. There are a number of these routes, however, by which the drug exerts a local effect, and most of the drug does not enter the systemic circulation (e.g., intrathecal, intraventricular, intraocular, intracisternal). Certain routes of administration may exert both local and systemic effects depending on the characteristics of the drug and excipients (e.g., subcutaneous, percutaneous, and rectal).

The choice of a particular parenteral route will depend on the required time to onset of action, the required site of action, and the characteristics of the fluid, among other factors.

The need for a rapid onset of action usually requires that an i.v. route be used, although at a certain stage of cardiopulmonary resuscitation, the need for a rapid effect may require the use of an intracardiac injection. The required site of action may influence the choice of route of administration (e.g., certain radiopaque dyes are given intraarterially near the site being evaluated; streptokinase is sometimes given experimentally into the coronary arteries close to coronary vessel occlusion during a myocardial infarction to [it is hoped] cause lysis of the thrombus and reestablish coronary blood flow).

The characteristics of the fluid (i.e., study drug) to be injected will influence which parenteral routes of administration are possible to consider. The compatibility of the fluid used must be evaluated with other fluids (e.g., saline, dextrose, Ringer's–lactate) that the drug may be combined with for administration to the patient.

There are certain clinical situations in which a parenteral route of administration is preferred to other possible routes. These include the following:

1. When the amount of drug given to a patient must be precisely controlled (e.g., in many pharmacokinetic studies), it is preferable to use a parenteral (usually i.v.) route of administration.
2. When the "first-pass effect" of a drug going through the liver must be avoided, a parenteral route of administration is usually chosen, although a sublingual route or dermal patch will also avoid the "first-pass effect."

3. When one requires complete assurance that an uncooperative patient has actually received the drug and has not "cheeked" it or otherwise rejected it (e.g., via emesis).
4. When patients are in a stupor, coma, or otherwise unable to take a drug orally.
5. When large volumes (i.e., more than a liter) of fluid are injected in peritoneal dialysis, hyperalimentation, fluid replacement, and other conditions. Drugs given in large volumes require special consideration of fluid balance in the patients receiving the large volumes.

Intravenous

The i.v. route is the most common means to introduce a drug directly into the systemic circulation. It has the following advantages:

1. Rapid onset of effect.
2. Usefulness in situations of poor gastrointestinal absorption.
3. Avoidance of tissue irritation if present with i.m. or other routes (e.g., nitrogen mustard).
4. More precise control of levels of drug than with other routes, especially for toxic drugs, where the levels must be kept within narrow limits.
5. Ability to administer large volumes over time by a slow infusion.
6. Ability to administer drugs at a constant rate over a long period of time.

It also suffers from these disadvantages:

1. Higher incidence of anaphylactic reactions than with many other routes.
2. Possibility of infection or phlebitis at site of injection.
3. Greater pain to patients than with many other routes.
4. Possibility that embolic phenomena may occur, either air embolism or vascular clot as a result of damage to the vascular wall.
5. Impossibility of removing or lavaging drug after it is given except by dialysis.
6. Inconvenience in many situations.
7. Possibility that rapid injection rates may cause severe adverse reactions.

For i.v. fluids it must be determined how the dose will be given (i.e., by bolus or slow injection, intermittent or constant infusion, or by constant drip) and whether special equipment will be used to control and monitor the flow. Drugs with short half-lives are usually given by a constant drip or infusion technique. All i.v. fluids given immediately subsequent to an i.v. drug must be evaluated for their compatibility with the study drug. Suspensions are not given i.v. because of the possibility of blocking the capillaries.

Subcutaneous

Drugs given by the s.q. route are forced into spaces between connective tissues, as with i.m. injections. Vasoconstrictors and drugs that cause local irritation should not be given s.q. under usual circumstances, since inflammation, abscess formation, or even tissue necrosis may result. When daily or even more frequent s.q. injections are made, the sites of injection should be continuously changed to prevent local complications. Fluids given s.q. must have an appropriate tonicity to prevent pain, and fluids given into the central nervous system must be pure and sterile to prevent neurotoxicity and infection. Care must be taken to prevent injection of the drug directly into veins.

The absorption of drugs from a s.q. route is influenced by blood flow to the area, as with i.m. injections. The rate of absorption may be retarded by cooling the local area to cause vasoconstriction, adding epinephrine to the solution for the same purpose (e.g., with local anesthetics), decreasing blood flow with a tourniquet, or immobilizing the area. The opposite effect may be achieved with the enzyme hyaluronidase, which breaks down mucopolysaccharides of the connective tissue matrix and allows the injected solution to spread over a larger area and thus increase its rate of absorption.

In addition to fluids, solid forms of drugs may be given s.q. This has been done with compressed pellets of testosterone placed under the skin, which are absorbed at a relatively constant rate over a long period.

Intramuscular

The i.m. route is frequently used for drugs dissolved in oily vehicles or for those in a microcrystalline formulation that are poorly soluble in water (e.g., procaine penicillin G). Advantages include rapid absorption in many cases, often in under 30 min. Other advantages of the i.m. route include the opportunity to inject a relatively large amount of solution and a reduction in pain and local irritation compared with s.q. injections. Complications include infections and nerve damage. The latter usually results from the choice of an incorrect site for injection.

Although the time to peak drug concentration is often on the order of 1 to 2 hr, depot preparations given i.m. are absorbed extremely slowly. Numerous physical–chemical properties of the material given i.m. will affect the rate of absorption from the site within the muscle (e.g., ionization of the drug, lipid solubility, osmolality of the solution, volume given). The primary sites used for i.m. injections are the gluteal (buttocks), deltoid (upper arm), and vastus lateralis (lateral thigh) muscles. The rate of drug absorption and the peak drug levels obtained will often differ between different sites used for i.m. injections. This is related to differences in blood flow among muscle groups (Evans et al., 1975). The site chosen for an i.m. injection may be a critical factor in whether or not the drug exhibits a therapeutic effect (Schwartz et al., 1974).

Intraarterial

Intraarterial injections usually require a surgical "cut-down" procedure before they can be given. This route requires highly skilled individuals to prevent a variety of potentially serious complications. These complications include thrombosis formation, arterial spasm, and the possibility of loss of blood supply distal to the site of injection. Its uses include injection of radiopaque contrast media and selected antineoplastic agents.

Intradermal

Intradermal injections are often used with allergy-testing materials used for diagnosis of types of allergies or for evaluating improvement after treatment. Small volumes (0.05 ml) of isotonic solutions are usually used and are placed into the skin so that a small wheal is formed (a small circumscribed transitory area of edema of the skin). If a wheal is not raised, then the injection has probably been given s.q. and must be repeated at another site or at a later time.

Intralesional

Intralesional administration is used for several drug groups, of which corticosteroids are the most common. This route is often chosen when topical agents either lack adequate potency or do not satisfactorily penetrate the epidermal skin barrier. Drugs given by this route may be used on their own or as an adjunct to topically applied drugs as therapy for many diseases. Long-term use of intralesional injections may cause systemic effects to occur (Amene, 1983).

Intrathecal and Epidural

Intrathecal injections of drugs (in isotonic fluids) are also referred to as subarachnoid injections. Drugs are placed in the cerebrospinal fluid in the subarachnoid space inside the spinal canal. Injections are often made between lumbar vertebrae 2 and 5. This route is used for numerous purposes, including induction of spinal anesthesia and treatment of leukemic foci in the central nervous system. The term "spinal" injection is colloquial for a subarachnoid injection.

Epidural injections are also referred to as peridural and extradural injections. Drugs are injected into the space surrounding the dura mater but within the spinal canal. Both caudal and lumbar approaches are used. Intraspinal is a general term referring to subarachnoid and epidural routes together.

Intraventricular, Intraperitoneal, and Intracardiac

For intraventricular injections, an indwelling catheter may be used with a reservoir to provide chemotherapeutic drugs to patients when the blood–brain barrier is intact. This system provides high local concentrations plus low systemic drug levels.

The intraperitoneal route is rarely used in humans but has been used to administer anticancer drugs for abdominal ascitic tumors. Intracardiac injections are for the most part used only during emergency cardiopulmonary resuscitation attempts. These injections may be made through an open or closed chest.

TOPICAL ROUTES OF ADMINISTRATION

There are numerous considerations of study design to deal with in using a topical route of administration that are difficult to adequately control. These potential problems are a major reason why double-blind well-controlled studies are less common in dermatology than in many other areas of medicine. A number of these considerations, which are difficult to control adequately, are the following:

1. Where on the body surface will the drug be applied? Should mucus membranes be avoided? Even on the skin surface, the absorption of a drug varies enormously between different sites and depends on clinical conditions (e.g., approximately 1% of topical hydrocortisone penetrates normal human skin on the forearm, but only one-seventh as much will penetrate the skin through the plantar foot arch, and 42 times as much will penetrate through scrotal skin; hydration of the skin increases absorption of hydrocortisone by about four- or fivefold; inflammation also markedly increases the skin penetration of hydrocortisone and most other topically applied drugs).
2. Will the drug be absorbed into the systemic circulation, and if so, what are the consequences for the patient and for the study?
3. How will the amount of drug dispensed be measured (e.g., length of a ribbon, size of skin covered, weight of drug container before and after application)?
4. If a percutaneous route is used (i.e., absorption of drug occurs through unbroken skin) with rubbing of an ointment or other form of drug, how will the rubbing be quantitated and controlled in terms of pressure and duration?
5. How will the effect of the drug be measured (e.g., by a clinical scale of several gradations, biopsy results, other techniques)?
6. At which of the following sites is the drug presumed (or known) to act: skin surface, stratum corneum, viable epidermis and upper dermis, glands, and/ or systemically?
7. How will the study be controlled, since clinical lesions vary markedly in intensity of symptoms and appearance from site to site within one patient as well as between patients? Although it is desirable for each patient to serve as his/her own control (e.g., by treating lesions on each arm or leg with different drugs), it is often difficult to accurately quantitate different lesions in one individual, though this often must be done.
8. Numerous other factors must be considered (e.g., vehicle used, appropriate form of drug).

Section II

Developing and Writing Clinical Protocols

14 Formulating an Approach to Developing a Protocol

A protocol is the written mechanism that describes how the study design will be implemented. There is no single approach that all individuals follow in developing a protocol for drug studies. Furthermore, the same individual will follow different approaches in developing different protocols. Nonetheless, there are a number of principles that are usually adhered to and a general approach that is often followed, although many variations are possible. The chapters in Section II describe this general approach and are presented with the assumption that individuals will generally need (or desire) to modify the proposed order of steps in preparing specific protocols to make this approach work more effectively for them. The stages or steps presented in Table 14.12 represent a sequence of activities that may be modified or reordered to effectively meet the requirements of specific situations.

One may begin to write a clinical protocol after many discussions among numerous individuals. Alternatively, the writing of a protocol may represent the initial groundbreaking in a new clinical area, and one can only rely on his/her previous experience without a background of recent discussions. The study may be modest in scope and conducted at one site, or it may be scheduled for several years and encompass many sites. Whatever the size of the projected study, and regardless of how much prior preparation has been done by the individual responsible for the

TABLE 14.12. *Factors in the development and writing of a clinical protocol*

1. Formulating an approach
2. Establishing criteria for patient inclusion
3. Identifying and choosing safety parameters
4. Modifying dosing schedules and developing compliance checks
5. Identifying, choosing, and evaluating efficacy parameters
6. Developing time and event schedules
7. Preparing, packaging, and dispensing study drugs
8. Preparing the introduction
9. Polishing the "boilerplate"
10. Regulatory, patent, and legal considerations
11. Ethical considerations
12. Completing and reviewing the initial draft
13. Improving the protocol
14. Preparing data collection forms
15. Instructions for patients, investigators, and study personnel
16. Continuation protocols
17. Comments on multicenter studies

protocol, there are many steps that must be considered. A thesis of this book is that the development of most protocols usually follows a similar series of steps, even though protocols are written in a highly diverse manner and are applied in different areas of medicine. It is assumed that a protocol is a self-contained document and does not need to refer to other protocols or texts for content.

The procedures described that are followed in developing a protocol have been arbitrarily divided into the 16 points (items 2–17) listed in Table 14.12. Each of the 16 topics is the focus of a separate chapter in Section II. The individual who is writing the protocol is also generally engaged in numerous other activities designed to initiate the protocol. A number of these activities are being considered and/or conducted at the same time that the protocol is being written. Many of these activities (e.g., interviewing potential investigators) are discussed in Section III of this book.

It is widely believed that a first-hand clinical appreciation of the disease being evaluated helps the author of a protocol to choose the most appropriate study design to address the objectives and the optimal parameters to measure the anticipated clinical changes. For this reason, there is a potential problem when trained scientists prepare protocols rather than medically trained individuals, since members of the former group lack clinical experience. Collaboration between a scientist and a clinician in the protocol development process, however, can almost always solve any study design issues that arise.

The style used in writing clinical protocols depends on the skills and personality of the person writing the protocol as well as the requirements (if any) of the institution at which the study will be conducted, the requirements of the sponsor (if any), and other factors. Thus, there may be stylistic constraints placed on the individual who is in the process of developing a clinical protocol. The presence and nature of any stylistic requirements should be determined before the writing phase commences.

15 Establishing Criteria for Patient Inclusion

Introduction • Characteristics of Patients • Characteristics of the Disease and its Treatment • Environmental and Other Factors • Results of Screening Examinations

INTRODUCTION

This chapter describes the various criteria that can be used for patient inclusion and exclusion. Inclusion criteria constitute the definition of patient characteristics required for entry into a study. Inclusion criteria may generally be used for patient exclusion as well as inclusion, since most criteria (e.g., age range of 18–65 years) establish both inclusion (18–65 years) and exclusion (lower than 18 or above 65 years) groupings. The single term "inclusion" is usually used in a general sense throughout this book to include the concept of "exclusion" as well.

If the limits for patient entry are set too broadly, then a heterogeneous group of patients may be enrolled. This may create a problem when the data generated are inadequate to address the study objectives. Under circumstances in which an excessively heterogeneous group of patients is enrolled, the interpretation and relevance of the study may be questioned. Conversely, if the limits of patient entry are set too narrowly, then it may be impossible to obtain an adequate number of patients to conduct the study. In addition, it may be difficult to compare data from such a population with data generated from a broader population (i.e., interpretation of the data may not be relevant for general clinical situations).

The advantage of using relatively "tight" entry criteria is that the study will be conducted with a more homogeneous population. This will often provide more meaningful data and interpretations, especially for Phase II controlled studies. Many of the criteria used to determine patient inclusion are listed in Table 15.13. These criteria have been arbitrarily divided into four groups: (1) characteristics of patients, (2) characteristics of the disease and its treatment, (3) environmental and other factors, and (4) results of screening examinations.

In determining the criteria to be used for patient inclusion, it is important to exclude those patients for whom the study will create unacceptable clinical risks. If patients with a given disease, state, or attribute are to be excluded from a study, then it is important to determine the procedures used to exclude these patients. For example, if all patients with a given disease are to be excluded from a study, it may be sufficient for the investigator to question all prospective participants as to whether they presently have the given disease. An additional question that may be posed by the investigator is whether the patient has ever had the disease. A further

TABLE 15.13. *Factors to consider as criteria for patient inclusion*[a]

A. Characteristics of patients
1. Sex
2. Age
3. Weight
4. Education
5. Race and/or ethnic background
6. Social and economic status
7. Pregnancy and lactation
8. Use of tobacco; ingestion of caffeine and/or alcohol
9. Abuse of alcohol or drugs
10. Diet and nutritional status
11. Physiological limitations and genetic history
12. Surgical, anatomical, and/or emotional limitations
13. Hypersensitivity to a study drug or test
14. Other drug and nondrug allergies
B. Characteristics of the disease and its treatment
1. Disease being evaluated
2. Concomitant drugs
3. Previous drug and nondrug treatment
4. Washout period of nonstudy drugs or nondrug treatments
5. History of other diseases
6. Present clinical status
7. Previous hospitalizations
C. Environmental and other factors
1. Patient recruitment and cooperation
2. Participation in another drug study
3. Participation in another part of this study or in any other study using this study drug
4. Institutional or environmental status
5. Occupation
6. Geographical location
7. Litigation and disability
D. Results of screening examinations

---

[a]This term is used to encompass criteria used for exclusion as well.

step is to request that a laboratory or other test be performed to document that the patient does not have the disease. The degree of documentation required for patients to enter the study may be set at whatever standard is deemed appropriate to insure that patients in the study do not have the excluded disease. The criteria established in most of the categories discussed in this chapter may be (1) ascertained by patient history as recounted by the patient or as noted in medical records, (2) observed by the investigator, (3) documented by scores on tests, or (4) confirmed by other professionals using clinical judgment. It may be important for key tests to be performed by independent investigators, laboratories, or groups to prevent bias from entering into critical measurements that affect patient inclusion. Inclusion criteria should be designed to eliminate (insofar as possible) hard-core nonresponders with the disease being evaluated. If this is not done, then no matter how well the study is designed and conducted in a large number of hard core nonresponders, the data obtained may actually represent a false–negative result.

CHARACTERISTICS OF PATIENTS

The first group of specific inclusion criteria to be discussed relates to characteristics of patients (Table 15.13).

Sex of the Patient

Certain studies are limited to patients of one sex by their objectives (e.g., prostate or ovarian evaluations). Women of child-bearing potential must be excluded from almost all clinical studies of investigational drugs until appropriate reproductive and teratological studies have been performed. Many Phase I studies, therefore, exclude all women. Inclusion criteria usually indicate which classes of women of non-child-bearing potential may be enrolled (i.e., women who are postmenopausal and/or those who have had a hysterectomy and/or those who have had a tubal ligation). In pediatric studies, females are often excluded once they have reached the menarche.

Age of the Patient

The ranges of patients' ages have been arbitrarily grouped into three categories: children (until age of majority), adults, and elderly.

A frequently discussed and debated question relates to the acceptable lower age limits for patients who are included in a drug study. Establishing a lower age limit depends on many factors such as the nature of the disease, adequacy of available treatment(s), evaluation of the study drug's safety and efficacy, guidelines of pediatric committees, and the views of the various ethics and administrative committees that must approve the protocol. If separate pediatric studies are being planned, then the investigator should review the various guidelines for conducting drug studies in children prior to writing the protocol (Food and Drug Administration, 1974, 1977a; American Academy of Pediatrics Committee on Drugs, 1977; Ryan, 1977; Working Party on Ethics of Research in Children—British Paediatric Association, 1980). With parental or legal guardian consent, minors below the age of 18 may be included in drug studies. Children from the age of about 7 to their majority (legal adult age) must give their "assent" (usually verbal and in the presence of a witness) to participate in a clinical study. In addition, the investigator must obtain the informed consent from the child's parent(s) or legal guardian.

It has been well known for many years that neonates, infants, and children respond to certain drugs differently than adults, primarily because of pharmacokinetic differences. Now there is increasing information indicating that older individuals also respond to some drugs differently than younger adults. The impact of these findings on the testing of investigational drugs is that early clinical studies usually exclude older individuals as well as children. Older individuals are gradually included in clinical studies as drug safety is more firmly understood and established. Separate studies targeted to the elderly age group are also performed on both investigational and marketed drugs. Definitions of elderly patients based solely on age are arbitrary and do not consider that chronological age and physiological age are often quite different in any one patient or within a group of patients.

In recent years, more attention has been directed towards the evaluation of drug effects in the older population as a result of the following:

1. An increased number of older people in society and projections for a steadily increasing percentage of older patients in the population.
2. A disproportionately high use of drugs in the older population.
3. An increased frequency of adverse drug reactions in the older population.
4. Differences in pharmacokinetics, pathology, and receptor sensitivity and/or density plus impaired homeostasis.

Drugs that are particularly important to evaluate in the geriatric population are those that (1) are widely used in the elderly, (2) affect the central nervous system, (3) have a low therapeutic ratio (i.e., the minimal dose that elicits clinically significant adverse reactions divided by the minimal dose that elicits a clinically significant beneficial effect), especially if the drug is eliminated via the kidneys or if there is a hepatic "first-pass" effect, and those that (4) change the body's homeostatic mechanisms (e.g., in hypertension).

It may be relevant to indicate the specific point in the study at which the age criterion applies. For instance, in a study with age inclusion of 16 to 70 years, an investigator may call the monitor and state that he has two prospective patients, one who was 70 last week and another who will be 16 midway through the study. It is desirable to have one standard to apply to all such situations. One valid standard is to specify that all patients must meet the entry criteria on the day that they officially enter the study, whether this is defined to be at screen, start of baseline, or treatment. It is the author's view that some leniency may be applied to the upper but not to the lower age limit.

Weight

In studies in which the patient's weight is of major interest, a detailed description of acceptable patient weight characteristics and history must be specified. Those characteristics would probably be utilized for efficacy determinations and are not discussed in this book. In studies that do not focus on weight characteristics, it may be necessary or prudent to exlude patients who fall outside general weight limits. In many studies, however, no guidelines or inclusion criteria need be presented. In studies of new investigational drugs, general prudence has often dictated that patients be relatively close (possibly ± 10%) to an ideal or average weight. As experience with a new drug increases, this requirement is generally loosened to ± 15% or ± 20% and then eliminated entirely. The concept of ideal weight has recently been criticized (Knapp, 1983), and it is possible that future drug studies may focus less on including individuals near their ideal weight and would only exclude extremely thin or obese patients.

There may be reasons relating to drug metabolism or the ability of the investigator or patient to adequately perform certain examinations or tests to exclude individuals of excessively high or low weights from a study. Individuals of certain weights outside the normal range may be required, however, in other studies such as those designed to evaluate questions relating to metabolism. The conditions under which a patient's weight is measured may be specified (e.g., noontime, prior to meal, in socks, after voiding).

In certain protocols, height may be viewed as a factor to be used in stratifying patients or considered in a manner similar to (or in additon to) weight.

Education

Although a patient's education is not specifically addressed in the inclusion criteria of most protocols, there are studies in which a patient's education may be a significant factor. To evaluate the effect of an investigational drug on a complex series of sophisticated psychological tests, it may be appropriate to include a criterion relating to the patients' education (e.g., being high school graduates). One variation of this criterion is to require patients to have an education "equivalent" to that of a high school graduate.

It is also possible that a clinical study objective may relate to evaluating patients with different educational levels. Thus, a predetermined number of patients may be required with specified levels of education. One example of this approach is in evaluating the comprehension and usefulness of patient package inserts in individuals with different levels of education.

Race and/or Ethnic Background

In certain clinical areas, such as in dermatology, the question of race may be important. In measuring the flare reaction to injected histamine, for example, it may be appropriate to limit a study to white individuals or to those blacks with pale-colored skin.

In other studies, the question of race may be the central focus of the study. For example, several studies have evaluated the responses of white and black individuals to antihypertensive medications. In this type of study, entry criteria may be established to include specific numbers of patients of each race. Another area where race is important is in evaluating diseases that are more (or less) prevalent in a given race (e.g., sickle cell anemia in blacks).

The ethnic background of patients may also be relevant in clinical studies in which a similar control population is desired. For example, many patients with the disease thalassemia are individuals whose families originate from the Mediterranean area around Greece or Italy. It may be relevant to require that the control population also have the same ancestry as the study group.

Social and Economic Status

The marital status of the patient may be used as a selection factor for some studies (i.e., single, married, divorced, or widowed), although this is not a common criterion for entrance into a study. In addition, the patient's income or economic status is only rarely included in an entrance criterion, although certain diseases and types of drug abuse are more common in specific social and/or economic groups.

Pregnancy and Lactation

Most clinical studies exclude women who are pregnant or lactating. The name of a specific urine or blood test to be used for confirming the lack of pregnancy is often indicated in the protocol. The protocol might contain a sample waiver of pregnancy form in the appendix if women of child-bearing potential are to be included in the study. An example of such a form is shown in Fig. 22.12. If the length of the study warrants, a second or even multiple repetitions of the pregnancy test may be included.

Information is sometimes presented in the protocol indicating the steps to be followed if a female patient becomes pregnant. These steps will probably include immediate discontinuation of the study treatment, medical supervision and examinations during the course of pregnancy, and evaluation of the newborn infant.

Specific studies may be conducted in women who are pregnant or lactating. Defining the limits of inclusion criteria for such studies requires extremely careful and cautious consideration of the patients to be studied and the objectives of the study. The ethical considerations must be carefully evaluated.

Ingestion of Tobacco, Caffeine, and/or Alcohol

Patients who smoke tobacco may be excluded from studies for a variety of reasons such as interference with ward procedures for inpatient studies, possible or demonstrated interactions of tobacco with the study drug, interactions with diagnostic or other tests, and the desire to control as many factors as possible that might influence results obtained in the study. One of the most well-studied areas of interaction between smoking and drugs involves altered metabolism of drugs in patients who smoke (Conney et al., 1977). Caffeine-containing drinks such as coffee, tea, and certain sodas may also have an influence on the adverse reactions noted with the study drug because of their stimulant effect and the variable amounts that patients use. These beverages also may affect performance on certain efficacy tests. Chocolates contain xanthines, and their consumption by study patients may also be regulated. During the study, the quantities of caffeine-containing drinks consumed can only be controlled to a variable degree if the study is conducted in outpatients but may be controlled to a more significant degree if inpatients are used.

Alcohol consumption is often regulated (i.e., an attempt is made to control the amount of alcohol consumed) in many or even in most studies. If this is an especially important factor to control, then periodic blood alcohol levels may be measured, and/or an inpatient study may be considered. Nonetheless, it remains a difficult (if not impossible task) to fully control this factor, even in patients who do not abuse alcohol.

Abuse of Alcohol or Drugs

One general definition of drug abuse is when a patient uses more than the recommended dose of a drug, uses the recommended dose for longer than the recommended period, or uses ethical (i.e., prescription) drugs that have not been therapeutically recommended and are not indicated. Thus abuse of alcohol by patients entering a clinical study is undesirable for numerous reasons, including a decreased reliability of the patient in following the protocol, increased possibility for drug interactions, and increased difficulty in clarifying adverse reactions.

A history of drug or alcohol abuse is generally important to probe for in the entry criteria. An important consideration in this regard is whether a positive history that is more than 6 (12, 18, or a more appropriate number) months in the past should be a basis for patient exclusion. Studies dealing with diseases having a high incidence in alcoholics (e.g., cirrhosis or pancreatitis) may have more lax entry criteria concerning alcohol abuse. Inpatient studies in alcohol abusers will provide more supervison of patients and may circumvent at least some of the potential problems that might be encountered in an outpatient study (i.e., patients consuming alcohol during the study).

It is a simple matter to write an exclusion criterion that excludes patients who abuse either licit or illicit drugs. It is a difficult matter, however, to truly know whether such individuals have, in fact, actually been excluded. After a definition of abuse has been established, a patient history, laboratory tests for evaluating liver function, and a urine drug screen are among the few methods or tests available to insure that such individuals are truly excluded from the study. These methods, however, are not completely effective.

Diet and Nutritional Status

There are many variations in a patient's diet and/or nutritional status that may be desired as either an inclusion or exclusion criterion. No attempt will be made to list all possible variations except to state that in developing a protocol it may be relevant to address this issue.

Bioavailability, biological activity, drug elimination, and toxicity of many drugs are known to be affected by food in general and by specific nutrients and chemicals. Clinically important drug–nutrient interactions have been reported for numerous combinations of drugs and specific nutrients. Many lists are available of the most common drug–nutrient interactions observed. The interactions may lead to effects primarily on the nutrient (e.g., folate deficiency caused by phenytoin) or the drug (e.g., decreased tetracycline absorption because of the calcium in ingested dairy products). In the former situation, drugs may affect nutrition through effects on taste, appetite, intestinal motility, and the absorption, metabolism, and excretion of nutrients.

Food or specific nutrients may interfere with the actions of a drug by numerous mechanisms such as altering the absorption of oral drugs and therefore the bioavailability of a drug by affecting gastrointestinal pH, secretions, osmolality, motility, and transit time. Food may also alter the ionization, stability, and solubility of a drug or form a complex with a drug in the gastrointestinal tract. The net effect of food on drug bioavailability cannot be predicted on a theoretical basis but must be determined through clinical experience and evaluation. Food may affect a drug's metabolism (e.g., through enzyme induction or inhibition) or excretion (e.g., by altering urine pH). An active substance in food may exert an agonistic or antagonistic pharmacological effect on a drug. Some of the well-known examples of food affecting drugs are (1) the divalent metal ions (primarily calcium) contained in dairy products, which can combine with tetracycline to form complexes that are poorly absorbed, (2) charcoal-broiled meat, which accelerates the oxidation of phenacetin, and (3) the normal deactivation of pressor amines such as tyramine by hepatic monoamine oxidase being blocked by the class of drugs known as monoamine oxidase inhibitors. When patients receiving monoamine oxidase inhibitors (usually for depression) ingest tyramine-containing foods, a fatal increase in blood pressure sometimes occurs in susceptible individuals.

When some drugs (e.g., lithium) are given with food, the absorption of the drug increases. This is usually because food delays gastric emptying or increases gastrointestinal transit times. These delays allow the drug to have a longer time of contact with the site(s) of absorption and/or permits more complete dissolution of the drug.

Patients who enter clinical studies may be receiving special diets for medical reasons (e.g., low sodium, low glucose) that may be adversely affected by certain drugs (e.g., those with high sodium or glucose contents). If the diet of a patient changes during a clinical study, it may have an influence on the therapeutic outcome (e.g., if a patient's diet changes during a study evaluating a hypolipidemic drug). The state of a patient's nutritional status may be important to qualify, since malnutrition and its associated deficiency disorders and diseases may affect drug activity and pharmacokinetics in multiple ways.

The dividing line between drug–drug interactions and drug–nutrient interactions is not always clear. For example, minerals and vitamins that are self-prescribed may be considered as either nutrients or drugs, depending on the dose taken, the need for a dietary supplement, and other factors. These substances sometimes interfere with drug absorption (e.g., iron salts reduce absorption of tetracycline).

Physiological Limitations and Genetic History

The criterion of physiological limitations refers to the use of results of certain tests as a basis of patient inclusion (exclusion). One methodology for implementing this concept is to include (exclude) patients when results of their physiological tests are within or outside established limits. This particular criterion overlaps with that describing clinical characteristics of the study disease, laboratory examinations, and other sections as well.

A genetic history can be used to concentrate on a patient's condition that is desired to be included as the focus of a study or as a characteristic to be excluded. There are genetic disorders known to affect drug responses (e.g., G6PD deficiency, porphyrias, hemoglobinopathies), and patients with these conditions are often excluded from studies in which adverse reactions would be predicted or anticipated on the basis of these genetic defects.

Surgical, Anatomical, and/or Emotional Limitations

It is relatively common to exclude patients who have had surgery within a specified period. Additionally, patients may be included (or excluded) because of anatomical characteristics (e.g., patients without a spleen or other organ). Anatomical limitations may be related to the disease being studied (e.g., amputation in diabetic patients, blindness caused by a specific disease) or to the patient's characteristics (e.g., body surface area above or below a given range).

Patients with clinically significant emotional problems or retardation are often excluded from clinical studies unless the study is designed specifically to include them. These groups usually require special consideration in obtaining informed consent and eliciting acceptable cooperation. Specific *DSM-III* categories (American Psychiatric Association, 1980) or other standard classification systems may be used to exclude (or include) certain groups of patients (e.g., those with organic brain syndrome).

Patients who have active suicidal tendencies are virtually always excluded from studies, although this is not always listed in the exclusion criteria. If a psychotropic drug is being evaluated, it is usually relevant to specify this exclusion criterion in the protocol.

Hypersensitivity to a Study Drug or Test

This is a standard exclusion criterion that is included in most studies. Patients with a higher risk of having a serious adverse reaction because of the likelihood of being hypersensitive to a study drug should be excluded. In addition, many clinical tests use chemicals or drugs, and these agents may also be a source of hypersensitivity reactions.

The investigator must probe for a history of hypersensitivity or allergic reactions to drugs chemically related to the study drug. Common chemical "relatives" are sometimes listed in the protocol or appendix to assist the investigator in obtaining this history.

Other Drug and Nondrug Allergies

Known allergies to drugs other than the study drug(s) and to nondrug materials may be relevant factors to insert as an inclusion criterion. Individuals with numerous allergies may or may not be desirable patients to enroll in a drug study.

CHARACTERISTICS OF THE DISEASE AND ITS TREATMENT

The following inclusion criteria relate to characteristics of the disease and its treatment.

Disease Being Evaluated

This is probably the most important entry criterion for studies involving patients as opposed to studies that involve normal volunteers. In defining the presence of a disease, one may focus on the basic lesion or the primary or secondary clinical features. As an example of this classification, the disease myelogenous leukemia can be used. The basic lesion in this disease is the presence of immature leukocytes, and the primary clinical features include fever, enlarged spleen, and anemia. Secondary clinical features include weakness and infections.

The specific (or general) diagnosis of the disease being evaluated will almost invariably be stated in the inclusion criteria, as will the basis on which the diagnosis is to be made. Determine whether there are standard sources of diagnostic criteria that can be utilized, such as guidelines promulgated by societies or national or international organizations. Two examples are *Primer on the Rheumatic Diseases* (Rodnan, 1973), which is prepared by a committee of the American Rheumatism Association of the Arthritis Foundation, and the *DSM-III*, which is prepared by the American Psychiatric Association (1980). Consider whether laboratory tests are mandatory, helpful, or not helpful in establishing the patient's diagnosis. The intensity or severity of the disease may be relevant for entry criteria, as may be the duration of the disease.

If there are specific tests that will be used to evaluate the primary or secondary characteristics of the disease being studied, then these tests should be utilized, if possible, to screen patients for the desired effect or response and to establish a baseline. Some of the qualifications of the stated disease that may be described in the inclusion criteria are listed in Table 15.14. These qualifications will probably be used for purposes of both inclusion and exclusion.

Concomitant Drugs

There are two major aspects to the issue of concomitant drugs in a clinical study. The first aspect is to determine which concomitant drugs are (or are not) permitted at the outset of the study. This issue is related to inclusion criteria and is discussed in this chapter. The other aspect relates to which concomitant drugs are (or are not) permitted during the conduct of the drug study. This latter question is discussed in Chapter 18.

It is generally desired to exclude patients using specific drugs or classes of drugs when an adverse interaction may occur. When it is important to eliminate the possibility of all drug–drug interactions, then no concomitant drugs should be allowed in the study. This is generally the case for pharmacokinetic studies, Phase I safety studies, and a number of Phase II efficacy studies. Allowing concomitant

TABLE 15.14. *Selected qualifications to use for diseases described in the inclusion or exclusion criteria*[a]

---

1. No qualifications presented
2. Disease present (or diagnosed) for at least ____months (years)
3. Previous hospitalization for this disease is (is not) required
4. The duration of hospitalization was no longer than (at least) ____days (weeks)
5. The number of hospitalizations was more (less) than ____during the last ____ weeks (months, years)
6. The disease is clinically stable (unstable)
7. A diagnosis of this disease has been previously made
8. The following characteristics are present at this time: ____, ____
9. Specific laboratory values measured at screen (and/or during the preceeding ____ weeks) were above (or below, or between) ____units
10. The disease is presently clinically characterized by the following signs and/or symptoms: ____, ____ with the following intensity____, ____
11. The disease has been characterized as ____with the following specific methods: ____, ____within the last ____months (years)
12. The patient has been diagnosed with____, ____tests (e.g., biopsy), within the last ____months (years)
13. The patient has been treated (or not treated) presently (previously) with the following drug(s) ____at the following dose (dose range)____, or nondrug modalities with the following characteristics: ____, ____
14. The patient did (did not) respond to the drug (nondrug) treatment described above, with the following results____

---

[a]Each disease described may be general (e.g., renal disease) or specific (e.g., glomerulo-nephritis).

drugs in a study increases the possibility of drug interactions confounding the results obtained, but it may be ethically unacceptable to evaluate the study drug as monotherapy.

If the study objective is to evaluate the effects of a test drug in patients already receiving a specific drug, then the inclusion criteria must reflect this as well as the parameters of the concomitant drug that will be controlled. Parameters that may be controlled include the name (generic or trade name) of the drug, dosage(s) permitted, frequency of dosing, duration of treatment, adverse reactions allowed (or required), and blood levels. The term "required" is emphasized, since a number of drug studies are designed to evaluate the effect of one drug on adverse reactions caused by a different (concomitant) drug (e.g., to treat emesis caused by *cis*-platinum or other chemotherapeutic drugs). Table 15.15 lists several variations of the criteria that may be established to delineate the types of concomitant drugs that either may or may not be allowed in a study. Combinations of these criteria are also possible to specify in the inclusion section of the protocol.

If any concomitant drugs are allowed at the outset of a study, then a policy for dealing with combination drugs should be considered. For example, if patients may receive one drug from a specified category or list as a concomitant drug, it must be determined how to classify the patient who is taking one combination drug. It may be desired to treat a combination drug as either one or two drugs (or more, depending on the specific combination). If some combinations but not others are

TABLE 15.15. *Options for describing concomitant drugs in the inclusion criteria*[a]

1. Patients may not take any drugs at the time of entry into the study[b] (e.g., in many pharmacokinetic studies and in studies of acute analgesia)
2. Patients may take specific antidisease drugs. The number of drugs and dose ranges may be specified, as may acceptable blood levels (e.g., in epilepsy, since it is not generally considered ethically acceptable to evaluate a newly developed drug as monotherapy)
3. Patients may take any number of drugs to treat their disease. Dosages may or may not be specified (e.g., in some Phase III and most Phase IV studies, where drugs are being evaluated under "normal use" conditions)
4. Patients may take any number of drugs for other diseases but not for the disease being treated with the study drug (this option is commonly used in many drug studies)
5. Patients may not take drugs to treat other diseases but must take a specific drug or drugs to treat the disease being tested with the study drug (in studies where specific drug interactions are being evaluated)
6. Patients may take drugs without any restrictions on the number, purpose, or dosage regimens (in a long-term study such as the Framingham study)
7. Qualifications for nonprescription drugs may be described separately from those for prescription drugs (where nonprescription drugs may cause interactions with study drugs or may influence the results noted with ethical study drugs)
8. Certain combinations (or variations) of the above options may be specified

[a]The length of the drug-free period should be specified for drugs that have been stopped prior to entry into the study. It may be relevant to specify different drug-free periods for different classes of drugs or for specific drugs.
[b]Patients should be carefully questioned about this point, since many patients state that they are not taking drugs when they are using oral contraceptives or a variety of over-the-counter (OTC) drugs on an occasional or chronic basis, such as laxatives, mild analgesics, and vitamins.

acceptable, then a specific listing of acceptable drugs may be appropriate. For concomitant drugs that are commonly given by more than one route of administration (e.g., corticosteroids), it may be relevant to specify separate criteria for each route (e.g., "No systemic corticosteroids may be used for 7 days, and no topical steroids may be used for 24 hr prior to the baseline").

It is important to clarify whether a concomitant drug may be taken to treat the disease or problem being studied, or whether the concomitant drug is limited to treating other diseases the patient may have. A study may become unacceptably complicated if a patient continues to take a concomitant drug to treat an unrelated disease and that drug also has an effect on the disease being studied. This situation could occur when diazepam is being used by a patient to treat anxiety and the patient enters a study evaluating muscle spasm. Diazepam will affect muscle spasm as well as anxiety. This type of potential problem should be considered and resolved prior to the initiation of a study.

If a patient is taking a concomitant drug that is allowed by protocol, the minimum length of time should be specified that each accepted drug or class of drugs must have been taken without dosage changes prior to entry into the study. This precaution is necessary to insure that patients are in a steady-state condition when initiating treatment with the study drug.

Previous Drug and Nondrug Treatment

There are often appropriate reasons to include or exclude patients from a study who have been treated previously with certain drugs or nondrug treatment (e.g., radiation therapy in patients with cancer). The various nondrug or drug treatments that may affect the study should be evaluated and a decision reached about whether to enroll patients who have ever been treated (or treated within some number of preceding weeks or months) with specific therapies.

Washout Period of Nonstudy Drugs or Nondrug Treatments

Whenever patients are being taken off one treatment and a different one is being initiated, a period of time must elapse to eliminate or minimize the influence of the original drug or treatment on the subsequent treatment. This interval is referred to as the washout or drug-free period. The plasma half-life of a drug is a useful tool to determine how long it will require for almost all of a drug to be removed from the patient's body. A period of five half-lives is usually adequate to allow for biological removal of the drug. The half-life of a drug in normal individuals, however, may be significantly prolonged in some patients (e.g., those with renal or liver disease) or shortened in other patients (e.g., those with induced microsomal enzymes in the liver). Another factor to consider is the duration of the biological effects of a drug. For example, the biological effects of reserpine on catecholamine depletion persist for a much longer period than the reserpine itself remains in the body.

The possible carryover or residual effect of a drug must be considered in determining an adequate washout period. In this situation, the effects of a previous treatment persist beyond the time of the drug's known biological activity. This carryover effect must be considered not only prior to initiating a clinical study but also between successive parts of the study, such as when a crossover design is used. If it is considered possible or likely for a carryover effect to occur, then a baseline period inserted between the two periods of a crossover will provide additional baseline measurements and also allow for an adequate washout period prior to initiation of the second part of the study.

Once an optimal period of time has been determined for the drug's washout period, it may not be clinically possible or acceptable to apply this time as a requirement for patient inclusion in the protocol. Many patients with numerous diseases cannot tolerate the necessary drug-free period required for an adequate washout of a drug. For example, many patients with Parkinson's Disease cannot be completely taken off L-DOPA for an adequate period to become drug-free prior to being tested with another drug.

One approach to this problem is to taper the concomitant drug gradually until it is removed and then to add the study drug. A second solution is to add the test drug in a gradually ascending dose at the same time (or before) the original medication is tapered. Thus, after a certain time period, patients will be completely weaned from their original drug and will be receiving the study drug. This latter approach has disadvantages in that it does not allow baseline measurements to be obtained during a drug-free period and allows for drug interactions to occur.

Another approach to this problem is to decrease the optimal drug-free period to an acceptable duration that will allow sufficient numbers of patients to be enrolled. Data obtained from patients with a shortened washout period may be analyzed separately from those with an acceptable washout period.

History of Other Diseases

A history of diseases other than the one(s) being studied may be considered as an entrance criterion in some studies. Certain patients should be excluded from a study because of safety considerations. For example, in the early stages of testing a new drug that affects the central nervous system, patients with a history of epilepsy may be excluded to prevent the possibility of the drug precipitating seizures. Apart from safety, the presence of certain diseases (e.g., renal failure) in patients may affect the quality and type of data obtained with a study drug. Data obtained in patients with renal failure or serious cardiovascular disease could adversely prejudice results of a study and give a new drug an undeserved "bad reputation."

Once sufficient information and experience with a new drug's use are obtained, however, then adequate provisions and precautions may be made for evaluating the drug in patients with various diseases. Thus, individuals with many specific diseases are generally excluded from early studies of a new drug's investigation until adequate data are obtained on how various types of patients are affected by the study drug. The history of other diseases may be qualified by whether patients have required hospitalization for one or more specific diseases. The means to qualify previous hospitalizations is discussed in the following section.

Previous Hospitalizations

Previous hospitalizations for a specific disease may be used as a general measure or indicator of a certain level of disease severity that may be relevant for the entrance criteria. The parameter of prior hospitalizations may be used to exclude some, but not all, patients with a specific disease. The duration of hospitalization also may be indirectly related to severity of disease and thus be used to qualify the criterion describing hospitalization [e.g., patients with a history of psychiatric disease requiring hospitalization within the last ____ months (years) will be excluded if the hospitalization lasted for ____ or more days].

Present Clinical Status

Patients with clinically unstable acute or chronic diseases unrelated to the study disease are usually not acceptable for entry into a study. Even patients with stable chronic diseases unrelated to the study disease are often excluded from a study, especially in Phase II.

For certain diseases or types of disease that are the focus of the study, it is not always straightforward to define which patients may be included. One approach to this issue is to state that patients with a certain disease must be excluded:

1. If they have been hospitalized for this disease within the last ____ months (years).
2. If they require treatment with ____.
3. If their disease has recurred more than ____ times in the past ____ months (years).
4. If their disease was originally diagnosed more than ____ months (years) ago.
5. If their disease is of an intensity more than or equal to ____ (describe a degree of intensity on a standard test, measure, or scale).

If patients with a relatively normal medical examination (except for the study disease) are desired, one may simply exclude all patients who presently have any clinically significant cardiovascular, renal, pulmonary, etc. disease. Various qualifications of this type of statement may be made (e.g., only specific diseases may be excluded instead of types or classes of diseases).

ENVIRONMENTAL AND OTHER FACTORS

The following inclusion criteria relate to environmental and other factors.

Patient Recruitment and Cooperation

If specific recruiting practices or specific sites for recruitment are to be used, information on patient recruitment may be incorporated into the protocol. Examples might include a provision that patients live within x miles or y hr by car of the study site. Another possible specification is that only patients who work in a given place or attend a specific school or clinic may be enrolled in the protocol. Also, the possible solicitation of patients by advertisements or by referrals from other professionals may be discussed.

Patients who are not likely to cooperate in a study because of their mental status or other factors may be excluded. Determining the degree of future cooperation in advance for the entire course of a study is virtually impossible for most (if not all) patients, but categories of patient types may be described that are expected to include a high percentage of noncooperative patients. Although patients in these categories may be excluded from the study, the value of this type of exercise is questionable. A more detailed discussion of patient recruitment is given in Section III of this book.

Participation in Another Drug Study

Some patients enroll in as many drug studies as they can for financial gain, to obtain temporary housing, or for other motives that are questionable. This is especially common in Phase I clinical studies. In Phase I studies (and often in

Phase II studies), it is therefore usually advisable to exclude any patient who has participated in another drug study within a specific period (e.g., 3 months). This is primarily to minimize the chance of any carryover effect from the preceding study, especially when the preceding study involved an investigational drug, a large proportion of the clinical pharmacology of which is unknown.

Participation in Another Part of the Same Study or in Any Other Study Using the Same Study Drug

It may be relevant to exclude patients who have participated in another part of the same study or in other studies conducted with the same drug. The pros and cons of each alternative relating to this point should be discussed among the individuals responsible for the protocol.

Institutional or Environmental Status

There are occasions when specific types of patient populations either are or are not desired, and the specific catchment areas that are (or are not) acceptable may be specified. Some studies use both inpatients and outpatients. Certain studies are conducted with patients who reside in institutions or nursing homes or who constitute a specific population (e.g., patients visited by a public health nurse). This may be an important or relevant factor in a number of protocols, especially those utilizing psychiatric populations, chronic care facilities, or debilitated populations.

In an outpatient psychiatric study, it may be desired to limit patient enrollment to any (or all) of the following catchment areas: office of a private practitioner, clinic of a general hospital, community mental health center, or other type of psychiatric clinic.

Occupation

It may be important to exclude patients engaged in occupations involving the use of dangerous machinery (including driving a car) from certain studies. This is especially relevant when it is expected that sedation or disorientation could result from use of the study drugs.

Other occupations may be relevant to identify as a specific inclusion criterion, especially if the study is conducted to address a question as it relates to workers (or patients) within a specified work group (e.g., farmers exposed to specific pesticides).

Geographical Location

In relation to patient inclusion, geographical location generally refers to the place where the patient lives and/or works. Studies may be limited to those patients who reside within a specified neighborhood or area in order to evaluate differences with another area. Studies may also be undertaken to evaluate patients who have lived in the same area for different periods of time.

Litigation and Disability

Some diseases are associated with a high incidence of litigation, such as cervical pain or back pain resulting from trauma. In cases where there may be secondary gain to the patient if he/she does not improve with treatment, the beneficial effects of a drug may be compromised or completely unobserved if a patient with pending litigation is entered into a study. Thus, criteria of patient inclusion are sometimes established that consider workman's compensation, disability benefits, and whether or not any litigation related to the disease is pending. In addition, a consultation with an attorney about the disease may be sufficient grounds to render the patient unacceptable for admission to the study.

RESULTS OF SCREENING EXAMINATIONS

Most patients receive a physical examination prior to entry into a clinical study. The inclusion criteria may list specific findings that either are not acceptable for entry (e.g., nystagmus, absent deep tendon reflexes) or are mandatory (e.g., specific skin lesions of defined size and severity). Another approach to specifying results of screening examinations that are required for entry into a study is to generally state that the results obtained must be clinically acceptable to the investigator.

A routine physical examination includes a neurological examination and measurement of vital signs. Nonetheless, protocols often discuss vital signs as if they were a separate event. Any aspect of the physical examination, such as the neurological examination, that is of particular relevance to the study may also be listed separately in the inclusion criteria. The details of how thoroughly the investigator is to conduct each of the screening examinations are usually indicated in the protocol and described in detail in data collection forms.

Screening examinations generally include safety evaluations that are also conducted during or after treatment, such as the ECG, EEG, and ophthalmological and laboratory examinations. Criteria for patient exclusion based on abnormalities in the hematological, blood chemistry, urinalysis, or other related tests may be specific (e.g., white blood cell count over $9,000/mm^3$) or general (e.g., "results must be clinically acceptable to the investigator").

Many normal volunteers will not have all clinical laboratory results within "normal limits." Thus, a rigid adherence to a criterion that insists that all laboratory values must be within normal limits will undoubtedly lead to a variety of problems with patient enrollment. Repeating laboratory tests in patients whose initial results were abnormal will often demonstrate that the repeated value is now within the normal range, although values of other tests that were originally within the normal range may have "crept" outside the normal range in the interim. Repeating baseline laboratory measures, both at the start and throughout a study provides a better perspective than relying on one set of data and is also one means of minimizing difficulties with variations in the data obtained. The author agrees with Joubert, Rivera-Calimlim, and Lasagna (1975) that a reasonable approach to obtaining "normal" individuals lies between the extremes of absolute rigidity and totally lax entry criteria.

The number of laboratory and other tests requested in the screening examinations will depend on both past experiences with the test drug(s) and expectations of potential problems. The tests requested should be adequate to include baseline values of important safety tests for each patient. As experience with a drug develops, the need for extensive clinical laboratory studies gradually decreases, although the need to monitor a specific laboratory test(s) may increase. A list of the most commonly utilized laboratory tests is presented in Table 17.17.

16   Identifying, Choosing, and Evaluating Efficacy Parameters

Types of Efficacy Criteria ● Clinical Scales, Visual Analog Scales,
Patient Diaries, and Drawings ● Other Factors Relating to Efficacy

TYPES OF EFFICACY CRITERIA

Although it is impossible to provide specific details in this chapter, there are a number of general considerations and principles that are discussed. The major efficacy measure(s) for most diseases are usually well established, but one must evaluate which tests will provide the most definitive data within the limits of the resources available to the study. For example, it might be desirable to obtain computerized tomography scans in a particular study but only financially possible to perform a clinical examination. It is almost always preferable to include direct validated measures rather than indirect measures of efficacy, whether they have been validated or not. If no direct efficacy measures are available to use in a study, then indirect measures must be used.

There are various types of criteria that may be used to measure efficacy (or safety) parameters.

1. Presence or absence (i.e., existence) criteria. This refers to a symptom, sign, lesion or other manifestation of a disease that is either present or not. Criteria and/or operational definitions may be established to define the existence of the effect.
2. Graded or scaled criteria. This refers both to scales of the types shown in Table 16.16 and to visual analog scales. Graded scales can be applied to subjective as well as to objective clinical symptoms and signs. A number of scales have become well established in clinical medicine (e.g., cardiac murmurs are graded from 0 to 6, neurological reflexes are graded from 0 to 4).
3. Relative change criteria. These criteria refer to measurements in specific tests that provide direct or indirect indications of efficacy.
4. Global criteria. This category involves the overall evaluation of a patient's disease or change in disease (e.g., severity of disease, global improvement). The individual factors that this aggregate evaluation is based on may or may not be specified. Specific (or general) criteria or a scoring system may also be developed to rate each of the factors.

One must determine the pros and cons of each efficacy measure incorporated into the study. The potential value of data obtained from each efficacy test added

TABLE 16.16. *Examples of grading systems used in clinical scales*

A. 1 = Not at all ____
    2 = Very little ____
    3 = A little ____
    4 = Mildly ____
    5 = Moderately ____
    6 = Quite a bit ____
    7 = Distinctly ____
    8 = Markedly ____
    9 = Extremely ____

B. 0 = Not assessed
    1 = Normal, not at all ____
    2 = Borderline ____
    3 = Mildly ____
    4 = Moderately ____
    5 = Markedly ____
    6 = Severely ____
    7 = Among the most severely ____

C. 0 = Absent
    1 = Slightly present or a suspicion of its presence
    2 = Clearly noticeable but mild and occurs not more than ____per ____
    3 = Clearly present and occurs from ____to ____times per ____
    4 = Definitely present and frequent
    5 = Continuous and gross

D. 0 = Absent
    1 = Rarely present (occurs less than ____times per ____)
    2 = Occasionally present (occurs ____to ____times per ____)
    3 = Often present (occurs ____to ____times per ____)
    4 = Always or almost always present (occurs more than ____times per ____or
        continually)

to the study must be evaluated against the increase it will elicit in time requirements, personal efforts, financial costs, and additional complexity of the study. At some point in virtually all studies, adding tests becomes counterproductive, and the study becomes inefficient.

CLINICAL SCALES, VISUAL ANALOG SCALES, PATIENT DIARIES, AND DRAWINGS

Clinical scales may be developed if no satisfactory efficacy measures exist. Scales may be established to describe subjective or semiobjective parameters in a fixed number of categories (usually from three to seven). The most common type of scale is a variation of the scale describing a parameter or question for which the response is normal or not present (score = 0), mild (score = 1), moderate (score = 2), severe (score = 3), or extremely severe (score = 4). Other variations are shown in Table 16.16. The individual scores from a number of separate categories are often added to derive a total composite score. One of the most important clinical scales used to measure efficacy is the clinical global impressions (CGI) scale. This scale provides a measure of the overall improvement or deterioration of a patient's condition and is completed by the investigator and/or the patient. It may also be used to evaluate safety and is described in more detail in the following chapter.

Another approach to the issue of developing efficacy measures where satisfactory ones do not exist is to develop a visual analog scale. Visual analog scales have been widely used in recent years to provide quantitative measures of subjective ratings. They are frequently used to measure the intensity of pain or quality of the patient's mood at a particular time. These scales may also be used to document changes over time when they are used on multiple occasions. Specific examples of parameters measured with visual analog scales include stress, anxiety, itch, hunger, alertness, and depression. Subjective ratings of clinical improvement (or deterioration) or the value of a specified treatment may also be measured with a visual analog scale.

Visual analog scales may be created to have patients evaluate a parameter between two fixed points that may be arbitrarily defined (e.g., 0–10, 1–100, "not at all"–"extremely") along a straight line with or without gradations or on a round dial (with or without gradation). A few examples are illustrated in Fig. 16.8. It is preferable to use a validated visual analog scale in a drug study unless the study is specifically designed to evaluate the validity of the scale. Certain parameters (e.g., pain) have been shown to be reliably measured with these scales. Sriwatanakul et al. (1983) evaluated five different visual analog scales to measure pain and observed that graded linear horizontal scales were more reliable and also were preferred by more patients than were the other scales they tested. In addition, they concluded that the visual analog scales yielded more accurate and more sensitive information on pain intensity than did descriptive pain scales.

Another potential source of efficacy data in certain studies is patient diaries. Data obtained from patient diaries provide the most important efficacy data in outpatient evaluations of antidiarrheal drugs (stool number and consistency) and antiepileptic drugs (number and type of seizure occurrences). If diaries are used by patients, then the diaries should be supplied by the investigator or sponsor to insure that each patient addresses similar questions and completes them in a similar manner. Instructions for using diaries should be reviewed with patients and, ideally, should be printed in the diary itself.

Drawings or figures may be utilized as a technique to collect data on efficacy, safety, or medical history. Patients may be requested to either fill in drawings, prepare drawings, or write something themselves. An example of the fill-in approach is the *McGill Pain Questionnaire*, in which patients are asked to indicate on both front and back drawings of a person exactly where their pain is located (Melzack, 1975). Serial drawings provide data on the effects of their therapy or course of disease. Many visual and ophthalmological tests involve the patient interpreting a visual design. An example in which patients are asked to provide written material is in Parkinson's Disease, where samples of the patient's handwriting over time are used as one indicator for evaluating therapy. Psychiatric evaluations of a patient's psychological state are sometimes based on interpretations of drawings prepared by the patient.

OTHER FACTORS RELATING TO EFFICACY

Many efficacy measures yield less objective data than one would ideally like to obtain. Subjective measures often depend on clinical evaluation or examination of the patient or on the investigator's interpretation of the patient's statements. Under these circumstances, it is generally desirable to have the same investigator perform the nonobjective measures throughout the study.

1.

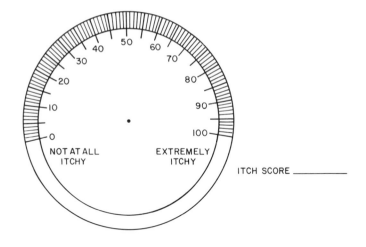

2.

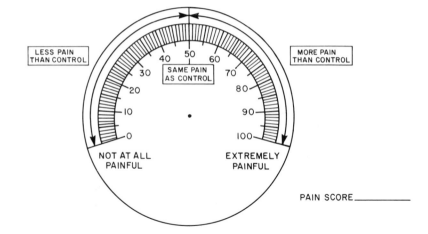

3.

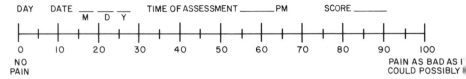

FIG. 16.8. Examples of visual analog scales.

It is also advisable for certain tests to be performed at the same time of day throughout the study. Whenever possible, key efficacy parameters should be measured at the times of both peak and trough blood levels. Most investigators are aware that cortisol levels (and certain other hormones) vary during the day and that the time of their collection must be specified and controlled. Many nonobjective or objective tests also vary or tend to vary during the day, sometimes in a predictable manner (e.g., morning stiffness in arthritis patients), and these tests should be performed at the same time(s) of day throughout the study.

The results of efficacy (or other) tests can be affected on occasion by extraneous factors that may easily be controlled. Examples include the physical position a patient is placed in for taking a test, having the patient relax (or exercise) for a given period of time prior to starting a test, having patients empty their bladders before a lengthy test, starting a test just prior or subsequent to mealtime, and conducting a test at various times of day during the course of the study. Many of these factors may be outlined or discussed in instructions that the investigator and/ or patient follows. Efficacy (and safety) tests should not be required more often during a study than necessary (and realistic) to accomplish the study's objectives. The schedule should be arranged to cause the minimum hardship or harassment to the patient and/or investigator.

It is sometimes relevant to enumerate the different individuals in the protocol who are permitted to perform certain tests for either one or for all patients. The qualifications of individuals conducting efficacy (or safety) tests in terms of degrees, certification, or training may be relevant to specify. Interrater reliability may be measured prior to the study to confirm the validity of having more than one individual conduct certain tests where individual technique, bias, or experience may be a factor.

The quality of life is an important parameter to consider in some clinical studies, but its measurement is fraught with problems. Some studies attempted to utilize entirely objective criteria, but the attempt to validate these methods failed. This failure suggested that objective methods are not entirely adequate to measure the quality of life. Subjective criteria, however, also have serious limitations. Using both types of criteria to measure the quality of life is a reasonable approach. The relative values of the use of objective and/or subjective criteria are discussed by von Kerekjarto (1982). Other broad categories used to describe or measure the quality of life include state of health, psychosocial status, and patterns of communication (Krauth, 1982). Each of these categories is further divided by Krauth, who indicates that it is necessary to weight the different criteria used and to combine ratings of both patients and physicians. He presents several variables that can be used to measure the criteria (once they are agreed on). The variables relate to the patient, to the therapist, and to the social conditions of the patient. All three of these variables are not static but change with time. He discusses many of the problems inherent in evaluating this difficult area.

17 | Identifying and Choosing Safety Parameters

Overall Assessment • Laboratory Examinations • Ophthalmological Examination • Procedures to Counteract Abnormal Laboratory Observations • Behavioral Rating Scales, Performance, Personality, and Disability Tests

OVERALL ASSESSMENT

Choosing the appropriate safety parameters for a clinical study depends on a number of factors. A selected list of examinations and tests commonly used to assess the safety of drugs is given in Table 17.17. The majority of these tests will not be conducted in most drug studies. An assessment of the quantity and quality of prior experience and previous data obtained with the drug is essential to enable one to decide which specific safety tests to incorporate in a drug study. The choice of safety parameters is governed by a need both to have data in areas where there are indications of potential (or actual) safety problems to monitor and also to have additional experience and data with a new drug. Until a sufficient body of safety data has accumulated, more laboratory parameters of safety are generally included than will be needed at a later date. The nature of the study and efficacy tests used may dictate that certain safety parameters should or should not be included (e.g., in testing a new anticancer drug, it may be necessary to perform a bone marrow biopsy and smear to confirm the lack of toxicity, and in assessing an agent in anesthetized patients, the appropriate tests to insure the patient's safety while under anesthesia must be performed). If, on the basis of preclinical pharmacological or toxicological data, any toxicity is either anticipated or considered possible, then an attempt should be made to evaluate patients for those possible problems. The anticipated use(s) of a drug will also influence which safety parameters are chosen for evaluation (e.g., ophthalmological tests would be included for drugs intended for ocular use).

After specific safety parameters are chosen, it is necessary to determine how thorough an evaluation of each parameter should be conducted. It is also possible that different types of examinations would be suitable at different points of the study. For example, a physical examination may be specified to include more or fewer measurements or facets, and a complete examination may not be necessary or even suitable during some periods of the study.

Vital signs may be measured with the patient in a supine, seated, and/or erect position. Both supine and erect positions are usually used if orthostatic changes are being evaluated. The need for such data will depend on the situation, but the

TABLE 17.17. *Selected list of examinations and tests used
to evaluate safety*

A. Clinical examinations
  1. Physical
  2. Vital signs (usually considered as part of the physical examination)
  3. Height and weight (state of dress is usually specified, e.g., in socks)
  4. Neurological or other specialized clinical examinations
B. Clinical laboratory examinations
  1. Hematology (see Table 17.18)
  2. Clinical chemistry (see Table 17.18)
  3. Urinalysis (see Table 17.18)
  4. Virology (viral cultures or viral serology)
  5. Immunology or immunochemistry (e.g., immunoglobins, complement)
  6. Serology (e.g., VDRL)
  7. Microbiology (including bacteriology and mycology)
  8. Parasitology (e.g., stool for ova and protozoa)
  9. Pulmonary function tests (e.g., arterial blood gas)
  10. Other biological tests (e.g., endocrine, toxicology screen)
  11. Stool for occult blood (specify hemoccult or guaiac method)
  12. Skin tests for immunologic competence[a]
  13. Drug screen (usually in urine) for detection of illegal or non-protocol-
      approved drugs
  14. Bone marrow examination
C. Probe for adverse reactions
D. Psychological and psychiatric tests and examinations
  1. Psychometric and performance examinations[b]
  2. Behavioral rating scales[c]
E. Examinations requiring specialized equipment (selected examples)
  1. Audiometry
  2. Electrocardiogram (ECG)
  3. Electroencephalogram (EEG)
  4. Endoscopy
  5. CT scans
  6. Ophthalmological[d]
  7. Ultrasound
  8. X-rays
  9. Others

---

[a]Examples are *Candida albicans*, tricophyton, and dinitrochlorobenzene.
[b]See Table 17.22.
[c]See Tables 17.20 and 17.21.
[d]See Table 17.19.

position of the patient for this examination, as well as the period of time desired
for stabilization, should be noted in the protocol.

There are certain parameters that may be viewed as being either safety or efficacy
parameters. The electroencephalogram (EEG) is an example, although there is
some controversy as to its true adequacy as an efficacy parameter. Nonetheless, it
is important to clearly establish in the protocol whether each parameter is being
incorporated in the protocol for safety or efficacy evaluations (or possibly both).

LABORATORY EXAMINATIONS

Clinical laboratory parameters must be specified individually in the protocol.
Abbreviations such as "SMA-6" or "SMA-12" are rarely acceptable (unless each

component is specified), since different laboratories include different tests in their "SMA-6" (or "SMA-12") battery, and using these abbreviations without an explanation will adversely affect the clarity of the protocol and possibly lead to the collection of data on different parameters at different sites. Other precautions to consider prior to initiating a study are to decide if (1) severely abnormal results should be routinely confirmed, (2) samples should be divided and sent to two separate laboratories when specified abnormalities are determined, (3) additional tests should be routinely requested if specified abnormalities are observed, (4) medical consultants should examine patients whenever severe abnormalities are observed, and (5) aliquots of known concentrations of standard drugs should be sent to laboratories for confirmatory measurements and interlaboratory evaluation.

Specific tests that may be used in hematology, clinical chemistry, and urinalysis are shown in Table 17.18, adult and pediatric behavioral rating scales in Tables 17.20 and 17.21, and psychometric and performance tests in Table 17.22. Common ophthalmological tests are shown in Table 17.19. Note that any of these tests could be utilized as measures of efficacy if they addressed the study objectives.

Choosing Laboratory Tests

There is no standardized series of laboratory parameters that are evaluated in all clinical studies, nor is there one standard that is applied to drugs that are in Phase I, II, or III. There are, however, loose standards and general guidelines for laboratory tests that are performed at each stage of clinical development.

In Phase I clinical studies, there is the greatest need to obtain a wide variety of laboratory evaluations as part of developing the safety profile on a new drug. This entails an evaluation of the basic hematology, clinical chemistry, and urinalysis parameters (Table 17.18). There will never be 100% agreement among investigators and/or clinical scientists as to which specific tests constitute a "basic" workup.

The number of normal laboratory values that is sufficient to collect on a new drug to demonstrate safety is impossible to specify. Numerous factors must be considered, such as the toxicological profile on other safety parameters and the expected use of the drug in patients. It is important to determine if a drug is to be used topically or parenterally, whether it is to be used in generally healthy patients or in seriously ill patients, whether it is a "me-too" drug or a totally novel drug chemically, and whether it will be life saving or provide a minimal therapeutic effect. The number of laboratory tests performed usually decreases as an investigational drug moves closer to the market, but one or more tests may be added to the list in Table 17.18 and studied in great detail.

Evaluations of virtually any biological fluid, tissue, or sense (taste, smell, hearing, sight, and touch) can be conducted to ascertain the safety of a drug. Captopril has been reported to affect taste in some patients, and there are many other examples involving drug-induced effects on one of the five senses. The choice of tests will depend on experiences with the drug and/or suspicions about possible problems. Hair analysis is a relevant test to detect the qualitative presence of certain toxic metals in individuals occupationally or otherwise exposed to heavy metals. For further information on evaluating drugs for teratogenic potential, drug dependence, and carcinogenicity, see Folb (1980).

Hematology

A basic hematology evaluation usually includes determination of hemoglobin, hematocrit, red blood cell (RBC) count, white blood cell (WBC) count, RBC indices [mean corpuscular hemoglobin (MCH), mean corpuscular hemoglobin concentration (MCHC), and mean corpuscular volume (MCV)], and platelets. Either a platelet estimate or platelet count may be obtained. The former measurement is less expensive and usually suffices to demonstrate a lack of drug effect unless there is a previous indication or current expectation of a possible effect on platelets. The WBC differential count is usually not required as part of a basic hematological workup unless a specific parameter of the differential count is being evaluated. Nonetheless, a WBC differential count is often obtained in Phase I and generally provides useful information. Other hematological parameters (some of which are indicated in Table 17.18) are not usually obtained unless there is a specific reason to do so. As experience with a drug develops, there is a progressively diminishing need for monitoring the parameters shown to be normal.

Clinical Chemistry

A measurement of renal function (creatinine and/or BUN) is an "essential" test for most clinical studies, as is the inclusion of at least one liver function test (SGOT, SGPT, LDH, CPK, GGT, and/or alkaline phosphatase). The specific tests chosen to be included in a study are somewhat dependent on both the investigator's and/or clinical scientist's experiences and the characteristics of the drug. Other important parameters to measure include serum electrolytes and at least some of the tests listed in Table 17.18.

Drug levels may also be measured in a clinical study. Drug levels are usually part of a pharmacokinetic analysis but also provide important safety data. This information would be particularly relevant in cases of suspected or actual drug overdosage, drug interactions, to correlate drug levels with toxic events, or in other situations (see Table 11.9). It must be clarified whether free levels of the drug or the salt will be measured by the laboratory.

The total amount of blood that may be taken from a patient in most drug studies should be limited to one unit (about 460 ml) per 8-week period. This figure represents the standard practice followed in blood banking, where an individual may donate one unit of blood every 8 weeks.

Urinalysis

Most clinical laboratories have established a standard battery of tests that includes most or all of the basic parameters listed in Table 17.18. If a dipstick is used to

TABLE 17.18. *Hematology, clinical chemistry, and urinalysis parameters usually evaluated during the development of a new drug*

A. Hematology
   1. Red blood cell (RBC) count
   2. Hemoglobin
   3. Hematocrit
   4. White blood cell (WBC) count and differential
   5. Platelet estimate or platelet count
   6. Red blood cell indices (MCV, MCH, MCHC)[a]
   7. Prothrombin (PT), partial thromboplastin time (PTT)
   8. Reticulocytes
   9. Fibrinogen
  10. Any additional tests suggested by previous data

B. Clinical chemistry
   1. Albumin
   2. Albumin/globulin ratio
   3. Alkaline phosphatase (and/or its isoenzymes)
   4. Amylase
   5. Bilirubin, total and direct
   6. Bicarbonate (carbon dioxide)
   7. BUN/creatinine ratio
   8. Calcium
   9. Chloride
  10. Cholesterol (and/or a lipid panel)
  11. Creatinine
  12. Creatine phosphokinase (CPK)
  13. γ-Glutamyl transferase (GGT)
  14. Globulin
  15. Glucose, nonfasting or fasting
  16. Glucose-6-phosphate dehydrogenase (G6PD)
  17. Glutamate oxalacetic transaminase (SGOT), now frequently referred to as aspartate aminotransferase (AST)
  18. Glutamate pyruvate transaminase (SGPT), now frequently referred to as alanine aminotransferase (ALT)
  19. Iron (and or other related parameters such as ferritin, total iron binding capacity)
  20. Lactic acid dehydrogenase, total (LDH, and/or its isoenzymes)
  21. Inorganic phosphorus
  22. Potassium
  23. Sodium
  24. Total iron binding capacity (TIBC)
  25. Total protein
  26. Triglycerides
  27. Urea nitrogen (BUN)
  28. Uric acid

C. Hormones and/or other chemical substances in blood

D. Urinalysis[b]
   1. Appearance and color
   2. Specific gravity
   3. Acetone
   4. Protein
   5. Glucose
   6. pH
   7. Bile
   8. Urobilinogen
   9. Occult blood

TABLE 17.18. *(continued)*

---

    10. Microscopic evaluation of sediment
        a. Red blood cells (number per high-power field)
        b. White blood cells (number per high-power field)
        c. Casts (describe and give number per high- or low-power field)
        d. Crystals (describe and give number per high-power field)
        e. Bacteria (generally rated as few, many, or loaded)
        f. Epithelial cells (number per low-power field)
  E. Other urine tests sometimes evaluated
    1. Creatinine (actual values are preferable to estimated values)
    2. Electrolytes (usually sodium, potassium, and chloride)
    3. Protein
    4. Specific hormones or chemicals
    5. Twenty-four-hour collections for specific evaluations

---

[a]MCH, mean corpuscular hemoglobin = hemoglobin divided by RBC count; MCHC, mean corpuscular hemoglobin concentration = hemoglobin divided by hematocrit; MCV, mean corpuscular volume = hematocrit divided by RBC count.

[b]Sample codes used to quantify several parameters in the urinalysis are the following. Protein, glucose, ketones, bilirubin: 0, none or negative; 0.5, trace or positive (qualitative); 1, + or 1 +; 2, + + or 2 +; 3, + + + or 3 +; 4, + + + + or 4 +. Epithelial cells, crystals, WBC, RBC, casts: 0, none or negative; 0.5, rare, occasional, few present, trace (1–5); 1, several, mild (6–10); 2, moderate (11–25); 3, many, much (26–50); 4, loaded, severe (>50). Bacteria: 0, none or negative; 0.5, rare, trace, occasional, few, several (1–10); 1, mild (11–50); 2, moderate (51–75); 3, many, numerous (76–100); 4, loaded, severe (>100).

test the urine for several parameters, it is useful to use one that measures occult blood, even if a microscopic examination will count the number of RBCs per high-power field. The means of obtaining the specimen should be indicated (i.e., normal voiding sample, clean catch, midstream, catheterization, suprapubic tap, or cystoscopy), especially in studies in which an antibiotic (or other relevant drug) is being tested.

The specific type of container used to collect blood and/or urine samples is sometimes indicated in a protocol, especially if a special anticoagulant or additive is required or if other specific conditions of sample collection and handling are required. It is generally not necessary to provide this information for commonly requested laboratory tests.

OPHTHALMOLOGICAL EXAMINATION

Various parts of the ophthalmological examination are shown in Table 17.19. The most important single ophthalmological test to evaluate patients for the presence of chronic drug-induced toxicity is the slit-lamp examination. Specific types of drugs with a known potential for ocular toxicity may require that special attention be directed to other examinations shown in Table 17.19 (e.g., the possibility of nystagmus with certain anticonvulsants). Most drugs that are to be taken systemically require at least some evidence of ocular safety prior to approval for marketing.

TABLE 17.19. *Procedures and tests performed in an ophthalmological examination*

1. Ophthalmological history (attention is paid to patient and family history plus the patient's diseases and drugs used)
2. Visual acuity (Snellen chart) corrected (i.e., with glasses if present)
3. External ocular examination (i.e., check for inflammation, ptosis, nystagmus, tearing, proptosis, and other abnormalities)
4. Extraocular muscle testing
5. Pupil size and evaluation (in darkened room with intense illumination)
6. Slit-lamp biomicroscopy (with dilated pupils)
7. Tonometry (Goldmann applanation tonometer and/or American Optical noncontact tonometer)
8. Ophthalmoscopy with fundus photographs (with dilated pupils)
9. Visual field testing and color vision testing
10. Gonioscopy[a]
11. Lacrimation[a] (Schirmer test)

[a]These tests are of minimal value in determining drug toxicity and are not recommended for routine inclusion in ophthalmological examinations to detect drug-induced toxicity.

PROCEDURES TO COUNTERACT ABNORMAL LABORATORY OBSERVATIONS

In evaluating the safety of drugs using laboratory or other tests, it is important to develop data that will establish the nature and magnitude of any issue or problem (real or potential) that arises with abnormal laboratory data. Data obtained must also measure the strength of the association between the drug and event noted or of the serial trends that are observed. While this information is being collected, the alternative courses of action in dealing with the issue or problem can be developed and evaluated. These countermeasures may take the form of (1) periodic monitoring [e.g., prothrombin (PT) or partial thromboplastin time (PTT) times for patients receiving anticoagulants], (2) cessation of drug treatment, (3) decreasing the dose or changing the dose schedule, (4) initiating countertreatment (e.g., antiarrhythmic drugs may be used to treat arrhythmias induced by a test drug), (5) specific antidotes may be used to counter or reverse drug effects (e.g., neostigmine may be used to reverse the neuromuscular blockade caused by nondepolarizing types of neuromuscular blocking drugs), (6) increasing surveillance of the patient, or (7) various other alternatives.

BEHAVIORAL RATING SCALES, PERFORMANCE, PERSONALITY, AND DISABILITY TESTS

A number of behavioral rating scales and psychometric and performance tests listed in Tables 17.20 to 17.22 are briefly described below. Since many of these scales and tests may be used to evaluate safety as well as efficacy, they are included in this chapter. The following comments on the tests provide only a few highlights; readers who are interested in more details are advised to obtain additional infor-

TABLE 17.20 *Adult behavioral rating scales[a]*

Scale	Scale rated by	
	Professional	Patient
1. Anxiety Status Inventory (ASI)	X	
2. Beck Depression Inventory (Beck)		X
3. Brief Psychiatric Rating Scale (BPRS)	X	
4. Carroll Depression Scale		X
5. Clinical Global Impression (CGI)	X or	X
6. Clyde Mood Scale		X
7. Covi Anxiety Scale	X	
8. Crichton Geriatric Rating Scale	X	
9. Depression Status Inventory (DSI)	X	
10. Hamilton Anxiety Scale (HAMA)	X	
11. Hamilton Depression Scale (HAMD)	X	
12. Hopkins Symptom Checklist (HSCL)		X
13. Inpatient Multidimensional Psychiatric Scale (IMPS)	X	
14. Nurses Observation Scale for Inpatient Evaluation (NOSIE)	X	
15. Plutchik Geriatric Rating Scale (PLUT)	X	
16. Profile of Mood States (POMS)		X
17. Sandoz Clinical Assessment—Geriatric	X	
18. Self-Report Symptom Inventory (SCL-90)		X
19. Wittenborn Psychiatric Rating Scale (WITT)	X	
20. Zung Self-Rating Anxiety Scale (SAS)		X
21. Zung Self-Rating Depression Scale (SDS)		X

[a]Standard abbreviations are used (See *ECDEU Assessment Manual for Psychopharmacology*, Guy, 1976). Additional tests are described in *Mental Measurements Yearbook* (Buros, 1972).

mation before choosing the tests that appear most relevant to be included in their particular protocol. Additional information may be obtained from the *ECDEU Assessment Manual for Psychopharmacology* (Guy, 1976), which was the source for many of the details listed in this section, *Mental Measurements Yearbook* (Buros, 1972), and psychiatrists, professional associations, and other sources. The two-volume *Mental Measurements Yearbook* contains numerous references and critiques of many of these and other related tests.

Unless otherwise noted, all of the adult and children's behavioral scales are given once pretreatment and at least once posttreatment. Investigators may schedule additional evaluations with these tests, but this is usually not done at less than weekly or biweekly intervals. Many tests provide data on both a total score and subtest (factor) scores. The specific subscale factors used for certain tests are listed. The times given to complete tests are subject to significant variation depending on the anxiety and characteristics of the patient and/or the experience of the professional. The times listed do not include either scoring or preliminary and/or necessary observations of the patient. Within each of the following three subheadings (Adult Behavioral Rating Scales, Pediatric Behavioral Rating Scales, and Performance Tests), tests are presented in alphabetical order. A few additional personality and physical disability tests are discussed at the end of this chapter.

Adult Behavioral Rating Scales

Anxiety Status Inventory

The Anxiety Status Inventory (ASI) scale is the professional-rated version of the Zung Self-Rating Anxiety Scale (SAS). Both tests (ASI and SAS) contain 20 items, each with a four-point scale, and are designed for use in adults diagnosed as having anxiety neurosis. Both assess anxiety as a clinical disorder rather than a "feeling state." The tests rate either the present time or the average status of the patient during the week preceding the evaluation. The ASI takes up to 15 to 20 min to complete and gives two scores: state anxiety and trait anxiety.

Beck Depression Inventory

The Beck Depression Inventory (Beck) test may be used to measure the depth of depression as a rapid screen for depressed patients. It is a self-rating scale of 21 items (13 in a shortened form), with each item rated on a four-point scale. It measures the immediate present and has been used in antidepressant drug studies. The original 21-item scale can be completed in about 10 min and the test is able to discriminate between anxiety and depression. No subtests are present in the Beck.

Brief Psychiatric Rating Scale

The Brief Psychiatric Rating Scale (BPRS) is used primarily in adult inpatients to evaluate treatment response in drug studies and in nondrug clinical treatment, but it is also use in some outpatient studies. Abbreviated instructions are printed on the form. Ratings are based on observations of patients. Originally developed for psychopharmacologic research, this test contains 18 symptoms, each rated on a seven-point severity scale. It requires approximately 20 min to complete and rates the period of time since the last test. If the test is being used for the first time, it rates the previous week. Five separate subscales are obtained: anxiety–depression, anergia, thought disturbance, activation, and hostility–suspiciousness.

Carroll Rating Scale for Depression

The Carroll rating scale for depression (52-item self-rating scale) is scored with yes or no answers by patients. It was designed to closely match the information content and specific items included in the Hamilton rating scale. It has been validated by comparisons with both the Hamilton Depression Scale (HAMD) and Beck and requires approximately 20 min to complete. Seventeen components of depression are measured.

Clinical Global Impressions

Although the *ECDEU Assessment Manual for Psychopharmacology* (Guy, 1976) provides a formal test for the Clinical Global Impression (CGI) Scale, numerous investigators have modified the three major questions as well as the scales used in order to fit this test to their own studies. The three questions, which may be applied in almost all Phase II and Phase III clinical studies, are:

1. Severity of illness. "Considering your total clinical experience with this particular population, how mentally ill (the investigator may substitute a more appropriate term if this is not applicable) is the patient at this time?"
2. Global improvement. "Rate total improvement, whether or not in your judgment it is due entirely to drug treatment."
3. Efficacy index. "Rate this item on the basis of drug effect only." This utilizes a rating of both efficacy and adverse reactions and divides the efficacy score by the adverse reaction score to form a ratio ("efficacy index").

Severity of illness is the only one of these three rated pretreatment. All three questions may be rated posttreatment, and additional ratings are possible during a study. The CGI measure, which is widely used in all types of drug studies, is generally well accepted.

A scale of two to nine gradations is usually used for questions 1 and 2, although five or so gradations are probably most common. A typical five-point scale for question 2 would be that the patient is rated as 1 (much worse), 2 (minimally worse), 3 (unchanged), 4 (minimally improved), or 5 (markedly improved).

Clyde Mood Scale

The Clyde Mood Scale test may be used as either a self-rated or observer-rated scale. It contains 48 items to measure mood and has been shown to be sensitive to drug effects. The test takes 5 to 15 min to complete and measures the immediate present in a patient or normal individual. The test gives six scores: friendly, aggressive, clear thinking, sleepy, unhappy, and dizzy.

Covi Anxiety Scale

The Covi Anxiety Scale is a global observer's rating scale of patient anxiety. There are three items that are each rated on a 0-to-5 scale. The test is simple to use and requires only a few minutes to complete.

Crichton Geriatric Rating Scale

The Crichton Geriatric Rating Scale test measures the level of behavioral function in elderly psychiatric patients using a five-point scale on 11 items. It rates either the present or the period within the last week and takes 5 to 10 min to complete.

Depression Status Inventory

The Depression Status Inventory (DSI) scale is the professional's version of the Zung Self-Rating Depression Scale (SDS). Each of the two scales (DSI and SDS) consists of the same 20 items rated on a four-point scale and is applied to adults with depressive symptomatology. The DSI is completed by the professional, and the SDS is completed by the patient. Both tests take about 5 to 10 min to complete. The DSI rates either the present situation or the last week prior to the test, and a total score is obtained.

Hamilton Anxiety Scale

The Hamilton Anxiety (HAMA) scale was designed to be used in adult patients who already have a diagnosis of anxiety neurosis rather than for making a diagnosis of anxiety in patients who have other problems. The test contains 14 items, each with a five-point scale, and is completed by a physician or psychologist. The test emphasizes the patient's subjective state. The two subscales determined are somatic anxiety and psychic anxiety.

Hamilton Depression Scale

The HAMD is one of the most widely used tests to quantitatively evaluate the severity of depressive illness in adults. The most widely used form of this test contains 21 items covering a broad range of symptomatology, with a three- to five-point scale for most items. The minimum time required to complete this test is usually 10 to 20 min, and it requires a skilled interviewer. Either the present time or the period within the last week is rated. Six subscales are obtained in the HAMD: anxiety/somatization, weight, cognitive disturbance, diurnal variation, retardation, and sleep disturbance.

Hopkins Symptom Checklist

The Hopkins Symptom Checklist (HSCL) is a scale that has been used to measure the presence and intensity of various symptoms in outpatient neurotic patients. It is a 58-item self-rating scale and has generally been replaced by the Self-Report Symptom Inventory (SCL-90). It measures the symptoms during the past week and requires approximately 20 min to complete. There are five subtests: somatization, obsessive–compulsive, interpersonal sensitivity, depression, and anxiety.

Inpatient Multidimensional Psychiatric Scale

The Inpatient Multidimensional Psychiatric Scale (IMPS) is used to measure psychotic syndromes in hospitalized adults capable of being interviewed. The 89 items are rated on the basis of a psychiatric interview. This test has been well validated and requires 10 to 15 min following a 35- to 45-min interview. There are 10 scores: excitement, hostile belligerence, paranoid projection, grandiose expansiveness, perceptual distortions, anxious intropunitiveness, retardation and apathy, disorientation, motor disturbances, and conceptual disorganization.

Nurses Observation Scale for Inpatient Evaluation

The Nurses Observation Scale for Inpatient Evaluation (NOSIE) (30-item test) is used by nursing personnel to rate a patient's behavior on the ward, with a five-point scale for each item. This test is widely used and is well accepted for adult inpatients. The test, which rates the most recent 3 days, is relatively easy to use and requires 3 to 5 min to complete. A revised NOSIE was validated in over 600 chronic schizophrenic patients aged 26 to 74. This test has also been validated in mentally retarded patients and gives seven scores: social competence, social interest, personal neatness, irritability, manifest psychosis, retardation, and total score.

Plutchik Geriatric Rating Scale

The Plutchik Geriatric Rating Scale (PLUT) (31-item test) is designed to measure the degree of geriatric functioning in terms of both physical and social aspects. The three-point scale for each item is completed on the basis of direct observation of the patient's behavior and takes 5 to 10 min to complete. The subscales measure overall dysfunction, aggressive behavior, sleep disturbance, social isolation, sensory impairment, work and activities, and motor impairment.

Profile of Mood States

Profile of Mood States (POMS) self-rating scale is used in both normals and psychiatric outpatients to evaluate feelings, affect, and mood. It has been widely used in drug studies. The 65 adjectives included in this test may be used to rate the present and/or previous week. This test requires from 5 to 10 min to complete and provides scores for six subtests: tension–anxiety, depression–dejection, anxiety–hostility, vigor, fatigue, and confusion.

Sandoz Clinical Assessment—Geriatric

The Sandoz Clinical Assessment–Geriatric (SCAG) test measures 18 individual symptoms plus a global rating using a seven-point scale similar to those used in the Brief Psychiatric Rating Scale. It measures the present period or that within the last week, requires about 10 to 15 min to complete, and does not contain subtests.

Self-Report Symptom Inventory

Each of the 90 items in the SCL-90 uses a five-point scale of distress. It was designed as a general measure of symptomatology for use by adult psychiatric outpatients in either a research or clinical setting. It rates either the present or previous week. It requires about 15 min for the patient to complete this form and about 5 min for a technician to verify identifying information. This test is sensitive to drug effects and may also be used with inpatients. Nine subscales are measured: somatization, obsessive–compulsive, interpersonal sensitivity, depression, anxiety, anger–hostility, phobic anxiety, paranoid ideation, and psychoticism.

Wittenborn Psychiatric Rating Scale

The ECDEU version [Wittenborn Psychiatric Rating Scale (WITT)] is a 17-item test shortened from the original 72-item test. All but one item use a four-point scale, and the test takes 5 to 10 min to complete. It is used in both in- and outpatients and rates either the present or previous week. This test is not intended to make diagnoses but to reflect changes within one patient and to provide a basis for comparing different patients. This test provides descriptive, as opposed to etiological or prognostic, information on patients and includes the following subscales: anxiety, somatic–hysterical, obsessive–compulsive–phobic, depressive retardation, excitement, and paranoia.

Zung Self-Rating Anxiety Scale

The SAS test requires approximately 5 to 10 min to complete. See Anxiety Status Inventory for details.

Zung Self-Rating Depression Scale

The SDS test requires approximately 5 to 10 min to complete. See Depression Status Inventory for details.

Pediatric Behavioral Rating and Diagnostic Scales

Many of the behavioral rating scales described for adults are not suitable for use in the pediatric population. Special tests have been designed, and a number of pediatric behavioral rating scales are presented in Table 17.21. General comments on these tests are presented below. A further description of rating scales used in pediatric drug studies is given in the *ECDEU Assessment Manual For Psychopharmacology* by Conners (1976). His article is a practical guide to identifying appropriate scales for a particular situation. Conners discusses the two broad

TABLE 17.21. *Pediatric behavioral rating and diagnostic scales*[a]

---

1. Children's Behavior Inventory (CBI)
2. Children's Diagnostic Classification (CDC)
3. Children's Diagnostic Scale (CDS)
4. Children's Psychiatric Rating Scale (CPRS)
5. Clinical Global Impression (CGI)
6. Conners Parent Questionnaire (PQ)
7. Conners Parent–Teacher Questionnaire (PTQ)
8. Conners Teacher Questionnaire (TQ)
9. Devereux Child Behavior Rating Scale
10. Devereux Elementary School Behavior Rating Scale
11. Dosage Record and Treatment Emergent Symptoms (DOTES)
12. Stereotyped Behavior in Retarded[b]

---

[a]Additional tests are described in *Mental Measurements Yearbook* (Buros, 1972).
[b]This test is described by Davis et al. (1969).

approaches of many pediatric rating scales as either "rating current behaviors, symptoms or states; or...describing basic traits, dispositions, and personality characteristics." The choice of one of these two approaches depends in part on the purpose of using a scale in a drug study. Three general purposes have been suggested for using a behavioral test (prediction, measurement of change, and classification). The choice of one of these three purposes usually implies that one of the two specific approaches implicit in the pediatric behavioral scales will be more appropriate:

1. To be able to predict something about a patient, choose a scale that rates basic traits.
2. To measure change in a patient, choose a scale that rates current symptoms.
3. To assess a patient's classification, choose a scale that rates either basic traits or current symptoms, depending on the purpose of the classification.

The type of patient population and the desired format of the test to be used in a study also influence the particular scale(s) chosen.

Conners (1976) reviewed six different scales (tests) for teachers and recommended two for use in drug studies (Devereux and Conners). Information on all six scales is available in his article. Three scales are described for parents to complete, and two of these are mentioned below (Devereux Child Behavior Rating Scale and the Conners Parent Questionnaire). There are a small number of child psychiatry rating scales that are available. Conners briefly described a few and stated that the scale reported by Davis et al. (1969) for use in retarded children was sensitive to drug treatment. A scale that can be used in a wide variety of pediatric inpatients is the Children's Behavior Inventory.

Children's Behavior Inventory

The Children's Behavior Inventory (CBI) is a 139-item, two-point (yes–no) scale to record maladaptive behavior in children aged 1 to 15 years. Relatively little training is needed to administer this test. It is easily used by nurses, teachers, graduate students, psychologists, and others. This test usually requires at least 2 hr of observation of the child, but better reliability is achieved if behavior is observed over an 8-hr period. Nine subtest scores are provided: anger–hostility, conceptual dysfunctioning, fear and worry, incongruous behavior, incongruous ideation, lethargy–dejection, perceptual dysfunctioning, physical complaints, and self-deprecation.

Children's Diagnostic Classification

Children's Diagnostic Classification (CDC) test may be used instead of the Children's Psychiatric Rating Scale (CPRS) to arrive at a diagnosis. This differs from the CPRS in that it is highly directed and leads the observer to a diagnosis. It rates the current status of the child and may be used at pretreatment and/or the termination of the study.

Children's Diagnostic Scale

The Children's Diagnostic Scale (CDS) is used in children up to 15 years of age to assist in the diagnosis and classification of the child's condition. It contains 13 items, eight of which have a seven-point scale. The others are specific diagnostic questions. It measures current status only and is mainly used at the start of a study, although it may be used at the termination of the study as well.

Children's Psychiatric Rating Scale

The CPRS is a comprehensive scale to assess a wide range of psychopathology in children up to age 15. It contains 63 items, with a seven-point scale derived from the Brief Psychiatric Rating Scale (BPRS). This test rates 28 items by direct observation of the child, based on behavior expressed during the interview, and rates other items based on the child's reports of events that occurred either over the preceding week or that occurred during the interview. Scores of 15 separate clusters of the rated items are provided as well as the overall score.

Clinical Global Impression

See adult behavioral rating scale description of the CGI.

Conners Parent Questionnaire

Conners Parent Questionnaire (PQ) is a 94-item checklist of symptoms that evaluates common behavior disorders using a four-point scale in children up to 15 years of age and takes 15 to 20 min to complete. It is used once pretreatment and may be repeated but is often replaced after the first use by the 11-item Conners Parent–Teacher Questionnaire (PTQ). There are eight subscales: conduct problem, anxiety, impulsive–hyperactive, learning problem, psychosomatic, perfectionism, antisocial, and muscular tension.

Conners Parent–Teacher Questionnaire

See descriptions above for Conners Parent Questionnaire and below for the Conners Teacher Questionnaire (TQ). The PTQ is used in conjunction with either the PQ or TQ and yields a total score only (i.e., no subscales are given). The PTQ takes about 5 min to complete and is not used pretreatment.

Conners Teacher Questionnaire

The TQ form was designed to obtain teacher evaluations of children up to age 15 in terms of their interactions with peers and their ability to cope with the school environment and requirements. There are 41 items, and the first 39 have a four-point scale. Question 40 deals with the teacher's evaluation of the child's severity of illness, and question 41 deals with global improvement in four different areas. This test is used once at pretreatment and as needed afterwards. It takes about 15 min to complete and covers either the present or any interval period up to a month. A shorter 11-item PTQ is often used after the initial use of the 41-item TQ. Teachers require some instruction in the use of this test. The five subscales included are conduct, inattentive–passive, tension–anxiety, hyperactivity, and social ability.

Devereux Child Behavior Rating Scale

The Devereux Child Behavior Rating Scale contains 97 items and is similar to the Devereux Teacher Scale. It is used for emotionally disturbed and mentally retarded children aged 8 to 12. Besides being easy to use, this scale is well researched and discussed in the literature. It requires 10 to 20 min to complete by clinicians, child care workers, parents, or others and gives 17 scores. There is a Devereux Adolescent Behavior Rating Scale for children from age 13 to 18.

Devereux Elementary School Behavior Rating Scale

The Devereux Elementary School Behavior Rating Scale is a widely used test incorporating 47 items that have a high test–retest reliability. It uses a checklist format and is easy to use (requires 10 min). There are 11 factor scores and three item scores. Conners (1976) believes that this might be the test of choice for teachers to complete in many drug studies.

Stereotyped Behavior in Retarded

The Stereotyped Behavior in Retarded test (Davis et al., 1969) has been reported to be sensitive to drug treatment in retarded and severely disturbed inpatients.

Psychometric and Performance Tests

The psychometric and performance tests presented in Table 17.22 may be grouped as being applicable for use in either children or adults. In children, the tests measure intellect (GOOD, Porteus Mazes, WISC, Peabody), achievement (WRAT), and motor performance (vigilance tests, reaction time). There are other tests that may be used to measure learning, although many of these tests utilize equipment and are not described. All of these tests (unless otherwise noted) are given once pretreatment, at least once posttreatment, and at additional times if desired by the investigator. The contribution of learning in the scores obtained at second and third testings is usually unknown. The methods used to motivate patients to perform to the best of their ability in all tests should be standardized and reported.

Bender–Gestalt Test

The Bender–Gestalt is a nonverbal performance test in which the individual copies a design shown on a card. It is often used to identify a problem of visual perception and/or motor performance or minimal brain dysfunction in children.

TABLE 17.22. *Psychometric and performance tests*[a]

Test	For use in	
	Adults	Children
1. Bender–Gestalt Test	X	X
2. Conceptual Clustering Memory Test	X	X
3. Digital Symbol Substitution Test	X	X
4. Embedded Figures Test	X	X
5. Frostig Development Test of Visual Perception		X
6. Goodenough–Harris Figure-Drawing Test (GOOD)		X
7. Peabody Picture Vocabulary Test		X
8. Porteus Mazes	X	X
9. Reaction Time	X	X
10. Vigilance Tests	X	X
11. Wechsler Adult Intelligence Scale (WAIS)	X	
12. Wechsler Intelligence Scale for Children (WISC)		X
13. Wechsler Memory Scale (WMEM)	X	X
14. Wide Range Achievement Test (WRAT)		X

[a]Additional tests are described in *Mental Measurements Yearbook* (Buros, 1972).

The scoring used for children (age 4 or 5–11 years) differs from that used for adults (age 15–adult). This test measures perceptual maturity, possible neurological impairment, and emotional adjustment in children. It measures maturation, intelligence, psychological disturbance, and cortical impairment in adults. The test requires 10 min to complete. Scores may fluctuate from test to test and thus must be cautiously interpreted.

Conceptual Clustering Memory Test

For the Conceptual Clustering Memory Test, patients are given a list of 24 specific words from a number of different categories such as birds, cars, or types of drinks. The words are presented one at a time over 2 min, after which patients are asked to recall as many of the specific words as possible. The test measures the total recall as well as the degree to which words of a specific category (e.g., birds) are recalled from the cluster of words given in that category (e.g., crow, dove, pigeon).

Digital Symbol Substitution Test

Subtest of the Wechsler Adult Intelligence Scale (WAIS), the Digital Symbol Substitution test measures sensory–motor integration and learning relationships of symbols. It has been used in many psychopharmacological studies. Patients are given different forms of this test at each session. The test requires the patient to match as many of 100 symbols to their respective numerals, found in a code key, as possible within 60 sec.

Embedded Figures Test

For the Embedded Figures Test, patients are shown a complex design and must identify as quickly as possible a simple figure that is "embedded" within the design.

Twenty-four embedded figures are included, and a maximum of 3 min is allowed for each one.

Frostig Developmental Test of Visual Perception

The Frostig Developmental Test of Visual Perception (FROST) measures the development of perceptual skills in children from 4 to 8 years of age or in older children with learning difficulties. It may be administered individually (requires 30–45 min) or to groups (requires 40–60 min).

Goodenough–Harris Figure-Drawing Test

The Goodenough–Harris Figure-Drawing Test is a brief (10–15 min) easy to use test for children 4 to 15 years of age to measure intellectual maturity.

Peabody Picture Vocabulary Test

The Peabody Picture Vocabulary Test is a rapid 10- to 15-min intelligence test for children aged 2.5 to 18 that is useful when there is inadequate time to give the WISC.

Porteus Mazes

The Porteus Mazes is a nonverbal test that has been shown to be sensitive to drug effects in both children (over 3 years) and adults. The test has three series of mazes to prevent score improvement on retesting with the same test. It requires about 25 min and provides both a qualitative and quantitative score.

Reaction Time

There are many different tests used to measure reaction time. These tests measure the period of time between the presentation of a stimulus to a patient and the onset of the resulting response. The signal is usually a visual or auditory stimulus, and the onset of a motor reaction, such as the lifting of a finger, arm, or leg or the pressing of a buzzer, is used to measure the speed of response.

In simple reaction times, a stimulus is presented that always requires the same response, even if the nature of the stimulus changes. A complex reaction time requires the patient to respond to some stimuli but not to others.

Vigilance Tests

Numerous tests have been designed to measure vigilance. In these tests, patients are requested to respond in some manner to certain stimuli or occurrences but not to others. The stimuli may be controlled to present minimally perceived signals that require vigilance on the part of the patient.

Wechsler Adult Intelligence Scale

The WAIS consists of 11 subtests—six verbal tests and five performance tests. This provides an age-related IQ in adults from 16 to 75 years of age, i.e., the test measures intelligence of the person in relation to his age group and not to the entire population. It may be used either as an initial assessment or as a tool to measure change. The test, which takes 40 to 60 min to complete, provides 13 scores in verbal and performance categories plus a total score.

Wechsler Intelligence Scale for Children

The Wechsler Intelligence Scale for Children (WISC) was extensively revised in 1974, and it became the WISC-R, which requires 40 to 60 min to complete. This widely used scale in children from 6 to 16 years of age may be used for either screening or baseline data or as a measure of change. There is a "preschool and primary scale of intelligence" version that may be used in children from 4 to 6½ years of age (requires 50–75 min). The WISC-R has six verbal and six performance subtests.

Wechsler Memory Scale

The Wechsler Memory (WMEM) Scale is a brief test that is used to measure memory deficits. There are two forms of the test, and they are generally alternated to avoid a training effect in children taking the test on two or more occasions.

Wide Range Achievement Test

The Wide Range Achievement Test (WRAT) is used in children from age 5 to adults in college. It assesses basic skills in reading, spelling, and mathematics. It is simple, easy to administer, and requires 20 to 30 min to complete.

Personality Tests

In addition to the above behavioral and performance tests, there are a number of well-known tests of personality that may provide useful information in a clinical study. The most well known of these tests is the Minnesota Multiphasic Personality Inventory (MMPI). This test consists of 550 affirmative statements to which a true or false response is given and requires about an hour to complete. It is given to adults over the age of 16 and is scored for 10 scales: depression, hysteria, hypochondriasis, psychopathic deviate, masculinity–femininity, paranoia, hypomania, schizophrenia, psychasthenia, and social introversion.

Disability Tests

When drugs are tested in geriatric or other patients who have a significant degree of disability, it is useful to insure that drug-induced changes do not affect their ability to function at their usual level of activity. This information is usually obtained by evaluating adverse reactions and physical examinations. But there are tests that directly measure and/or assess the patients' activities of daily living. These tests can provide an estimate of change that may not be specifically noted on evaluating adverse reactions or physical examinations. Some of these tests include the Northwestern (University) Disability Test and the Activities of Daily Living Test.

The Northwestern Disability Test measures the patient's ability to walk, dress himself or herself, eat, perform personal hygiene, and speak. Each of these categories is scaled with 5 to 10 explicit gradations that are described in reasonable detail (e.g., grade 4 for walking: Sometimes walks alone. Walks short distances with ease; walking outdoors is difficult but often done without help; rarely walks longer distances alone).

The Activities of Daily Living Test is often modified from study to study. A representative example includes six activities (walking, sitting, standing, putting on shoes and socks, getting into or out of a chair or car, and sleeping) that are each graded on a five-point scale. Grade 1 is normal, i.e., able to perform the activity without limitation, impairment, or discomfort. Grades 2, 3, and 4 represent mild, moderate, and severe impairment and/or discomfort, and grade 5 indicates that the patient is unable to perform the activity.

18 Modifying Dosing Schedules and Developing Compliance Checks

Modifying Dosing Schedules • Patient Compliance

MODIFYING DOSING SCHEDULES

There are two general approaches for developing dosing schedules for a clinical protocol. The first approach is to establish the dosing schedule to be used on the assumption that each patient behaves as an ideal patient and that no complications will occur that require modification of the dose. The second approach is to provide information that describes what the investigator and/or patient should do when everything is not proceeding according to the protocol plan and dosage modifications are required. The first aspect was discussed in the chapter on choosing a study design, and the second is briefly reviewed in this section.

Modifications or variations of dosing that are permitted by protocol could be included in the type of table illustrated in Tables 10.5 and 10.6. Examples of situations that might require dosage modification include adverse reactions, abnormal laboratory or clinical examinations, blood or urine study drug levels outside an acceptable range, exacerbation of the disease, remission of the disease, missed appointments, and missed doses. It is impossible to describe fully each of these potential problems in a protocol. The protocol should describe whether dose changes are acceptable and, if so, whether fixed dose increments (or ranges) or unrestricted dose adjustments may be used and whether any restrictions will be imposed on the total number or frequency of dose adjustments. The general or specific criteria that the investigator must follow to alter the dose of the study drug are usually stated in the protocol.

In some cases, dose adjustments must be made in the prescription of concomitant medications rather than in the dose of the study drug. Criteria for dose adjustments of concomitant medications must also be established. See Table 18.23 for a list of some of the options used to control dosages and use of concomitant drugs during a study. For example, in the area of epilepsy, blood levels of concomitant antiepileptic drugs are often monitored. If these levels fall outside the normal therapeutic range (or possibly change by a specific percentage from the baseline value but still remain within the therapeutic range), it may be desirable to adjust the dose to try to bring the blood level within the normal range. Laboratory data, however, are not infallable, and a repeated determination to confirm the accuracy of the abnormality is often important to obtain. In the case of an abnormal value, the need to

TABLE 18.23. *Options for controlling concomitant drugs during the study*

---

1. No drugs other than the study drug may be used for any reason
2. Other drugs are permitted only to treat adverse reactions
3. All patients must continue their specific antidisease drug(s) at their initial (fixed) dose
4. Same option as 3, but the concomitant drug's dose may be adjusted by the investigator according to criteria described in the protocol
5. Same option as 3, but the concomitant drug's dose may be self-adjusted by the patient according to general (or specific) criteria
6. Patients may be given one (or more) drug from a list of standard antidisease drugs if it is necessary for them to receive adjunctive treatment
7. Medications used prior to the study to treat other diseases or problems will be permitted during the study, and the dosages used may (may not) vary
8. Concomitant drugs are allowed to treat the disease being studied, but no concomitant drugs may be used to treat other diseases
9. In the case of a disease exacerbation or in the case of a medical emergency unrelated to the disease, other drugs may be used, and the patient may remain in the study
10. No restriction on other drug therapies will be made either for the study disease or for other diseases
11. Use of nonprescription drugs may (may not) be restricted; any restrictions must be specified
12. Certain combinations (or variations) of the above options may be specified, including qualifications of the frequency, per-dose amount of drug, total daily (weekly) dose amount, or other factors

---

repeat the test may be specified in the protocol. A further complication may ensue if an abnormal laboratory value is reported in an outpatient study after the patient has returned home and the patient lives a great distance from the study site. The patient may be requested to go to another laboratory to have the required test performed. This situation may also be resolved by establishing criteria based on whether the abnormal blood level value of the drug is accompanied by adverse reactions (presumably from too high a blood level) or seizure exacerbations in studies on antiepileptic drugs (presumably from too low a blood level). If either of these clinical observations is made, then dosage adjustments would occur immediately, without a requirement to confirm the blood level abnormality.

PATIENT COMPLIANCE

Why and How Patients Do Not Comply with a Study

There are many reasons why patients may not comply with the requirements of a protocol. These may relate to the characteristics of the study design, study drug, individual patient's personality, relationships with study personnel, or other factors. Some of these reasons are listed in Table 18.24.

The quality of most outpatient studies is enhanced by incorporating a test or tests for compliance in the protocol. A compliance test with follow-up questioning of noncompliant patients may uncover a reason for diminished compliance that could be addressed in a protocol amendment (or new protocol). The revised protocol

TABLE 18.24. *Selected reasons for poor patient compliance*

---

1. Study requirements for patients are too complex, too demanding, too painful, and/or too stressful
2. Study requirements are inadequately understood by patients; instructions provided to patients may not be clear
3. Poor rapport exists between patients and investigator or other study personnel
4. Patients may have to wait excessively long to see relevant individuals at their study visits
5. Inadequate incentives are present for patients to be motivated to participate as directed (e.g., the patients' disease may be asymptomatic as in some patients with hypertension, or the drug may be used on a prophylactic basis)
6. Study drug[a] is difficult to swallow because of its large size or other characteristics
7. Study drug has an unpleasant odor or taste
8. Study drug causes adverse reactions
9. Study drug is not adequately effective
10. Study drug (or concomitant drugs) are too expensive
11. Transportation to the study site may be too expensive or too difficult
12. Taking time from one's occupation may create unacceptable difficulties
13. Personal problems or other factors not related to the study may adversely affect the patient's compliance (e.g., patient went on a trip and forgot to bring the study drug)
14. Too many drugs are being prescribed for the patient

---

[a]Study drug refers to either active drug or placebo.

would enable data to be collected that would have a greater chance of meeting the study objectives.

Information on why protocol compliance was inadequate might assist in the interpretation of the data. A number of the ways in which patients fail to comply with a study are listed in Table 18.25. These illustrations of decreased compliance are broadly divided into those related to the study drug and those related to other aspects of the study.

Tests to Measure Patient Compliance

There are a variety of tests to measure patient compliance, and a number of them are listed in Table 18.26. Most of these tests do not yield precise and accurate data, and their reliability may usually be challenged. The most simple and open approach to measuring compliance is to ask the patient a direct question such as "Are you taking all of your medicine?" or "Have you missed taking any of your medicine?" or, somewhat indirectly and possibly in a less threatening manner, "Are you having any difficulty remembering to take your medicine?"

The most commonly used measure of compliance apart from direct questioning is probably that of the pill count. The actual number of tablets or capsules in the drug container used by the patient are counted at each (or selected) clinic visits, and the expected number to be used is also determined. The ratio of actual pill use divided by expected pill use (times 100) gives a figure that may be referred to as percent compliance. Any drug refills obtained by the patient must be considered in calculating the actual number of pills used, and any changes in the dose prescribed must be considered in calculating the expected number of pills to be used.

TABLE 18.25. *Selected ways in which patients fail to comply with a protocol*

A. Noncompliance primarily related to the study drug
  1. Patients do not fill their prescriptions for study drug
  2. Patients do not take the study drug as directed; patients take
    a. Too few doses per day, but at the correct times
    b. Too few doses per day and at irregular times
    c. Irregular numbers of doses per day
    d. Correct number of doses per day, but at incorrect fixed times (i.e., in relation to meals or over too short a period)
    e. Too many doses on some days
    f. Irregular number of tablets per dose
    g. No doses on some days and a correct or incorrect pattern on other days
  3. Patients may prematurely discontinue the drug (this is especially significant if antibiotics or some other classes of drugs are prematurely stopped)
  4. Patients place the drug in their "cheek" (for inpatient studies) and then discard the dosage (or otherwise improperly ingest the medication)
B. Noncompliance unrelated to the study drug
  1. Patients may not adhere to the clinic visit schedule, may not contact the clinic as directed (e.g., for adverse reactions), or may fail to bring their drugs, diaries, or biological samples (e.g., urine) to clinic
  2. Patients may not properly complete patient diaries or other materials
  3. Patients may not maintain a diet, exercise program, or other outpatient aspect of the study

---

TABLE 18.26. *Tests for compliance*

---

1. Question directly at an interview or via a questionnaire
2. Perform pill counts of study and possibly nonstudy drugs
3. Measure drug levels in blood, urine, or other biological samples
4. Measure markers attached to drugs (or placebo); evaluate markers in biological samples collected from patients
5. Conduct unannounced visits to each patient's home to obtain biological samples
6. Determine the number of prescriptions filled and also refilled at pharmacies (i.e., the total quantity of drug dispensed is calculated)
7. Determine the amount of drug dispensed from mechanical drug dispensers
8. Measure physiological markers if they provide an indication of compliance (e.g., heart rate in patients receiving propranolol)
9. Evaluate patient diaries for completeness and adherence to instructions (i.e., accuracy)
10. Screen urine samples for drugs prohibited by protocol (e.g., caffeine and nicotine, if relevant)
11. Measure attendance at clinic and posttreatment visits (i.e., the number of missed and cancelled appointments)

Care must be used in determining these figures, since patients often switch medicines between bottles (e.g., a "purse" bottle may be created by the patient), which could affect the numbers counted. Some protocols are written to exclude some or all of a patient's data from analysis if the patient's percent compliance falls below a defined level and to discontinue patients who are unable to offer a satisfactory explanation of their failure to comply adequately with the study.

It is usually assumed that patients who ingest their study medication as prescribed are also compliant with other aspects of the protocol, but this is certainly not always the case. There are many means by which patients may "cheat" on pill counts, and it is difficult to accurately determine the degree of compliance based on pill counts alone. If the patient does not bring his/her medications to the clinic or office visit, a definite plan should have been evolved to deal with the situation. The patient may be asked to count the number of pills at home and to telephone the information to the investigator, but this is not a wholly satisfactory method since it alerts the patient to the attention paid to pill counts and may make the patient feel that he/she is being watched too closely. In fact, all pill counts should be conducted out of the patient's sight. Another alternative is to omit performing the pill count in question and to give special attention to the pill count at the next visit. This option is reasonable if there are several pill counts scheduled during the study, but if the instance in question represented the only pill count in the study, then requesting the patient to return to the clinic the next day or having a member of the study team visit the patient's home should be considered. Mailing drugs to patients or to the study site is not generally advocated except when absolutely necessary and under carefully controlled conditions.

If the study drug is obtained at a local or another pharmacy rather than through the investigator, records may be requested of the number and amount of refills obtained by patients. A sample pharmacy record that may be used if a pharmacy is involved in the study is shown in Fig. 18.9. Many variations of this form are possible.

A more precise assessment of patient compliance than pill counts is to measure the level of the drug in blood, urine, or other biological fluids or samples. This assumes that an assay method is available to measure drug levels. If drug levels are being evaluated to check for compliance and a placebo is being used in the drug study, then some type of marker may be incorporated into the placebo (and/or the active drug as well) so that the compliance of all patients may be assessed. Detectable labels that can be added to placebos or to drugs for which no suitable assay exists include quinine, sodium bromide, and riboflavin. If the drug is excreted or eliminated via the urine, then fluorescing agents may be used as markers, and urine samples collected for evaluation.

Samples must be obtained from patients at a time when the drug is still present in adequate amounts to be measured. This may pose problems for drugs with short half-lives unless their metabolites may also be measured and will be present in sufficient quantities at a time when the samples will be collected. Samples may be assayed immediately or refrigerated or frozen for subsequent assay.

The interpretation of drug levels in biological samples may be viewed in either qualitative or quantitative terms. In qualitative terms, the test result is scored as present or absent, and in quantitative terms, the precise level is measured and evaluated. In evaluating the quantitative levels of drugs and comparing different patients, it is important that each patient have ingested his/her most recent dose at the same time interval prior to the taking of the biological sample.

A problem may arise in interpreting blood level data if the study drug has a short half-life. For example, consider three patients who took their study drug at the same time on the day of their clinic visit: one patient had not taken the drug

Sample Pharmacy Record

PROTOCOL NO: __ TITLE OF STUDY:

Patient Initials _____ Patient No. _____

Complete the following information and use a new line each time study medication is dispensed or returned.

TREATMENT ____

Date Drug Dispensed or Returned	7 Digit No. on Bottle (Or Other Code)	Quantity Dispensed (No. of Tablets)	Quantity Returned (No. of Tablets)	Initials of Pharmacist	Comments

FIG. 18.9. Sample pharmacy record indicating the type of information that could be maintained on all study patients.

since his/her last clinic visit, the second patient had only taken the drug for the day preceding the present visit, and the third had taken all of the prescribed drug. The problem would be that all three patients might have the same blood level recorded on the day of the clinic visit, and the data would therefore be misleading in terms of measuring patient compliance. One approach to evaluating the possibility of patients not taking drug between clinic appointments is to visit the patient's home at an unannounced time to collect a blood, urine, saliva, or other biological sample. This method may only be used if the patient has previously agreed to participate in this program and has indicated this agreement in the informed consent. This technique is only feasible if patients live relatively close to the study site and resources are available for personnel to visit each patient and to collect and analyze samples.

Drug bottles containing either the precise number of pills for a daily dose or a standard number of pills may be placed into a mechanical device, sometimes called a "medication monitor." In inpatient studies, the patient may be advised to operate this machine to obtain medication but is not informed that the number of bottles is being monitored. The number of bottles of study drug dispensed to a patient may be easily determined, although it is a separate question whether all doses of the study drug dispensed were actually ingested.

In certain studies, physiological markers provide an indication of the degree of patient compliance. A well-known example is that of measuring heart rate in patients receiving β-adrenergic receptor-blocking drugs. If the heart rate is not in the expected range, and the patient is receiving a dose shown to decrease heart rate, then this is indirect evidence of a lack of compliance if there were no other reasonable explanations for the "elevated" heart rate.

Another means of estimating compliance is by evaluating patient diaries. Both the frequency (i.e., the number of times an entry was made compared to the number of times an entry should have been made) and the quality of the entries may be evaluated. The quality of the entry might be judged by whether the study drug was taken as scheduled and whether all requested information was filled out (e.g., daily evaluations of the patient's pain). The desirability of incorporating one or more of these methods into a protocol must be evaluated for each clinical study.

A urine screen can be used to generally confirm that patients being screened or entering the baseline period of the study are not using illicit drugs or drugs contraindicated in the protocol. It can also be used on a scheduled or random basis during the study to confirm that patients are not using illicit or unacceptable drugs. The urine screen is limited in that it is unable to detect positive compliance with the protocol and only measures certain aspects of compliance failure. If a urine test will be conducted at unannounced times in the study, then this point must be mentioned in the informed consent.

The number of drugs tested in the urine screen is generally determined individually for each study, since there is a wide variety of possible drugs that may be measured. The choice of drugs to screen will be based on their relative importance for the study plus the cost and reliability of the methodology. Results of urine screens are usually best viewed in qualitative (i.e., present or absent) rather than quantitative terms. The identification of specific drugs in a patient's urine may help in explaining unusual adverse reactions, laboratory abnormalities, or other events. Urine screens may detect the presence of the study drug. If the urine screen is able to detect the presence of the study drug, and this is reported as an unknown drug that is present or as a false–positive for another drug, then it could essentially unblind a double-blind study. To prevent this situation from occurring, data from urine screens may be reported to a nonblinded monitor rather than to the investigator. If a sample of the test drug is put in urine at a physiological concentration and sent to the laboratory, the possibility of cross reactivity with known drugs may be assessed prior to initiation of the study.

Improving Patient Compliance

In order to counteract the possibility of poor compliance adversely affecting the data obtained in a study, there are a number of steps that may be taken at the outset of a study. These steps are summarized in Table 18.27 and generally address potential reasons why poor patient compliance occurs. Thus, a study that avoids situations in which poor compliance occurs has a good chance of minimizing this problem. Additional discussions on patient compliance are found in articles by Blackwell (1972*b*), Hussar (1980), Pearson (1982), and Peck and King (1982).

TABLE 18.27. *Methods of improving compliance*[a]

---

1. Simplify the demands of the protocol on patients
2. Minimize the number and duration of unpleasant or painful tests
3. Maintain relatively frequent contact with patients, especially at emotionally or physically difficult periods for the patient; contact the patient prior to scheduled visits
4. Allow for flexible dosing regimens to deal with adverse reactions, toxicity, and unanticipated situations
5. Provide the patient with appropriate information on the study and strive for a positive physician–patient relationship
6. Avoid making the patient feel guilty about poor compliance and provide positive feedback to all patients
7. Establish a therapeutic goal in conjunction with the patient and assess the patient's progress towards that goal
8. Plan patient visits at a mutually convenient time and insure that the patient has a minimal delay in waiting to see the physician or staff
9. Allow for and encourage patients to participate in their own care (e.g., with self-monitoring of their disease and treatment)
10. Involve the patient's spouse, family, or support group in the clinical study

---

[a]This table does not include a number of methods used in general medical practice, where different factors must be considered and different techniques exist to improve compliance (e.g., switching patients to a different drug or manipulating factors that are not permitted in most protocols).

*General Organization of Time and Events Schedules • Defining Periods
and Times of a Time and Events Schedule*

GENERAL ORGANIZATION OF TIME AND EVENTS SCHEDULES

Time and events schedules (or charts) are synopses of all planned events that
will transpire during a study, although the information and categories incorporated
into these schedules may either be highly specific or general. Table 19.28 lists
many of the common categories included in the "events" part of the schedule, and
Table 19.29 lists the various table headings and descriptions of "time" that are
often used. A sample time and events schedule is shown in Table 19.30. This was
the schedule used in a double-blind add-on crossover study of cinromide (an agent
tested for antiepileptic activity) versus placebo (Spilker et al., 1983).

The time and events chart should be organized to present a complete profile of
the overall study. In many studies it will be advantageous to construct a second,
more detailed time and events chart in which one part of the study can be more
fully delineated. This is usually presented as a separate schedule. An alternative
form of the time and events schedule is to list events that will occur at each hour,
day, and/or week of the study as opposed to putting them in a chart (Table 19.30).

In determining the frequency of drug dosing and the intervals between doses, it
is often appropriate to choose conditions that are similar to those under which the
drug will eventually be used. For example, if the study drug is intended to be given
four times a day (q.i.d.), then a dosing schedule and time and events chart can be
prepared to indicate that patients are to be dosed at equal intervals during the
waking period (e.g., 7 A.M., noon, 5 P.M. and 10 P.M.) rather than every 6 hr
around the clock. This would not apply to certain drugs (e.g., some antibiotics),
where around-the-clock dosing is desired. Likewise, drugs given two or three times
a day in a study can be ingested at times that will mimic eventual clinical use
rather than being given at equal intervals throughout a 24-hr day. This approach
yields information that is more relevant to the eventual clinical use of the drug than
would information obtained from equally spaced doses, which would significantly
differ from those of the intended use.

It is sometimes possible to collect information via telephone conversations with
patients or even via the mail. Under carefully designed conditions, this type of
data collection may replace visits to the clinic and may be noted by different
symbols or by footnotes in the time and events schedule.

TABLE 19.28. *Selected events that may be included in a time and events schedule*[a]

---

1. Clinic (physician) visit
2. Screening interview
3. Informed consent
4. Medical history
5. Physical examination (complete)
6. Physical examination (abbreviated)[b]
7. Vital signs and weight (single test at each time point that is marked)
8. Vital signs and weight (multiple tests at each time point that is marked)
9. Neurological or other specialized examinations
10. Clinical laboratory battery (each test, such as hematology, clinical chemistry, and urinalysis, may but need not be listed separately)
11. Biological samples of study drug (usually collected in blood or urine)[c]
12. Biological samples of concomitant drugs
13. Admit patient to research facility
14. Randomize patient to treatment group
15. Adverse reaction probe
16. Electrocardiogram (ECG) (12 lead)[d]
17. ECG (lead II)
18. ECG (24-hr Holter monitor)
19. Other safety measurements
20. All efficacy measurements (usually listed separately)
21. Drug administration
22. Dosage record of the study drug
23. Dosage record of concomitant drugs
24. Pill count or other compliance check(s)
25. Nurse's evaluation
26. Patient's global evaluation
27. Physician's global evaluation of disease severity
28. Physician's global evaluation of improvement
29. Release from research facility
30. Study discontinuation record
31. Patient discharged from study

---

[a]Footnotes may be used to qualify or detail any notations. The categories used to denote time are shown in Table 19.29, and a sample schedule is shown in Table 19.30. It may be relevant to indicate when many of these procedures and tests will be conducted relative to meals, expected peaks and troughs of blood levels, or other factors.

[b]This may be described and defined in the text and/or in a footnote. Both categories of physical examination may be listed in the time and events schedule, as with ECGs.

[c]Samples should be obtained at times of peak, trough, or at multiple time points on the drug concentration curve.

[d]It is often useful to obtain an ECG at the time of peak plasma levels in addition to pre- and posttreatment, when blood levels of the study drug would generally be low or absent.

DEFINING PERIODS AND TIMES OF A TIME AND EVENTS SCHEDULE

The various periods of a study may be denoted as screen, baseline, treatment, and posttreatment, but various other terms are also used (see Table 19.29). The manner in which the duration of each study is divided and described varies. A study may be numbered sequentially from the start of screen (day 1) through to day *n* for posttreatment. One alternative is to begin each new period of a study as day 1 (day 1 of baseline, day 1 of treatment, etc.). In this latter example, the

TABLE 19.29. *Possible headings and subheadings for the time component in time and events tables*

Possible major study period headings	Possible subheadings for each of the study periods
1. Screen[a] 2. Baseline[b] 3. Dose ascension 4. Treatment[c] 5. Taper 6. Posttreatment (follow-up) 7. Dose period 1 to n[d] 8. Optional visit(s) 9. Extended baseline[f]	Day, hour, and/or minute specified from 0 (or 1) to n for entire study or from 0 (or 1) to n for each period of the study.[e] Other variations of specifying the time in a study are possible.

[a]Negative numbers may be used when convenient; e.g., screen may occur during days − 7 to − 1, baseline from days 1 to 10, treatment from day 11 to day 30, and follow-up from day 31 to day 35.

[b]Also referred to as the "stabilization phase" of a study.

[c]Also referred to as the "maintenance phase" of a study.

[d]Each dose period may represent a new dose, a new group of patients who are dosed, or a different period of the study.

[e]Subheadings of year, month, and/or week may also be used. See text for a discussion of the use of "0" times.

[f]This variation may be used if it will allow for specific measurements or parameters to return to a given value or range of values (e.g., between the two legs of a crossover study). It also may be used for other specific reasons.

maximum duration or range of time that can elapse between the last day of one period and the first day of the following period should be established and indicated in the protocol. A third alternative is to number the time allotted to screen as day − x to day − 1 and to begin baseline on day 1 and continue numbering the days sequentially through treatment and posttreatment. Other possible methods of numbering the weeks, days, or hours of a study are possible.

In some studies there is notation of a day "0." If so, it must be made clear whether day "0" represents a full 24 hr or possibly an instant through which the study passes as it goes from day − 1 to day 1. Day 0 may also be a variable part of a 24-hr day rather than a complete day, depending on when day 1 begins. For example, patients may complete their screen or baseline on day 0 and start treatment on day 1, which begins immediately after screen or baseline. The designation of time must be clarified when patients are given their first dose (possibly in the clinic) immediately after the completion of screen or baseline. The principle described for day 0 also applies to hour 0 or week 0. It is the author's view that there are certain studies in which inclusion of a day 0 or hour 0 is appropriate (e.g., if screen and/or baseline will be initiated and completed in 1 day, and the following part of the study will begin the next day). When a "0" time is included in a study, it is imperative that it be clearly defined.

It is often relevant to consider whether each day of the study begins (1) at 12:01 A.M., (2) at another fixed time of day, or (3) whether it begins at a different time

TABLE 19.30. Study time and events schedule

Event	Screen	Period 1 baseline A		Period 2 treatment A							Period 3 baseline B			Period 4 treatment B							Period 5 follow-up	
Weeks:		2	4[a]	5	6	7	9	12	15	16[b]	17	18	20[a]	21	22	23	25	28	31	32[b]	33	36
Admission criteria	X																					
Informed consent	X																					
Medical/seizure history	X																					
Physical exam	X								X										X			
Neurological exam	X								X										X			
Investigator's assessment	X	X	X	X	X	X	X	X	X		X	X	X	X	X	X	X	X	X		X	X
Vital signs	X	X	X	X	X	X	X	X	X		X	X	X	X	X	X	X	X	X		X	X
Electrocardiogram (ECG)	X	X	X						X	X	X								X	X	X	
Electroencephalogram (EEG)	X								X	X			X						X	X		X
Laboratory																						
Hematology	X	X	X		X	X		X		X	X	X	X			X	X	X		X	X	X
Blood chemistry	X	X	X			X		X		X	X	X	X			X	X			X	X	X
Urinalysis	X	X	X			X				X		X	X			X				X	X	X
Pregnancy test (when applicable)	X	X	X			X				X		X	X			X				X		X
AED plasma levels[c]	X	X	X	X	X	X	X	X	X	X	X	X	X	X	X	X	X	X	X	X	X	X
Adverse reactions	X	X	X	X	X	X	X	X	X	X	X	X	X	X	X	X	X	X	X	X	X	X
Dosage record	X	X	X	X	X	X	X	X	X	X	X	X	X	X	X	X	X	X	X	X	X	X
Seizure record	X	X	X	X	X	X	X	X	X	X	X	X	X	X	X	X	X	X	X	X	X	
Physician's global evaluation										X										X		
Study discontinuation record																						X

[a] Dosage ascension of test medication initiated. Week numbers refer to end of week.
[b] Dosage taper/discontinuation of test medication.
[c] AED, antiepileptic drug.

for each patient (which is then fixed), depending on when each patient reaches a certain point in the protocol. For example, a patient may complete his/her screen examination in the morning or afternoon and immediately begin drug treatment. Day 1 may be defined as beginning with this treatment. Another possibility is for drug treatment to be withheld for all patients until the day after the screen (or baseline) examinations in order to start dosing all patients at the same time on day 1. If a patient takes some of the first day's doses at the end of screen, either the numbering of days will be variable from patient to patient or different patients will take a different number of doses on day 1 in order to have day 2 begin at 12:01 A.M.

The numbering of days will probably not pose any significant problems in a long-term study, but in a study in which important measurements are made during the first few days of the study or several times during day 1, it is generally mandatory to apply the same definition of day 1 to all patients. There are many situations that may arise in which the numbering of days (hours) may become quite complex, and complications in the numbering system may develop. If one patient requires a longer washout of preexisting drugs than another patient before entering the study, or if patients may remain in screen (or baseline) until they qualify to enter the baseline (or treatment), the acceptable lengths of each period as well as its numbering must be specified.

Another aspect of numbering in a study arises in the association of clinic visits and study weeks or months. The clinic visit may always occur at the start, middle, or end of each specified week, or it may occur at any time during each specified week. Each of these possibilities is commonly used. There is no preferred method in the author's view, but consistency and clarification are necessary goals in writing the protocol. The numbering of study weeks (or months) may have a significant impact on how much drug is to be dispensed at each clinic visit and how data collection forms may best be organized and prepared.

A time and events schedule of theoretical times (e.g., day 1 to x, week 1 to y, or month 1 to z) is usually written in a protocol (see Table 19.30) since the exact dates that the study will be conducted are usually unknown when the protocol is written. The theoretical dates must be associated with real times (e.g., August 4–17, July–November) prior to initiation of the study. If all patients start a protocol at different times, then this process must be individualized for each patient. Studies may be quite flexible in this regard (e.g., patients may come to clinic each month at a "convenient" time) or quite rigid (e.g., unless patients arrive at a certain time on a certain day, the value of the data obtained will be compromised or lost entirely). In the latter case, the timing of the study must be established after consideration of weekends, holidays, vacations, availability of staff and necessary equipment, plus other factors required to conduct the study such as the scheduling of all necessary tests. In clinical studies in which the initiation of drug therapy is determined by the patient and not by the investigator (e.g., when certain symptoms or signs occur, the patient immediately begins drug treatment), there will have to be special consideration given to devising an appropriate time and events schedule.

20 Preparing, Packaging, and Dispensing of Study Drugs

Preparing Study Drugs • Packaging Study Drugs • Dispensing Study Drugs • Assigning Patient Numbers

PREPARING STUDY DRUGS

After the study design and dosing schedule have been developed, the optimal means of preparing, packaging, and dispensing the study drugs may be determined.

The protocol does not generally include information on the procedures used to manufacture the study drug. Details are included (if relevent) that relate to the final preparation of the drug, if any procedures have to be performed (e.g., drug must be mixed or thawed), at or shortly prior to the time of its administration. Each of the ingredients in the formulation of study drugs may be listed in protocols, as may a description of pertinent storage and handling information (e.g., if the drug must be kept frozen).

In specifying the characteristics of the placebo medications to be used, there are several factors that may be considered. These are indicated in Table 20.31. Since some dyes that color drugs may elicit adverse pulmonary responses, and a number of dyes used to color gelatin capsules, tablets, and solutions are not standard or accepted in all countries, this factor may be relevant to consider. The use of lactose in a placebo or active drug may cause diarrhea and gastrointestinal distress in patients with lactose intolerance. If the study involves a group of patients among whom the expected incidence of lactose intolerance is anticipated to be higher than that in the general population, an alternate excipient for the placebo and/or active drug may be desired. If a solid form (tablet) of the active drug has a distinct taste, then it and the matching placebo could both be coated to mask differences in taste. Another option might be to put the manufactured (marketed) drug, either whole or ground up (if it is in tablet form), inside a capsule (usually opaque) and to use a matching placebo capsule. This technique has been successfully used but requires prior demonstration of dissolution characteristics that meet USP standards and also a submission to regulatory authorities [i.e., Food and Drug Administration (FDA) in the United States].

Patients' responses to placebo have been reported to be sensitive to color, size, form, and number of placebos taken. For example, blue placebo capsules have been associated with sedative effects, red and yellow placebos were associated with stimulant effects, capsules were believed to be more potent than tablets, and larger capsules were perceived to be of a larger drug strength (Jacobs and Nordan, 1979; Buckalew and Coffield, 1982).

145

TABLE 20.31. *Factors to consider in establishing placebo characteristics[a]*

1. Overall visual appearance
2. Surface and internal color
3. Size
4. Shape
5. Taste on licking and chewing
6. Smell
7. Weight
8. Presence of dyes[b]
9. Presence of lactose[c]
10. Printing, scoring, or stamping on the surface
11. Finish of the surface
12. Surface and internal texture
13. Floating and dissolution characteristics
14. Viscosity

[a]These characteristics of placebo medication are intended to be evaluated in comparison to the active drug. The influence of placebo color on specific patient responses is discussed in the text. Not all of these factors will be relevant for all placebos.

[b]This factor may be important for patients who are susceptible to allergic reactions to specific dyes (e.g., yellow tartrazine dyes).

[c]This factor may be important for patients who are lactose intolerant.

PACKAGING STUDY DRUGS

Numerous options to consider in choosing a method to package drugs are listed in Table 20.32. If a pharmacist at the study site is chosen to package and/or dispense study drugs, confirm that the individual chosen has had prior experience with research protocols, especially if a complex packaging scheme is used. Also, determine the number of pharmacists that will be involved (and in what capacity) at each stage of the study. Discuss with the relevant pharmacist how the randomization code will be utilized in packaging the drug and what type(s) of dispensing container(s) may be used to maintain the integrity of the drug. It is generally believed that the number of problems in conducting a study often increases when too many individuals are involved. The optimal number of individuals to be involved in conducting a study should be determined (insofar as possible) prior to the study.

Study drugs and matching placebos may sometimes be obtained directly from the manufacturer. Printed markings on the drug's surface must not be present if a placebo is to be used. Obtain placebos that are identical to the study drug in color, size, appearance, weight, taste, and even floating and dissolving characteristics (see Table 20.31). If placebos are not virtually identical to the active drug, then the value of a study is in jeopardy of being compromised. Karlowski et al. (1975) reported that many patients broke the study's blind by tasting the contents of the capsules. The authors described the significant impact that this event had on the data obtained.

TABLE 20.32. *Options to consider in determining the details of packaging study drugs*

1. Will the sponsor, investigator, pharmacist, independent contractor, or another group package the study drug(s)?
2. When will the study drug be packaged relative to the shipping and starting dates of the study?
3. Will study drug(s) be prepackaged by a sponsor or investigator prior to a study or packaged from bulk supplies after a patient is screened and evaluated?
4. Will drug packages be prepared for specific patients, and how will randomization codes be utilized in the packaging?
5. Should drug containers be made of plastic or glass; should the color of the container be amber or clear; and, should the top be a screw cap or a child-resistant cap? Other relevant questions about the containers may be posed.
6. How much study drug should be put into each container to fulfill protocol requirements?
7. How much extra study drug should be put into each container to allow for missed or delayed appointments or other contingencies (as well as inserting a few extra tablets or capsules to make a pill count easier to conduct)?
8. Should a separate backup medication bottle be prepared for each patient in case of loss or damage to the original or in case of a missed or delayed appointment?
9. How many extra sets of medication should be packaged to allow for patient dropouts, broken bottles, and additional or replacement patients?
10. Should drug be packaged by unit dose or unit of use?
11. Should patients be given the same number of capsules (tablets) at each dose during dose ascension?
12. If an active control is used that looks different from the study drug, or if different sized capsules will be used to make up certain doses of the study drug, how many different types of placebos will be necessary to maintain the blind, and how will the placebos be packaged?
13. If bottles are prepackaged, how should they be grouped for packaging and placement into cartons (e.g., should all bottles for one patient or for one treatment period be grouped together, or should another schema, be utilized)?
14. Storage conditions of the drugs may require careful consideration for each point of their journey.
15. How will drugs be shipped to study sites?[a]

[a]See Table 22.41.

In addition to rigid glass and plastic containers, flexible packaging materials are also used to package drugs. Flexible materials primarily include the use of thin plastic or cellulose films and aluminum foils. Films and laminates are used to make blister packs (push through and peelable), strip packs, sachets, and other packages that can be used for unit-dose (contains one dose) packaging of solid or liquid drugs. In unit-of-use packaging, each package contains the proper amount of medication for one course of therapy (e.g., 20 tablets in a package labeled day 1 A.M., day 1 P.M., etc. to day 10).

Improper packaging of a drug can adversely affect a study in many ways:

1. If the package is permeable to moisture or gases, it may diminish the stability of a drug or allow volatile components to be lost. Plastics are well known to be permeable to water vapor, volatile oils, flavorings, some components of creams, and glues used for attaching labels to the container.

2. If the components of the drug container closure or seal interact with the drug, then the drug may leach out certain components from the container closure or seal, or an actual chemical reaction may occur. Teflon®-lined closures are usually more inert than closures made of rubber.
3. The opposite phenomenon may occur if the seal, closure, or container absorbs certain chemicals from the drug product.
4. Photosensitive drugs must be protected from light by the container, and it may also be necessary to keep the container in a dark place.

Once the drug package is opened, there are an entirely new group of potential problems that may adversely affect the study. Most of the potential problems that relate to study medication will be directly or indirectly caused by inappropriate actions of individual patients (e.g., placing containers on a radiator, allowing excessive amounts of moisture or light to reach the drug) and should not affect the entire study.

In determining the most appropriate packaging scheme, an intellectual trial-and-error exercise may be performed in which various possible problems that could occur during the study are considered. It will be useful to discuss the pros and cons of several alternative approaches before one is adopted. Some of the more common packaging schemes are presented in Table 20.33, and information that may be printed on the labels is illustrated in Table 20.34. If the container is too small to accommodate a label with all required information, the following is sufficient for open-label studies: (1) proprietary name, (2) generic name, (3) lot or control number, (4) name and place of business of manufacturer, packer, or distributor. All other required information must appear on the outer container or in a package insert.

The expiration date of an investigational drug is often not placed on the label, since the drug would have to be returned to the sponsor or discarded if the expiration date were reached. If the data on expiration are maintained by the sponsor or manufacturer, then appropriate assays may be performed to extend the expiration date. It is desirable for all unused drug to be returned to a sponsor to have complete accountability.

All ingredients must be listed on the label for products that are not taken by mouth (e.g., otics, topicals, injectables, and ophthalmics). The percent labeled strength must also be shown on labels for injectable drugs. Preservatives and alcohol plus their percent strength must always be shown.

It is important not to label bottles "Treatment A" or "Treatment B" in double-blind trials if the bottles are kept by blinded personnel. In a medical emergency, the code must be broken for one patient, and thus the entire study will be unblinded. Labeling bottles as "Treatment A," etc. also may serve to bias the investigator into believing that treatment A is either better or worse than treatment B and behaving differently towards different patients depending on which treatment they are receiving.

TABLE 20.33. *Common packaging schemes*[a]

1. Each dose for each patient is placed in a separate bottle
2. All doses for one patient for a given time period (day, week, month) are placed in a separate bottle
3. All doses for one patient for an entire study are placed in a separate bottle
4. Each patient is assigned (but not dispensed) a bottle or bottles of medication for the study; i.e., a drug bottle remains in a pharmacy or at another controlled site for the duration of the study. Patients may obtain drug from the pharmacy or from the nurse for an inpatient study
5. Each patient receives additional medication in his/her bottle to allow for a missed or delayed appointment and/or to make a pill count to evaluate patient compliance easier to conduct
6. Each patient receives a backup bottle of medication for the study to allow for loss or damage to the original bottle or for a missed or delayed appointment
7. Each patient is given two bottles for a given time period or for the entire study, and the patient takes an equal number of capsules (tablets) from each bottle every time a dose is taken
8. Each patient is given two bottles of two different dosage strengths of one drug, and the patient takes medication as prescribed
9. Each patient is given or assigned two bottles for each dose. The entire contents of one pair of bottles are ingested at each dose
10. Bulk bottles are supplied to the investigator or pharmacist to be packaged into one of the above schemata
11. All bottles in an open-label study contain an identical number of capsules and label except for their code numbers. A calculated number of bottles are given to the patient at each visit to last until the next visit
12. Other variations of the above packaging schemata are possible

[a]Although these schemata are described for drugs put into bottles, drugs may be packaged in blister packs (push-through or peelable), paper envelopes, weekly or daily "medication sets," or other containers. Parenteral drugs are often packaged in ampuls, multidose vials, prefilled syringes, minibags, or other containers for bolus injection or constant or intermittent infusion.

In double-blind drug studies with ascending doses, when it is not known how many doses will actually be used in the study, there is an option that may be useful in packaging individual-dose bottles. Both study drug and placebo are packaged, one bottle for each dose, by the sponsor in a double-blind fashion and sent to the investigator's site. Additional placebos are provided and subsequently added to each bottle prior to dosing at the investigator's site to provide the same total number of pills in each bottle. Thus, patients always receive the same number of pills at each dose. This technique has the advantage that one or more active (or placebo) pills may be removed from all containers to be used for the next dose and replaced with placebos if the next dose to be given must be adjusted downwards or kept the same (assuming that the next series of drug bottles to be used contained a higher dose). In this manner, the patient always receives the same total number of pills at each dose, which is generally preferable in double-blind studies.

Alternatively, one could prepackage all likely doses that would be anticipated to be used or initiate and conduct a new study to explore a selected portion of the entire dose range in more detail. Since these alternatives are both expensive and wasteful of drug, a simpler solution is to package all patient's drug bottles at the study site from bulk supplies. This solution, however, requires using an unblinded

TABLE 20.34. *Information that may be placed on study drug labels*[a]

1. Study name and drug code number, lot (batch) number, formulation number, and form
2. Drug name for open-label studies, plus active and inactive ingredients (including percent strengths of alcohol and all preservatives)
3. Patient number and group number
4. Study day, week, or month number (e.g., month 4 or week 5)
5. Proper name of the day, week, or month (e.g., April 2–17)
6. Dosing period number or test day number
7. Time of dosing (e.g., Take one tablet at 8 A.M. and one at 8 P.M.)
8. Storage instructions
9. Dosing instructions, indications, and contraindications
10. Investigator's name and telephone number
11. Name and address of manufacturer or product license holder
12. Blank space for investigator or pharmacist to write on. The blanks may be for the patient's group, initials, name, number, and/or date or other data
13. Total number of tablets (capsules) in the container
14. Weight of drug (both for each capsule and for the total net weight)
15. Volume of contents (e.g., total number of milliliters for a liquid)
16. Statement: "Caution, New Drug, Limited by Federal Law to Investigational Use Only." Other warnings or precautions may be listed
17. Date of expiration
18. Other information may be placed on study drug labels

[a]A tear-off portion may be attached with the same (or different) information to place in the patient's data collection form, pharmacy book, or in another place. A third part of the label (attached to the second part) may be prepared with coded information identifying the contents of the bottle. This portion of the label could be opened and examined if the blind had to be broken for a medical emergency.

individual at the study site, whereas the first option described above avoids this necessity.

The term "triple-blind" study has been used in both a positive and negative sense. The positive definition refers to a double-blind study in which the study monitor or monitoring group (as well as patient and investigator) remains blind to patient randomization and to any interim results of the study. The negative definition relates to a situation in which errors have occurred in packaging the drug so that neither the investigator, patient, nor monitor (or sponsor) knows what drug is in each package, and thus the container dispensed contains an unknown drug or dose. When data from these patients reach a statistician in a randomized order, a "quadruple-blind" study results.

DISPENSING STUDY DRUGS

The same person who packages the study drug may dispense it, but this is usually not done. A number of common methods of dispensing and handling study drugs are listed in Table 20.35. If the drug is prepackaged with a tear-off portion of the label, then at the time that the drug is dispensed, this portion may be placed either in the patient's data collection form or in another denoted place.

The tear-off portion of the label may contain duplicate information to that attached to the bottle or container as well as a third part to tear open in case of a

TABLE 20.35. *Common methods of dispensing and handling study drugs*

1. Investigator (or research coordinator under the supervision of the investigator) dispenses the study drugs
2. Pharmacist dispenses the study drugs
3. Nonstudy drugs permitted by protocol are dispensed by investigator, study pharmacist, or obtained independently by the patient
4. A log may be used by either the investigator or pharmacist to record the number of bottles (pills) dispensed and number of pills returned (see Fig. 18.9)
5. Returned drugs should be stored according to instructions given in the protocol. Prior to the return of the drug to the sponsor, empty or partially filled containers may or may not be combined and the empty containers discarded
6. Returned drugs should be disposed of by the sponsor or appropriate individuals in accordance with Federal and other guidelines as specified in the protocol and/or in other documentation

medical emergency. The third part discloses the patient's treatment. If a pharmacy is involved in dispensing drugs, then a log book or other system should be used to keep relevant information on drugs dispensed. Figure 18.9 illustrates an example of one type of logbook form that may be used by a pharmacy.

ASSIGNING PATIENT NUMBERS

There are several methods of numbering patients in protocols, and the specific method used can provide information about the patient and assist in referring to patients and the data. In a multicenter study, for example, patients can be assigned numbers as in the following:

Method A: 1 to 30   Patient numbers reserved for site 1
           31 to 60   Patient numbers reserved for site 2
           61 to 90   Patient numbers reserved for site 3
           etc.
Method B: 101 to 130 Patient numbers reserved for site 1
           201 to 230 Patient numbers reserved for site 2
           301 to 330 Patient numbers reserved for site 3
           etc.

In method B, the specific site may be more easily identified than in method A as soon as the patient number is referenced. Another approach used is to assign codes to each site, such as letters, as in method C below:

Method C: A1 to A30   Patient numbers reserved for site 1
           B1 to B30   Patient numbers reserved for site 2
           C1 to C30   Patient numbers reserved for site 3
           etc.

Method B is the most preferable of these three possibilities from the standpoint of data analysis and ease of communication.

It is desirable to be able to easily associate the name of each specific study site with a range of patient numbers assigned to that site regardless of the method that is used to assign patient numbers. Examples of common schemes used to assign specific patient numbers to specific sites for ease of recall include numbering the sites in order by listing the investigators' last names alphabetically or by listing the cities (or hospital names) of the investigators alphabetically. For instance, if a study is being conducted by three investigators (Drs. Brown, Jones, and Smith) it would be reasonable to assign patients numbers 100 to 199 to Dr. Brown, 200 to 299 to Dr. Jones, and 300 to 399 to Dr. Smith.

If the study is to be conducted at only one site, then it may be useful to number patients on the basis of the criteria used (if any) to assign them to groups. For example, patients may be assigned to two (or more) groups based on a characteristic of their disease, such as its severity, or based on a characteristic used to stratify patients, such as age, race, or weight. Numbers could be assigned based on patient characteristics using either method B or C above. Furthermore, both site and patient or disease characteristics may be combined in assigning numbers. One example, shown below, used the first number to identify the site, the second for the disease intensity (1, mild; 2, moderate; 3, severe), and the last two for patient numbering. Many variations on these few examples are possible.

Method D: 1,101 to 1,160 Patient numbers at site 1 with a mild intensity of disease.

1,201 to 1,260 Patient numbers at site 1 with a moderate intensity of disease.

1,301 to 1,360 Patient numbers at site 1 with a severe intensity of disease.

2,101 to 2,160 Patient numbers at site 2 with a mild intensity of disease.

2,201 to 2,260 Patient numbers at site 2 with a moderate intensity of disease.

2,301 to 2,360 Patient numbers at site 2 with a severe intensity of disease.

etc.

21

Preparing the Introduction

In writing an introduction to a protocol, it is the author's view that the purpose or intent of the protocol should be described as specifically as possible. Although the length of the introduction may vary from a single paragraph to many pages, it should be sufficient to meet its objectives. Some of the possible goals for the introduction are to:

1. Present preclinical and clinical data on a new drug that is being evaluated with the present protocol.
2. Present the background of a hypothesis that is being tested with the present protocol.
3. Present the background for a new methodology that is being evaluated or is being used to test a new drug with the present protocol.

Specifically, one must present what is considered to be adequate information on the safety, efficacy, and any other relevant aspects of the study drug(s). Various points to consider for inclusion in an introduction are listed in Table 21.36.

TABLE 21.36. *Information that may be included in a protocol's introduction*[a]

1. Synopsis of the disease to be studied
2. Background of standard drugs or other current therapy used to treat the disease
3. Limitations of currently available drugs and/or other treatments
4. Background of the drug(s) being studied in the present protocol:
Chemistry
Pharmacology
Toxicology
Pharmacokinetics
Clinical safety
Clinical efficacy
5. Rationale for the present study
6. Other information

[a]Include published (or unpublished) references that support the material presented.

22

Standardized Information Across Protocols (Polishing the Boilerplate)

Introduction • Protocol Format • Protocol Content
• Administrative Elements

INTRODUCTION

The term "boilerplate" refers to sections of information that are similar from protocol to protocol. Standardizing the format and content of these sections can save time for individuals who prepare numerous protocols. The term "standardization" does not mean that these parts of the protocol are identical in various protocols but that their format is often similar, and the material in the section can usually be easily modified to fit the specific nature of a new protocol. The various sections of the protocol that may be standardized are listed in Table 22.37.

PROTOCOL FORMAT

Title Page

There are many variations in the information presented on a title page. Table 22.38 presents a list of information that is usually present and also information that is sometimes present. Sponsors of clinical studies have usually established a preset format for the title page.

Table of Contents

This is an optional feature of a protocol, but it is often helpful, especially in longer protocols with distinct sections. A sample listing of possible items to include is shown in Fig. 22.10.

List of Abbreviations

If numerous abbreviations are used in the protocol, then it is useful to provide a listing. As a general rule, abbreviations should be limited to a relatively small number of commonly accepted ones.

References and Appendices

The need for references and appendices varies widely from study to study. Their usefulness in a protocol is dependent in part on the personal style of the individual

TABLE 22.37. *Protocol format, contents, and administrative elements that may be relatively standardized*

A. Protocol format
   1. Title page
   2. Table of contents
   3. List of abbreviations
   4. References and appendices
B. Protocol content
   1. Patient enrollment and duration of the study
   2. Location of study site
   3. Factors to control within or outside the study environment
   4. Shipping of drugs to and from the study site
   5. Obtaining, handling, and shipping biological samples
   6. Defining the time of patient entry and completion
   7. Eliciting and categorizing adverse reactions
   8. Missed appointments
   9. Patients lost to follow-up
   10. Patient discontinuation
   11. Early study discontinuation
   12. Medical emergencies
C. Administrative elements
   1. Administrative responsibilities of the investigator
   2. Informed consent
   3. Institutional approval
   4. Confidentiality of data
   5. Collection and processing of data
   6. Publishing of data
   7. Monitoring of the study
   8. Protocol amendments

TABLE 22.38. *Information listed on the title page of a protocol*

A. Usually present
   1. Title of study
   2. Name and address of investigator(s)
   3. Name and address of sponsor (if any)
B. Sometimes present
   1. Office and home telephone numbers of investigators
   2. Names of monitors
   3. Addresses and telephone numbers of monitors
   4. Date of issue of protocol
   5. Signatures of investigators plus date of signing
   6. Signatures and titles of individuals that have approved the protocol plus date of signing
   7. Signatures of monitors plus date of signing
   8. Specific information related to the study drug, such as IND number, NDA number, specific project or sponsor code numbers
   9. FDA Phase (I, II, III, IV) of the clinical study
   10. Person to contact in case of a medical emergency
   11. Statement of confidentiality
   12. Anticipated starting and completion dates for the study
   13. Other information

writing the protocol as well as on the requirements of the sponsoring institution for sponsored studies. There are few rules that can be used to evaluate the need for appendices, since styles and "accepted practice" differ so radically in this regard. Some individuals attempt to place all material suitable for an appendix into the data collection forms, whereas others prefer to include all tabular information and "fine" details of a protocol into an appendix. Table 22.39 lists numerous items that may be placed into appendices.

Material such as tables of male and female weights and/or other data needed to conduct the study should be readily available to study personnel conducting the study. These data may be placed either in the protocol or data collection forms and should not merely be referenced. Additional details of tests or procedures can be placed in appendices.

PROTOCOL CONTENT

Patient Enrollment and Duration of the Study

Some protocols explicitly state the expected or desired rate of patient enrollment. Protocols may also include an anticipated starting and/or completion date. These points depend on many factors and often have to be modified both prior to a study and during its conduct. It is the author's opinion that indicating these projected time points serves little purpose in a protocol. Realistic dates and rate of patient enrollment can be best determined through discussion and close collaboration of all people involved in the initiation and conduct of a study.

Location of Study Site

Although most studies are conducted at a hospital, laboratory, clinic, or professional office, studies may also be conducted at the patient's home (e.g., to evaluate intermittent positive-pressure breathing apparatus in patients with chronic obstructive lung disease), workplace, or other sites. More than one physical location may also be used to conduct a "one-site" study (e.g., an investigator with three offices). If so, it may be relevant to indicate which parts of the study are to be performed at each location or whether each location will serve as a "complete site."

Factors to Control Within or Outside the Study Environment

There are a number of factors relating to the study environment that should be controlled if that is considered to be appropriate for the study (Table 22.40). Some of these factors relate to behavioral aspects of the patients, whereas others relate more to the patient's environment. The quality and/or quantity of these factors may be controlled. The potential for caffeine-containing drinks, alcohol, or tobacco to affect the results of the study should be considered. An attempt to control these

Sample Table of Contents

FIG. 22.10. Sample table of contents, indicating topics that may be included.

TABLE 22.39. *Information that may be included in the protocol's appendix[a]*

A. The patient
   1. Sample copy of the informed consent
   2. Sample copy of the pregnancy waiver form
   3. Operational definitions to be used (e.g., for describing a patient's disease)
   4. Classifications to be used (e.g., diagnostic classifications)
   5. Instruction form to be given to or read to the patient
B. Study and other drugs
   1. Names and dosages of standard drugs (e.g., drugs that are acceptable for use by patients)
   2. Names of drugs chemically related to the study drug. Patients allergic to one of these drugs are often excluded from the study to avoid a hypersensitivity reaction.
   3. Additional chemical, pharmacological, clinical, or other information
   4. Package insert(s), either actual (for marketed drugs) or tentative based on current information (for investigational drugs)
   5. Details of drug preparation, packaging, and labeling
   6. Management of overdosage
C. Conduct of the study and tests used
   1. Types and details of equipment to be used in various tests
   2. Information about clinical, physiological, or pharmacological parameters (e.g., height and weight charts)
   3. Lists of specific laboratory parameters to be measured and other information related to these parameters (normal values)
   4. Details of efficacy parameters to be measured
   5. Details of how certain tests of efficacy and/or safety information will be performed
   6. Rating scales used for efficacy or safety parameters
   7. Description of how information on adverse reactions will be obtained
   8. Operational definitions of adverse reaction intensities and a description of how adverse reactions are to be related to study drugs
   9. How to collect, store, and handle biological samples containing study and/or other drugs
  10. Description of assay procedures
  11. Samples of patient diaries, self-completion forms, or related material
  12. Other instructions for the investigator and/or research coordinator (e.g., procedures manual)
D. Data handling and statistics
   1. Randomization code for open-label or single-blind studies
   2. Details of how certain calculations will be performed during the study
   3. Details of statistical tests to be used to analyze the data
   4. Tables of random numbers or other mathematical information to be used in the study
   5. Latin-square designs to be used for open-label or single-blind studies
   6. Sample data collection forms—either selected forms or the entire data collection form
E. Management and administration of the study
   1. Glossary of terms
   2. Contractural agreement between investigator and sponsor
   3. Government regulations—printed as excerpts, in their entirety, or paraphrased
   4. Sample release form to obtain, and potentially use, photographs of the patient
   5. Any forms required by the sponsor IRB, or institution[b]
   6. Other responsibilities of the investigator

[a]Many materials could be placed into more than one category. The five major categories listed were chosen to simplify the organization of this table.
[b]See Fig. 33.18.

TABLE 22.40. *Selected factors within or outside the study environment that may be controlled by protocol*

1. Activity: type and amount[a]
2. Exercise: type and amount
3. Diet and availability of food and snacks between meals
4. Nutritional status
5. Fasting
6. Fluid intake
7. Conversation
8. Visual stimuli
9. Auditory stimuli
10. Tactile stimuli
11. Stress (may be controlled to some degree through the inclusion criteria)
12. Contact with other patients and number of patients per room
13. The size, design, and contents of the room in which the study is to be conducted and/or in which inpatients are housed
14. Number and nature[b] of personnel conducting the study
15. Type and amount of tobacco, caffeine or other xanthine (e.g., chocolate), and/or alcohol use or consumption

[a]For example, how long are inpatients allowed to remain in bed.
[b]For example, age, sex, experience, formal training, personality, other commitments, and other factors may be relevant.

factors may be made during the conduct of the study in addition to the time of patient enrollment (i.e., limiting the inclusion criteria to patients with acceptable personal habits).

Shipping of Drugs to and from the Study Site

Procedures on shipping drug supplies to and returning them from the study site are not usually described in detail in a protocol. There are occasions, however, when a description of this activity is useful (e.g., for drugs that must be shipped in a frozen state). The address to which returned drugs should be sent after completion of the study is often listed in the protocol. General information on the documents that must accompany the shipment may also be included in the protocol. Other aspects of drug shipments are included in the following section, which deals with the shipping of biological samples.

Obtaining, Handling, and Shipping Biological Samples

Various fluids or tissues (e.g., saliva, feces, cerebrospinal fluid, biopsy material) may be collected in clinical studies for later analysis of drug levels or assessment of drug effects. Instructions for collecting, processing, storing, and handling such samples may be explicitly described. These could include information on the (1) specific materials used to collect samples, (2) procedures and specific equipment used to process the samples (including model numbers or design characteristics of equipment if relevant), and (3) previous training of the individuals who will collect, handle, examine, or otherwise deal with the biological materials.

In some studies, a central laboratory will be used to analyze samples. Information on the packaging and shipping of samples may be listed (see Table 22.41) whenever biological samples are to be sent from the site of collection to another location.

Defining the Time of Patient Entry and Completion

It may be relevant to define the precise point at which a patient is formally entered into a study. Entry occurs at different points in various studies (e.g., at the start or completion of screen or baseline or at the start of treatment). It may be important to clarify this point to enable a clear determination to be made of the precise number of patients entered into a study. In general, formal entrance into a study occurs at the initiation of an active baseline or treatment.

It also is relevant to define the point at which a patient is considered a "complete" patient. This is important from the perspective of data analysis, since data from "complete" and "incomplete" patients are generally analyzed separately. The time at which a patient is defined as complete often occurs at some point prior to the end of the study and may also be used as a criterion for replacing patients who have been prematurely discontinued (i.e., a protocol may state that patients who are discontinued prior to a given week will be replaced).

Eliciting and Categorizing Adverse Reactions

Adverse reactions were defined in terminology in the frontmatter as the physical and psychological signs and symptoms of the patient that may or may not be related

TABLE 22.41. *Information on shipping biological samples*

Item	Details and/or example
1. Package description	Use styrofoam containers (_____ × _____ × _____ cm) with minimum wall thickness of _____cm
2. Packing materials	Fill to _____% of volume and add _____kg (pounds) of dry ice. Do not put filler material between samples and dry ice
3. Labeling of package	"Plasma (or other) samples, perishable, rush. Send to: _____."
4. Contact with center (person) receiving the samples	Notify site and contact _____(person) 1 week (day) prior to shipping at telephone number _____.[a] Also contact this person just after the package is sent
5. Shipping samples	Use _____carrier only,[b] and request their _____ service. Send sample either collect or prepaid
6. Date of shipping	Send the package only on a Monday, Tuesday, or Wednesday and no less than 3 days before a holiday
7. Confirmation of receipt	Determine how to confirm arrival and who will trace package if it does not arrive on time

[a]Inform this individual of the carrier used, the bill of lading number, and the time of day to expect arrival.
[b]Both the type of carrier (air, truck, boat) and the specific company may be specified.

to the study drug. Adverse reactions are either predictable or unpredictable, based on the known properties of the drug. Operational definitions of each anticipated adverse reaction or at least of those most frequently expected in a study may be established prior to the study. This would clarify the differences in definitions for adverse reactions that are similar in nature (sleepy, drowsy, fatigue) but that may be used differently by different investigators in a multicenter study (or even in a study conducted at one site). Adverse experiences are defined as the group of adverse reactions plus all other medical events that occur during the study, such as illness or trauma, even though these latter events are generally believed to be unrelated to the study drug(s). Laboratory abnormalities are generally considered to lie within the definition given of adverse reactions but are sometimes treated as an independent class of abnormalities.

A basic question to address in discussing the recording of adverse reactions experienced by the patient is whether to probe for their presence or whether to record only those that are spontaneously reported. Spontaneously reported adverse reactions are of two basic types. In one type, patients are not given any instructions about reporting adverse reactions, and in the other type, patients are instructed to report any and all adverse reactions. Collecting only spontaneous reports has the disadvantage of probably underestimating the true incidence of adverse reactions, since many patients are reluctant to volunteer this information. Moreover, since patients differ in their willingness to volunteer information, collecting adverse reactions in this manner introduces another source of variation into the study. This source of variation may be controlled by standardizing the means of probing for adverse reactions. If adverse reactions are to be probed for, then this probe may take place whenever certain events occur (e.g., dose changes) or at fixed points in the protocol (e.g., once per hour in a single-dose study).

Three approaches to probing for adverse reactions will be described. In the first, the investigator reads a long list of possible adverse reactions, and the patient responds to those that are felt or experienced. This approach has a disadvantage in that it tends to elicit a greater number of adverse reactions than do the two other methods described below, because reading a list is suggestive to the patient and thus may magnify the true incidence of adverse reactions. A second approach is to read an abbreviated list of the most commonly observed adverse reactions that have been associated with the study drug.

It is the author's view that a third, or "neutral," approach to probing the patient about adverse reactions is the one that should most frequently be used. The presence of adverse reactions may be elicited using the same question for all patients, phrased in the same manner and tone at all times. This helps to insure uniformity among patients and treatment periods. One straightforward means of achieving this goal is to formulate a simple question with minimal connotations that can be used as the initial question at all evaluation points in a study. An example of this type of simple question is: "How have you felt since your last clinic visit?"

The question "How do you feel?" is considered too general and a cliché and will rarely elicit as accurate a response as desired in all patients. Patients also tend to be more open about adverse reactions with nursing staff than with physicians unless the patients are carefully questioned or probed. This may in part reflect the patient's desire not to "disappoint" the physician with "bad news" about the drug.

The general question used to probe for adverse reactions should be phrased to avoid direct reference to the study drug. This is because patients often attribute adverse reactions to non-drug-related events and may not associate their adverse reaction with a drug. Thus, they may be reluctant to volunteer important information about signs and symptoms in responding to a question that directly relates to a drug, such as "Have you had any problems caused by the drug?" The period of time that is relevant for the physician to include in his questioning should be described in the protocol or data collection forms (i.e., is the probe intended to elicit those adverse reactions that are presently experienced or felt within the last *x* days or weeks or since the last probe).

Adverse reactions that have previously been reported by the patient should be probed each time a formal probe is conducted. This will allow their duration, intensity, and other characteristics to be followed in time. The degree to which this "reprobe" should be formalized must be determined by the individuals writing the protocol.

Intensity of the Adverse Reaction

If a positive response is elicited to the introductory question, the investigator should probe further to determine (1) the intensity of the symptom, (2) the time of onset, (3) its total duration, (4) whether the adverse reaction is still present, and (5) the frequency of its occurrence. The relationship of the adverse reaction to the study drug or study schedule should be probed (e.g., a headache may be caused by fasting that is part of the study schedule).

The intensity of the adverse reaction should be characterized and then classified into clearly defined categories. One system uses the terms mild, moderate, and severe for describing the intensity of the adverse reaction. The definitions of these terms and the relationship to study drug may be described as follows:

1. Mild. The adverse reaction does not interfere in a significant manner with the patient's normal functioning level. It may be an annoyance.
2. Moderate. The adverse reaction produces some impairment of functioning but is not hazardous to health. It is uncomfortable and/or an embarrassment.
3. Severe. The adverse reaction produces significant impairment of functioning or incapacitation and is a definite hazard to the patient's health. This category includes adverse reactions that include or lead to (1) death or decreased life expectancy, (2) a life-threatening event, though acute and without permanent effect, (3) prolonged inability to resume usual life pattern, or (4) impairment of ability to adequately deal with future medical problems.

These three categories (mild, moderate, severe) are based on the investigator's clinical judgment, which in turn depends on consideration of various factors such us the patient's report, the physician's observations, and the physician's prior experience.

A different system for assessing the severity of adverse reactions was proposed by Tallarida et al. (1979). They used seven categories for their assessments instead of the three described above.

Relationship of an Adverse Reaction to Study Drug

In evaluating whether an adverse reaction is related to a specific test drug, one should consider the following points:

1. Previous experience with the drug and whether the adverse reaction is known to have occurred with the drug.
2. Alternative explanations for the adverse reaction, such as the presence of other drugs, illness, new illness, nondrug therapies, diagnostic tests, procedures, or other confounding effects.
3. Timing of the events between administration of the drug and the adverse reaction.
4. Drug levels and evidence, if any, of overdosage.
5. Dechallenge, i.e., if the drug dose was decreased or the drug was stopped, what happened to the adverse reaction?
6. Rechallenge, i.e., what happened if the drug was restarted after the adverse reaction had disappeared?

This information may be used to characterize the relationship of drug and adverse reaction into one of any number of predetermined categories. Between three and five categories are usually used to describe the attribution of a drug with an adverse reaction. An example of a three-category system is: (1) probably related, (2) probably not related, or (3) unknown.

This last category may be used when there are insufficient data available to make a judgment about the first two categories. It may also be used when there is equally strong evidence pointing towards both of the other two possibilities.

Definitions are given below for a five-category system that may be used to classify the relationship between adverse reactions and drug.

These are adapted from Karch and Lasagna (1975).

1. Definite. A reaction that follows a reasonable temporal sequence from administration of the drug or in which the drug level has been established in body fluids or tissues; that follows a known or expected response pattern to the suspected drug; and that is confirmed by improvement on stopping or reducing the dosage of the drug, and reappearance of the reaction on repeated exposure (rechallenge).
2. Probable. A reaction that follows a reasonable temporal sequence from administration of the drug; that follows a known or expected response pattern to the suspected drug; that is confirmed by stopping or reducing the dosage of

the drug; and that could not be reasonably explained by the known characteristics of the patient's clinical state.

3. Possible. A reaction that follows a reasonable temporal sequence from administration of the drug; that follows a known or expected response pattern to
   the suspected drug; but that could readily have been produced by a number
   of other factors.
4. Unknown. Relationships for which no evaluation can be made.
5. Not related. A reaction for which sufficient information exists to indicate that
   the etiology is unrelated to the study drug.

The three-category system is preferable in the author's view for Phase I and
early Phase II studies, since it is usually unethical to rechallenge a patient with a
drug that has caused a suspected effect, especially if the effect was severe in
intensity. Also, little information is available about a new drug at this stage of
development, and it is therefore difficult to know if the adverse reaction is typical
of the drug or has been previously observed. Although the three-point scale could
theoretically be used in all phases of drug development, the five-point scale provides
a more complete description of adverse reactions that occur in studies conducted
in late Phase II through Phase IV. There may be practical reasons, however, to
utilize the same system throughout all phases of a drug's development.

It is common for the nature, frequency, and/or intensity of adverse reactions to
change significantly when the personnel reporting and evaluating them also changes.
Blanc et al. (1979) have shown that trained investigators often disagree with each
other on the relationship between a drug and an adverse reaction. This factor may
have a significant effect on the outcome of the study and supports the view that it
is preferable to have a single investigator collect adverse reaction information on a
single patient (and preferably on all patients) throughout a single study.

After the information described above on adverse reactions is collected, the
investigator must determine the treatment (if any) that will be initiated. The action
taken by the investigator is generally one of those shown below.

Actions Taken by Investigators After Observing Adverse Reactions

Seven common steps (or lack of steps) are taken in response to adverse reactions:

1. None.
2. Increased surveillance of the patient to monitor the adverse reaction.
3. Counteractive medication or treatment.
4. Changing the dose of drug in question.
5. Both 3 and 4.
6. Drug administration is suspended.
7. Drug administration is discontinued.
8. Other.

The possible approaches listed above relate to how the investigator treats the
patient. The investigator must also notify his Institutional Review Board (IRB) and

either the Food and Drug Administration (FDA) (for unsponsored studies) or the sponsor if serious adverse reactions are observed. Sponsors then have the responsibility of notifying the FDA and of deciding whether the adverse reaction will have any influence on the conduct of the study. There are several alternatives for sponsors (or investigators) to consider in this regard. These are listed in Table 22.42.

A more sophisticated approach to the evaluation of adverse reactions has been proposed by one group of authors in three joint publications (Kramer et al., 1979; Hutchinson et al., 1979; Leventhal et al., 1979). The algorithms they propose are an attempt to relate more accurately the adverse reaction with the drug as definite, probable, possible, or unlikely. It is the author's view that this approach, although elegant, is not practical in most clinical studies. Another scale, based on 10 questions, was proposed by Naranjo et al. (1981) primarily for postmarketing surveillance and Phase III clinical studies. Their questions require a large body of information to be available about the study drug and thus are not particularly useful for Phase I and II studies.

Two new forms have been prepared to record "adverse health events." They are called Systematic Assessment for Treatment Emergent Events (SAFTEE) Form-GI (General Inquiry) and Form-SI (Systematic Inquiry). These forms are available from Jerome Levine, M.D. or Nina Schooler, Ph.D. at the address given below Table 26.54. The following major items of information are solicited on each adverse event reported:

1. Date of onset (month and day are used if the event first occurred in the interval evaluated; if the event occurred prior to the interval evaluated, "00/00" is used).

TABLE 22.42. *Alternative actions (relating to a study) for severe adverse reactions[a]*

---

1. No further action is required
2. Notify the FDA
3. Notify the IRB (a sponsor may confirm with the investigator that this task has been performed)
4. Advise other investigators in a multicenter study
5. Advise other investigators working with the drug but using other protocols
6. Revise the informed consent at all sites using the involved protocol or at all sites studying the drug
7. Modify the involved protocol and submit it to the sponsor and IRBs for approval
8. Modify all protocols using the drug and submit them to the sponsor and IRBs for approval
9. Initiate another study or studies to evaluate the questions raised
10. Suspend the study at the site(s) using the involved protocol or at all sites studying the drug
11. Discontinue the study at the site(s) using the involved protocol or at all sites studying the drug
12. Consult an expert or convene a panel of experts to discuss the problem and/or issues raised
13. Suspend further development of the drug
14. Discontinue further development of the drug

---

[a]Alternative actions to consider in treating the patient are discussed in the text.

2. Duration (recorded in days within the current assessment period).
3. Pattern (continuous, intermittent, or isolated).
4. Current status (ongoing problem or resolved, with or without sequelae).
5. Severity (five grades of intensity are used; this factor is assessed by the investigator through observation and/or the patient's report).
6. Functional impairment (five grades of impairment are used for describing the activities of daily living or of specific activities affected. This factor is assessed by the investigator through observation and/or the patient's report).
7. Contributory factors (one or more possible causes may be checked; seven possible causes plus "other" are listed).
8. Relationship of drug to event (this category differs substantially from usual definitions; it is used to give the reason(s) why the investigator believes that the adverse reaction may be drug related even if caused by a concomitant drug: six categories plus "other [specify]" and "not applicable" are listed).
9. Action taken (seven possible actions plus "other [specify]" and "don't know" are listed).
10. Comments, descriptors, and additional specification (allows for text to be written into the form).

It is not possible to state at this time whether the SAFTEE forms will be widely used in clinical studies and replace previous measures of adverse reactions developed by the government: Dosage Record and Treatment Emergent Symptoms (DOTES), Treatment Emergent Symptom Scale (TESS), and Self-Rating Treatment Emergent Symptom Scale (STESS). It is the author's view that the SAFTEE forms appear to be preferable to the older scales described.

Missed Appointments

When a patient does not keep a scheduled appointment, the missed tests may be either deleted and not made up or rescheduled, either as soon as possible or at a later and more convenient date. It is also possible to discontinue the patient from the study or to contact the monitor to discuss possible options. It is best to indicate the accepted procedure(s) in the protocol as well as the procedure to reintegrate the patient into the protocol schedule (i.e., when the tests scheduled at a patient's missed appointment are to be omitted as opposed to being rescheduled).

To minimize the occurrences of missed appointments, one may follow any or all of the following procedures: (1) give printed cards to patients with the date of their next visit when they complete one clinic visit, (2) contact the patient by telephone (or, less desirably, by letter) shortly (1 or 2 days) prior to the scheduled visit, and (3) provide transportation to the study site on the day of the appointment. In addition to these techniques, many of those described as methods to improve patient compliance may also have a role in decreasing the incidence of missed appointments.

Patients Lost to Follow-up

In long-term studies in which patients are being followed for a significant period, it is important to establish a system to maintain information on where patients live. This may require making periodic telephone calls or writing letters to patients. The question of how assiduously to search for patients who appear to be lost to follow-up must be addressed, as well as how to treat incomplete patient data. Large registries of mortality information and other sources may be utilized to search for missing patients if the need is present and resources are available. Tables 22.43 and 22.44 indicate a number of public and private agencies and businesses that may be contacted for information in addition to potential personal sources of information known to the patient, whose identity may be established by the investigator at the start of a clinical study (relatives, friends, employers). Additional information (social security number, driver's license number) that may be useful if a search has to be undertaken may also be requested. Middle-class patients are generally easier to locate than lower-class patients. Drug addicts are extremely difficult to locate.

TABLE 22.43. *Agencies and organizations that provide information[a] on patients lost to follow-up*

1. State Department of Motor Vehicles
2. State vital records offices
3. Social Security Administration
4. Veterans Administration
5. Internal Revenue Service
6. National Academy of Sciences and the Medical Follow-up Agency
7. National Research Council
8. Equifax Services (McLean, VA)
9. Westat (Rockville, MD)

[a]The information provided either relates to the patient's present location or to medical data such as vital statistics. Some of these agencies will not supply information to the public.

TABLE 22.44. *General sources for obtaining information on patients lost to follow-up*

1. Employers	12. Public utility records
2. Relatives	13. Religious affiliations
3. Friends and acquaintances	14. Tax records
4. Landlords	15. Voter registration
5. Former neighbors	16. Birth and death records
6. Schools	17. Credit transactions
7. Union office	18. Insurance applications
8. Associations or clubs	19. Mortgages
9. Medical groups (e.g., Health Maintenance Organizations)	20. Post office change of address forms
10. Criminal and traffic records	21. Private detectives
11. Occupation licensing records	

Patient Discontinuation

The reasons why patients are discontinued from clinical studies include (1) noncompliance in taking the study drug, (2) failure to adhere to the protocol, (3) failure to return for a specific number of clinic visits, (4) severe adverse reactions, and (5) abnormalities on physical, neurological, laboratory, or other examinations judged clinically significant. Patients may request to be discontinued from a study at any time without stating any reason, and this must be indicated in the informed consent. These and other reasons for discontinuing patients are listed in Table 22.45. If a patient is unable to take the study drug for valid reasons (e.g., unrelated medical problems), the length of time that a patient may discontinue taking the study drug and still remain in the study should be indicated. Special precautions relating to sudden withdrawal of medication must be provided in the protocol.

In addition to describing reasons (i.e., criteria) for patient discontinuation in the protocol, the basis for replacement of discontinued patients should be discussed. One may intend to replace all or none of the patients who do not complete a study or only those patients who do not complete the study for specific reasons (e.g., for reasons unrelated to the study). These and other options are listed in Table 22.46. Some investigators, scientists, and statisticians believe that noncompliant individuals should not be discontinued from a study, since the reason(s) for their noncompliance may relate to difficulties with the drug. These reasons might include (1) difficulty in swallowing a large capsule, (2) requiring a large number of pills to be ingested, or (3) the study drug having a bad odor.

A specific list of all tests and procedures to be conducted at the time of patient discontinuation is usually determined prior to initiation of the study and included

TABLE 22.45. *Possible reasons for patient discontinuation*[a]

---
1. Adverse reactions, either severe in intensity or including specific reactions that, according to protocol, require discontinuation
2. Abnormal laboratory values, either severely abnormal or including specific abnormalities that, according to protocol, require discontinuation
3. Lack of efficacy of the treatment
4. Improvement, resolution, or severe deterioration of disease being studied
5. Deterioration of patient's medical condition unrelated to disease being studied
6. Patient moved from area
7. Failure of patient to return for an appointment or for a specified number of appointments
8. Failure of patient to continue to meet criteria for continuation in protocol
9. Failure of patient to maintain an established standard of compliance
10. Decreased patient cooperation
11. Use by patient of a nonapproved drug or treatment
12. Pregnancy (observation and follow-up procedures must be initiated)
13. Any combination of the above
14. Withdrawal of patient's informed consent
15. Death

---

[a]The tests that should be performed in patients at the time of discontinuation (or as shortly thereafter as possible) should be detailed in the protocol.

TABLE 22.46. *Options concerning replacement of patients who discontinue treatment*

1. Do not replace any patients who discontinue treatment with the study drug
2. Replace all patients who do not complete the entire study
3. Replace all patients who do not complete at least a defined portion of the study (e.g., day *x* or part A)
4. Replace all patients who discontinue treatment for prespecified reasons (e.g., protocol violations)
5. Replace all patients who discontinue treatment until a defined minimum number of completed patients is reached
6. Replace patients who discontinue treatment at the investigator's and/or monitor's discretion

in the protocol. Before patients are discontinued because of abnormal laboratory values, it is usually important to repeat the test to confirm the presence and magnitude of the abnormality. If relevant, biological samples (e.g., blood, urine) may be divided and sent to two different laboratories to confirm the abnormal results as well as to evaluate the reliability of the original laboratory. In monitoring the progress of the abnormal laboratory value and its return to normal, it may be useful to continue sending divided samples to two separate laboratories.

Early Study Discontinuation

There are a number of situations based on ethics, accepted clinical practice, and statistics in which discontinuation of a study must be considered. It may be appropriate to consider and indicate at least some of these reasons in the text of a protocol (obviously, not all of the possible reasons could be envisioned or described). A study may be stopped early for either positive or negative reasons.

Negative reasons for discontinuing the study include (1) observation of serious adverse reactions or other abnormalities (in laboratory examinations or vital signs) that increase the risks to an unacceptable level for at least some of the patients to continue the study, (2) failure to enroll an adequate number of patients, (3) failure of the investigator and/or staff to maintain adequate clinical standards, (4) failure of the investigator and/or staff or patients to comply with the protocol, (5) termination of the study drug's development by the sponsor, (6) unacceptable changes in personnel or facilities at the investigator's site, and (7) determination that no statistically significant result can be obtained.

There are a number of positive reasons for discontinuing a study early. The major reason is that a beneficial effect of treatment is observed that raises unacceptable ethical concerns for patients who are not receiving this treatment. If early termination for ethical reasons is considered possible at the outset of a clinical study, then criteria should be established to define conditions under which the study would be discontinued. If the study is to be terminated early according to the criteria established, one must consider whether the data will be adequate to convince virtually all or at least the overwhelming majority of statisticians and clinicians of the conclusions. Criteria should be developed that will be impeccable from both a statistical and a clinical viewpoint. If either is not fully achieved, then the value of the study may be mitigated, and its potential to influence the treatment of future patients lost or at least compromised. If one is to err in choosing whether or not to stop a study, then to complete the study is preferable. Another way of expressing this concept is that if there is doubt about terminating the study, it should continue. An example of a study that was discontinued early for appropriate and proper reasons is the collaborative β-blocker heart attack trial study (β-Blocker Heart Attack Study Group, 1981).

The decision to stop a study should not be made solely by those concerned with its conduct. Impartial experts, such as a panel of outside consultants, may also be involved in the decision. There is a basic difference insofar as early termination is concerned between studies evaluating problems with severe clinical consequences (i.e., seeking to reduce mortality of a life-threatening disease) and those studies seeking to reduce relatively minor clinical problems (e.g., topical itching). Presumably, everyone would agree that the former types of study should be intimately concerned with the question of early termination prior to study initiation, whereas the latter type of study can deemphasize the question (unless unusual drug toxicity has been previously observed or is anticipated). The question of how much attention to give to early study discontinuation arises in the "gray area" between these two extremes.

Physicians involved in either a sponsored or unsponsored double-blind controlled study do not generally participate in the discussions about its early discontinuation. They must remain blind to patient randomization and should not be made aware of results of interim analyses. If they are cognizant of one treatment being markedly and significantly better than another, it may be ethically difficult for them to continue treating seriously ill patients with a less effective drug (or placebo).

In conclusion, every clinical study may be stopped early for negative reasons, but only some studies are liable to be stopped early for positive reasons. Those latter studies should be identified in advance, and criteria established under which the study will be terminated. Special considerations relating to the procedures for prematurely terminating a study are discussed in Section III of this book and in a publication by Klimt and Canner (1979).

Medical Emergencies

If treatments for study drug overdosage are known or are being developed, they may be outlined or discussed in an appendix to the protocol. For double-blind studies in which patients may be receiving placebo or one of multiple drugs, a rapid means of breaking the blind must be devised. This may take the form of sealed information kept in the investigator's possession or coded labels that are placed in the data collection forms (e.g., as tear-off portions of the label attached to the drug dispensed). Other forms of breaking the blind are possible, including direct contact with the monitor for sponsored studies. Day and nighttime telephone numbers of monitors should be given to investigators. Patients participating in drug studies may be given a wallet card with relevant drug and study information plus day and nighttime telephone numbers of the investigator(s) that can be used in case of emergencies.

The presence of standard resuscitation equipment (e.g., "crash cart") to be located at the study site may be specified, as well as details of any other emergency equipment deemed important. The presence of adequately trained staff to deal effectively with medical emergencies must be ascertained at prestudy site visits. This includes consideration of adequately trained staff coverage at all hours that inpatients are present at the study site and the distance and time to a hospital if the study will take place at a different type of facility.

ADMINISTRATIVE ELEMENTS

Administrative Responsibilities of the Investigator

The administrative responsibilities of an investigator for a clinical study vary enormously between studies. A number of aspects of this function, however, are common to all studies. These and other aspects must be discussed prior to the study by the investigator and sponsor (if any) or by the investigator and his/her colleagues who will assist with these responsibilities. Many of the responsibilities are listed in Table 22.47. One of these responsibilities includes the preparation of a final study report for the IRB and sponsor (if any). There may be various rules of the institutions involved regarding the format and/or content of this report. Information that is generally included in this report is listed in Table 22.48.

Informed Consent

Each investigator in the United States should be familiar with the Federal guidelines relating to the obligations of obtaining a patient's informed consent

TABLE 22.47. *Administrative responsibilities of investigators*

---

1. Appropriate interactions with the IRB (Ethics Committee) and other groups that must approve the protocol
2. Careful record keeping on the patient's medical chart and data collection forms
3. Maintenance of "good clinical practices" according to institutional, Federal, and other regulatory guidelines
4. Periodic reporting to the IRB (and sponsor, if any) of the status of the study
5. Adherence to the protocol
6. Reporting of all serious adverse reactions or other events to the IRB, sponsor (if any), and FDA if no sponsor is involved
7. Preparation of a final study report for the IRB and sponsor
8. Retention of either original or copied data collection forms according to Federal regulations[a]
9. Keeping all data related to the study accessible to the monitors

---

[a]For investigational drugs, this period is 2 years past the approval of a New Drug Application (NDA) or discontinuation of the investigational drug.

TABLE 22.48. *Information to include in the investigator's final study report*[a]

---

1. Overall opinion and summary of experiences with the study drug, especially in terms of relevant safety and efficacy parameters, plus a comparison with standard drugs
2. Interpretation of laboratory test values outside the normal range
3. Description of any protocol deviations and the reasons for them
4. Discussion of specific experiences with each patient
5. Conclusions
6. Optional items to include in this report:
   a. Introduction and rationale of the study
   b. Time and events schedule
   c. Dosage regimen
   d. Demographics of the patients
   e. Incidence of adverse reactions
   f. Plasma or other drug levels
   g. Any other data or comments that are considered relevant

---

[a]Usually sent to the IRB and sponsor (for sponsored studies) within _____ (e.g., 3 months) of study termination. Some sponsors request the investigator's final study report to be written before the study's blind is broken.

(Food and Drug Administration, 1981*a*) and the procedures under which this obligation is conducted. A summary of the points included in the Federal regulations is presented in Table 22.49. Investigators in other countries must familiarize themselves with the relevant laws of their locale. The protocol may state that the purpose of the study will be explained to the patient in the presence of a witness (plus the parent or legal guardian for pediatric studies) and an informed consent obtained. Although a witness is only required (in the United States) if the informed consent is obtained orally or in a summary written form, including a witness in the informed consent procedure is generally prudent. The elements necessary to include in an informed consent are listed in Table 22.49, and a sample (generic) informed consent is shown in Fig. 22.11 A sample form used to obtain a pregnancy waiver from women of child-bearing potential is illustrated in Fig. 22.12.

In addition to the various comments and types of information presented in the sample informed consent (Fig. 22.11), there are numerous other aspects of particular studies that may be included. Several of the additional comments that may be included in specific Phase I, II, III, or IV studies are listed below, and a few optional comments are included in Fig. 22.11. Informed consents are written in either first, second, or third person (e.g., I understand that blood will be taken . . . , you will have blood taken . . . , blood will be taken . . .). Informed consents may also combine different writing styles (i.e., first-, second-, and/or third-person descriptions) in different parts of the consent form. There is no single universally accepted rule as to which style is preferable. The language used should be readily comprehended by the patients enrolled and avoid sophisticated scientific and legal terms. It may be useful to have the sample informed consent read by lay people to review it for comprehensibility. The group of lay people chosen should have the same educational background as the patient population to be tested.

TABLE 22.49. *Elements of informed consent*

An informed consent must be written by the investigator, approved by the IRB (or Ethics Committee), signed by the subject (patient or volunteer) or authorized representative, and witnessed

The points below must be included in all informed consents:
1. A statement that the study involves research, an explanation of the purpose of the research and the expected duration, a description of the procedures, and identification of any procedures that are experimental
2. A description of any reasonably foreseeable risks or discomforts to the patient
3. A description of the benefits to the patient or to others that may be expected from the research
4. A disclosure of appropriate alternative procedures or courses of treatment, if any, that might be advantageous to the patient
5. A statement describing the extent, if any, to which confidentiality of the records identifying the patient will be maintained and that FDA may inspect the records
6. For research involving more than minimal risk, an explanation as to whether any compensation will be paid, whether any medical treatments are available if injury occurs, and what those treatments are. Information should also be provided on how further information about this study may be obtained
7. An explanation of whom to contact for answers to questions and whom to contact in the event of a research-related injury
8. A statement that participation is voluntary, that refusal to participate will involve no penalty or loss of benefits to which the patient is otherwise entitled, and that the patient may discontinue participation at any time without penalty

Additional elements of informed consent that must be present when appropriate:
1. A statement that the particular treatment or procedure may involve risks to the patient or to the fetus (if the patient is pregnant) that are currently unforeseeable
2. Anticipated circumstances under which the patient's participation may be terminated by the investigator
3. Any additional costs to the patient resulting from participation in the research
4. The consequences and procedures for withdrawing from the research
5. A statement that significant new findings (such as new hazards) developed during the research will be provided to the patient
6. The approximate number of patients in the study

Examples of Statements That May Be Included in Informed Consents

1. An infection or blood clot in the arm could possibly develop from the needle that will remain in your arm on days ____and ____.
2. Your participation in this study will not result in any direct medical benefit to you personally.
3. During this ____week study you will remain in the ____hospital (medical school) for ____consecutive ____(e.g., Friday) nights and will remain there until approximately ____P.M. on ____(the next day), at which time you will be released. You are expected to return at ____(time) every ____and ____.
4. The estimated amount of radiation you will receive during this study from the radioactive drug is ____rads (total body dose). The following scale of radiation doses is provided for comparative purposes.

(text continues on page 177)

Sample sections to include in an informed consent

Full Title of Protocol: _____

Name of Patient: _____

Date of Birth: _____ *Age:* _____ *Sex:* _____

Address: _____

Telephone: _____

1. *Purpose of the Study*

Drug A is an experimental drug developed by _____ Corporation and being evaluated for use in _____ disease. It has been tested extensively in animals to show this effect as well as to demonstrate that it is a safe drug. Initial human studies, conducted in ____normal volunteers, have demonstrated that Drug A is generally safe at the doses that will be tested in this study. At these doses, only mild adverse reactions (side effects) were observed. At ____ times higher doses, a number of other side effects were observed. This study on Drug A will last for ____ (days, weeks, months), and the purpose is to (1) evaluate its effectiveness in _____ disease, (2) evaluate the tolerance of patients to therapeutic doses of Drug A, and (3) study blood levels of the drug. Two previous efficacy studies have demonstrated that Drug A has been effective in _____ disease and was well tolerated.

This study has been approved by the _____ Medical University Institutional Review Board, which is an "Ethics Committee" charged by the U.S. Department of Health and Human Services to insure that the rights of human subjects are protected. The study is under the direction of Dr. _____.

2. *Procedures to be Followed*

In this study you will be examined in these offices at ____ to ____ day (week, months) intervals over a total period of ____ days (weeks, months). During the study you will have 2 to 4 samples of your blood taken for tests on Days ____, ____, ____, and ____, 2 urine tests on the same days, an electrocardiogram (ECG) on Days ____ and ____, physical examinations on Days ____ and ____, ophthalmological (eye) examinations on Days ____ and ____, plus the following tests to measure your _____ disease: ____ (Days...), ____ (Days...) etc.

This study is a double-blind study of ____ patients, lasting ____ weeks (months). The study will compare Drug A with a placebo. This means that you will not know whether the pill that you are given to take during the study will be Drug A or a pill that looks identical to Drug A, but which is inactive. You will have to take this pill ____ times a day (at ____, ____, and ____o'clock) and will not know whether you have received Drug A or the placebo until after the study is completed. The doctor and staff also will not know which of the two drugs you have been given. The identity of the pill can be determined immediately if any medical problem develops and it becomes important to learn which drug you have been given.

You will (will not) continue to take any other drugs you are presently taking to treat _____, but you cannot change the dose of this other drug during this study.

FIG. 22.11. Sample sections to include in an informed consent. See text for additional statements that could be included.

3. *Risks*

Drug A is a new drug and there is limited information available on its effects in humans. This drug has been previously studied in ____ people and the most commonly observed adverse reactions at the doses you may receive were _____, _____, and _____ of _____ intensity. At higher doses, the following adverse reactions of _____intensity were observed: _____, _____, and _____. If these or other adverse reactions occur and become intolerable or severe the dose will be reduced or completely stopped.

There is a remote chance that you will experience an allergic reaction to the drug, such as a skin rash, hives or possibly a more serious problem such as breathing difficulties or shock. It is not possible to predict in advance if any of these problems will develop, but if they do, you will be promptly treated.

Blood will be drawn at each clinic visit (a total of ____ blood drawings will be made over ____ months). The procedure of taking blood may cause local discomfort, bruising, swelling and rarely a local infection.

4. *Benefits*

This drug is being studied as a potential treatment for _____ disease. It is therefore possible that it may improve your conditon. Of course, this cannot be guaranteed or promised and you may not receive the experimental treatment.

Optional: If you do not receive the experimental treatment during this study, then you will have an opportunity to receive this treatment within ____months after this study is completed.

5. *Alternative Treatments*

There are other drugs used to treat _____ disease. These drugs are: _____, _____, and _____. If you wish, Dr. _____ will explain the benefits and risks of receiving treatment with any (or all) of these drugs. In addition to drugs, _____ disease may also be treated by the following non-drug methods: _____, _____, and _____. Dr. _____ will also discuss these treatments with you if you wish. You also have the alternative of not being treated. The possible consequences of this action can also be discussed with you.

6. *Confidentiality of the Records*

Your medical records that are related to this study will be maintained in confidentiality. The sponsor (_____ Co.) may examine your medical records, as long as your name cannot be identified from these records.

Your records from this study may be submitted by _____ Co. to the Food and Drug Administration (FDA), but your name will not be able to be identified from such records. No identity of any specific patient in this study will be disclosed in any public reports or publications. The FDA has the right upon proper judicial order to review pertinent medical records and other data with your name identified. They are required by law, however, to handle this information in a confidential manner.

7. *If Problems Develop*

If any serious problems develop you will receive prompt and appropriate medical attention. It is agreed that the facilities of _____ Hospital will be made available to you. Reasonable medical treatment will be free when provided through the facilities of _____ Hospital. Financial compensation is not available for medical treatment elsewhere, loss of work, or other expenses.

8. *Financial Considerations*

After participating in this study, you will be given $____. If you do not complete the study then you will not receive this money. To help pay for your transportation and meals, you will also be given $____ per clinic visit.

Optional: 1. There will be no financial benefits to you or your family for participating in this study.

2. If you complete at least half of the _____ week (month) study then you will receive one-half the usual amount of money (i.e., you will receive $_____).

3. If you do not complete the study, payment will be prorated, based on the percent of the study that you have completed.

9. *Obtaining Additional Information*

You are encouraged to ask any questions that occur to you at this time or to ask questions at any time during your participation in the study. You will be given a copy of this agreement for your own information. If you desire more information at a later date you may call _____ at _____ (during daytime hours) or _____ (at night).

10. *Basis of Participation*

You are free to withdraw your consent to participate in this study at any time. If you choose to do so, your rights to present or future medical care by Dr. _____ or at _____Hospital will not be affected.

11. *Signature*

I have read the above information and have had an opportunity to ask any questions and all of my questions have been answered. I consent to taking a medication called _____. I fully understand that its use in humans is limited and that its safety and effectiveness have not been fully established and that there is a risk of adverse reactions to the drug. I have been given a copy of this consent form.

Signature _____ Date _____

(Patient)

Signature _____ Date _____

(Parent or Legal Guardian)

I, the undersigned, have fully explained the relevant details of this study to the patient named above and/or the person authorized to consent for the patient. I am qualified to perform this role.

Signature _____ Print _____ Date _____

(Investigator) Name

Signature _____ Print _____ Date _____

(Witness) Name

Address of Witness _____

(*Important Note:* For all women of child-bearing potential who are entering this study, include discussion of the Pregnancy Waiver Form and request agreement to its terms, signified by the patients signature on the form.)

Sample Pregnancy Waiver

For Females Only

The following procedures will be read and explained to all prospective study patients of child-bearing potential:

(a) Patient is not known to be pregnant based upon results of the screening pregnancy test.

(b) Pregnancy tests will be administered at specified intervals (see protocol) during the study, and again at the end of the study.

(c) Patients who are physiologically capable of becoming pregnant will voluntarily sign a statement (see below) indicating their intent not to become pregnant during the course of the study, and they will agree to employ contraceptive methods acceptable to the investigator during the course of the study period.

(d) Should a patient become pregnant during the study, active drug treatment will be immediately discontinued. Monthly or bimonthly monitoring will be conducted by an obstetrician/gynecologist and pediatrician for up to two months following the end of pregnancy to assess the development of the fetus/infant.

VOLUNTARY STATEMENT OF INTENT TO AVOID PREGNANCY

I, _____ (print name) understand the above statements. Furthermore, I agree to attempt to avoid pregnancy while I am participating in this study. Should I have sexual relations during this period, I will employ a contraceptive method that has been approved by my physician. I will immediately contact Dr. _____ if pregnancy is suspected. I am aware that I may decline to sign this statement and that my refusal to sign will have no effect on the further treatment of my disease at this clinic.

DATE _____   SIGNATURE _____
                                                          Patient
DATE _____   SIGNATURE _____
                                                          Witness

FIG. 22.12. Sample form that can be utilized as a pregnancy waiver for women of childbearing potential who enter a drug study. This form would be used in conjunction with the informed consent.

One dental X-ray = 0.2 to 0.5 rads

Fluoroscopic examination = 10 rads/min

Abdominal X-rays (upper GI series) = 20 rads

Normal chest X-ray = 0.01 to 0.05 rads

Background radiation from natural sources = 0.1 to 0.5 rads/year

5. This study is to evaluate the drug in a broad population of patients with ____disease.

6. During this study you will be under the medical supervision of Dr. ＿＿. Other professionals may be designated by Dr. ＿＿to assist or act in his/her behalf.

7. Because blood samples are being taken during this study, you should not volunteer to donate blood for at least two months after participation in this study.

8. During this study your urine will be collected at random and unannounced times. It will be checked to confirm that you have not taken any drugs that are not allowed in the study.

9. If we are unable to contact you directly during this study, we want to obtain your permission to contact your family, friends, employers, or other sources so that we may reach you to learn about your medical status.

10. You may be given a blank medication at random periods throughout this study and for durations that will not be told to you. This medication is called a placebo. Your chances of receiving a placebo are one in ＿＿.

11. We would like to visit you at your home one time during this study in order to obtain a blood (urine or other) sample. We will not contact you prior to our visit.

12. This drug has already been approved for marketing and is sold only with a doctor's prescription.

13. The purpose of this study is to gather information on the benefits and problems associated with this drug.

14. This study is a continuation of the study "[Protocol Title]" in which you previously participated. The purpose of the present study is to evaluate long-term effects of ＿＿in patients who have benefited from this drug. This study will last for ＿＿months (years).

Additional Information That May Be Incorporated into Informed Consents

Discuss placebo medication and estimate the chances for any patient to receive a placebo. If the patient receives a placebo in the study, what are his/her possibilities of receiving the active drug at a later date? If a patient receiving placebo may receive the active drug after the "end" of the original study, it must be clarified whether the "end" represents the termination of the patient's participation, the completion of all patients' participation, or the conclusion of the analysis of the data indicating that the drug does in fact possess clinically significant efficacy. The distinction among these three time points for providing active drug to patients may be several months or years and would have great significance for a patient who is considering enrollment in a long-term study.

There are a variety of nondrug factors in many Phase II or III studies that may have a marked influence on the outcome of a study. Two such examples are the diet followed in a study testing a lipid-lowering drug and the amount of bed rest in patients receiving a drug to modify acute back pain. If these factors are included in an informed consent or are personally discussed with patients at the start of a study, there is a reasonable chance that their inclusion may modify patient behavior, yet it may not be desired to standardize these nondrug treatments within the study design. Under such conditions, investigators should be instructed how to approach these topics with patients in order to minimize the effect that patient-induced changes in diet, behavior, activity, or other factors will have on the study as well as to minimize the variations that will occur between different sites.

For studies of long duration, the patient may be requested to maintain periodic (e.g., annual) contact with the clinic for a certain number of years even if he/she is no longer actively participating in the study. In the event that this contact is not maintained, the patient should be informed that the center reserves the right to locate the patient in order to determine his/her medical condition or vital status.

Length of an Informed Consent and Other Considerations

The sample informed consent shown in Fig. 22.11 is longer than the majority of such forms used. The inclusion of any of the specific points described above will make the form even longer. Although this may seem to be excessively long, the information may be read at a leisurely pace by the patient. The patient will also be given a copy to refer to at a later time. Epstein and Lasagna (1969) reported that there was an inverse relationship between the length of the informed consent form and the comprehension of the form by the patients. They suggested that brief information be presented. The informed consents they compared, however, differed almost exclusively in the amount of information on risks that were presented by the drug (aspirin, in their study). Only a brief statement of aspirin's use was also included. Since there are new Federal regulations requiring the presentation of additional information to the patient, and since the present sample form does not overly emphasize the risks inherent in the hypothetical study, the relatively long form is not considered to be a drawback to obtaining patient participation as long as the patient is able to understand the language used. The author agrees with Epstein and Lasagna that an excessive amount of peripheral risk information (e.g., all of the unusual adverse reactions reported for the drug) is unwarranted.

The regulations governing informed consents do not cover many of the nuances relating to the individual who actually obtains the informed consent. For example, if a nurse, research coordinator, or other individual obtains the informed consent but is not able or qualified to discuss the details of the protocol or alternative treatments, then the signed consent form may not be legally valid if it is ever challenged. Variations on the traditional means of obtaining informed consents are discussed by Hassar and Weintraub (1976). They suggest that (1) holding a group meeting of patients, (2) testing patient comprehension, and (3) including relatives in discussions of informed consent are among the techniques that can improve patient comprehension of the benefits and risks inherent in a study.

An informed consent does not have to be obtained if (1) the patient is confronted by a life-threatening situation necessitating use of the study drug, (2) the patient is unable to communicate, (3) there is insufficient time to obtain consent, and (4) there is no alternative method of acceptable treatment available.

Under certain circumstances it is necessary to prepare a new or revised informed consent for patients in a study. Many of the reasons why a new (or revised) informed consent may be required are listed in Table 22.50. Informed consents are prepared by the investigator and not by the sponsor. The sponsor, however, will usually review the consent form to insure that it satisfies Federal regulations.

Institutional Approval

Each protocol should indicate that institutional approval will be obtained prior to initiation of the study. The processes followed in having a protocol approved are shown in Fig. 22.13. The institutional approval is given in the United States by an IRB and in the United Kingdom by an Ethics Committee. Protocols of both medical devices and biologicals (e.g., vaccines) that are regulated by the FDA must have IRB approval. The IRB must have at least five members, at least one of whom is unaffiliated with the institution on whose IRB he/she sits. The IRB may not be composed entirely of men or of women or of individuals of only one profession. At least one member must be active in a nonscientific area. The IRB maintains responsibility for the continuing review of the clinical study.

Physicians who maintain a private clinical practice or who work outside a formal institution often have access to an IRB. If they do not, they should determine how they may become associated with one. The obligations of an investigator towards the IRB should be well known by each investigator. These obligations include filing periodic reports, advising the IRB of any changes in the protocol (significant changes such as those listed in Table 22.51 will require IRB approval), and advising them of any serious adverse reactions.

In certain institutions, investigators must have a protocol approved by more than one committee (e.g., IRB, Departmental Committee, and the Clinical Research Unit Committee that has responsibility for the site where the study will be con-

TABLE 22.50. *Conditions under which a new or revised informed consent is often obtained*

1. Results of interim analyses demonstrate that some or all patients are at a greater clinical risk if they continue with their present treatment, but the study is not to be terminated early
2. Severe adverse reactions that are probably or definitely drug-induced are observed, which place some or all patients at greater clinical risk
3. Significant beneficial effects of one treatment are observed in an interim analysis that place patients receiving the other treatment at a clinical disadvantage, but the study will not be terminated early
4. A decision is reached by the sponsor of an investigational drug to discontinue future development of the drug
5. Any of the statements in the informed consent have significantly altered since the statement was signed, and the alteration is believed to have a potential impact on the patients' well-being
6. A new investigator has replaced the original investigator
7. A major change in the site or its facilities has occurred that is believed to have a potential impact on the patients' well-being

ducted). A written copy of the IRB approval must be obtained by the investigator (and also by the sponsor for sponsored studies) before a protocol may be initiated. There are publications that have assessed the performance of IRBs (Gray et al., 1978), evaluated the consistency among different IRBs (Goldman and Katz, 1982), and evaluated their influence on research design (Allen and Waters, 1982). A general synopsis of their functions is included in a brief article by Brown (1979).

Confidentiality of Data

There are several types of confidentiality associated with clinical studies. Confidentiality relates to information supplied by the sponsor to the investigator and to the IRB plus information contained in the patient's medical record. Standard statements may be drafted to describe the confidentiality of patient data and information supplied to the investigator. These may be included in the protocol or put in a letter or statement that is sent by a sponsor to the investigator. If a letter is sent to the investigator, the letter will state that information supplied about a specific drug must be kept confidential. A witnessed signature by the investigator may be requested, and if so, it could be affixed to a copy of the letter, which is then returned to the sponsor. The sponsor may indicate in its letter some of the reasons for requesting confidentiality (e.g., to protect patient rights).

Confidentiality statements relating to patient information must be consistent with FDA regulations and with IRB and sponsor's policies. The rights of the sponsor to consult source documents such as electrocardiograms (ECGs), X-rays, laboratory reports, and workbooks in order to document or verify final data collection form entries (within reasonable institutional, regulatory, and ethical constraints) may be stated in the protocol and/or in the informed consent. These original data should have the patient's name removed and replaced with the patient's assigned number in the study and also the patient's initials, as a check that the patient's number has been transcribed correctly. Under certain conditions, the FDA has the right to see patient data with the patient's full name. This fact must be indicated in the informed consent.

Collection and Processing of Data

Each protocol usually indicates how data will be collected, processed, and analyzed. In addition to the major procedures and approach that will be followed, the primary evaluations and statistical methods to be used may be indicated. Some protocols present this information in a general manner, whereas others are highly specific and detailed. The organization and content of this section of the protocol are generally discussed with the individuals who will be responsible for processing and analyzing the data. The protocol will often indicate which evaluations are to be performed during the conduct of the study and to what degree the data obtained will influence the study design and completion of the study. Any calculations or interim analyses that will be performed during the study may be described in detail

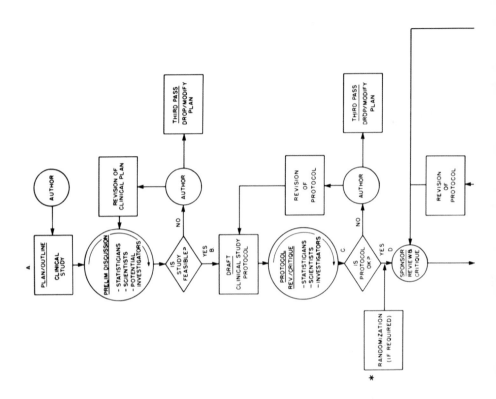

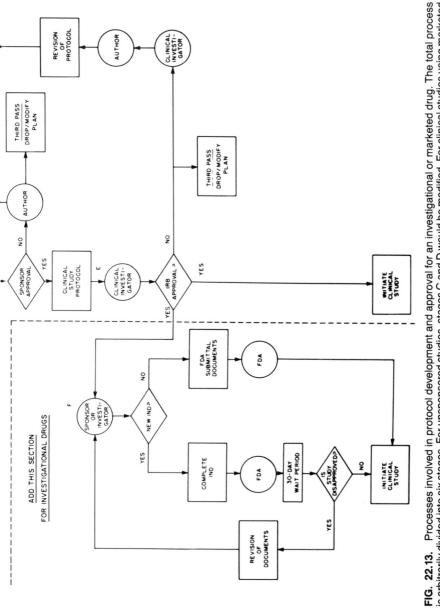

FIG. 22.13. Processes involved in protocol development and approval for an investigational or marketed drug. The total process is arbitrarily divided into six stages. For unsponsored studies, stages C and D would be modified. For clinical studies using marketed drugs without an IND, the last stage (F) would be omitted. Each IRB in a multicenter study must approve any changes made to the protocol.

TABLE 22.51. *Protocol changes that must be submitted to an IRB for approval*[a]

1. An increase in drug dosage or frequency of dosing or a change in the method of drug administration. This generally includes any change in drug formulation, since the bioavailability of the drug may be affected
2. Significant increases in the number of patients to receive the study drug. A 10% or greater increase is considered "significant" by some individuals
3. Use or inclusion of new groups of patients whose concurrent medical condition might significantly affect the scope and/or validity of the protocol
4. Use or inclusion of new groups of patients for whom special considerations are warranted in terms of care or other factors
5. Use or inclusion of new groups of patients whose concurrent therapy might confound study interpretation

[a]Each IRB may require submission of other protocol modifications for approval in addition to or in lieu of those listed in this table.

along with an indication of how the results will be used. A discussion on data analysis is presented in Chapter 38.

Publishing of Data

Procedures relating to publication of study results are described in some protocols. If the study is sponsored, the submission of a copy of the proposed publication (abstract or complete article) to the sponsor is usually requested a specific number of weeks prior to submission to the journal or society. If the study is multicentered, it may be appropriate to indicate whether a joint publication is planned and/or whether each site may publish its own data individually. Additional details relating to publication of articles should be reviewed at the roundtable meeting held prior to the study's initiation (see Chapter 34 for a discussion about this meeting). Even if a monograph is intended to be prepared to promulgate the data obtained, serious consideration should be given to publishing an article in a journal as well.

Monitoring the Study

The general methods to be followed for monitoring a sponsored study should be defined, including whether monitoring will be conducted by the sponsor, an independent group, and/or representatives of a contract organization. A contract organization usually acts as a "middleman" between the sponsor and investigator. Indicate that the monitoring will be conducted via periodic visits at the study site and by telephone contact on a scheduled or "as-needed" basis. The nature of the monitor's function as well as the tasks that the monitor performs are not usually detailed in a protocol. These aspects of the study are discussed more fully in Chapter 36.

Protocol Amendments

The procedures by which a protocol may be amended are sometimes included in the body of the protocol. The criteria for determining which protocol changes must be submitted for IRB approval are listed in Table 22.51.

23 Regulatory, Patent, and Legal Considerations

Regulatory Considerations • Patent Considerations • Legal Considerations

REGULATORY CONSIDERATIONS

Before protocols of investigational drugs may be initiated, a thorough evaluation of regulatory considerations must be conducted. This should be initiated as early in the protocol's development as possible, since there may be regulatory constraints that either preclude or have a significant impact on the initiation or conduct of the study. The vast number of potential regulatory problems and situations does not allow for more than a brief comment on this important area.

Sponsoring institutions of drug studies usually have individuals or complete departments concerned with regulatory affairs and are able to address the various issues raised. Investigators who initiate an unsponsored study should seek a review at an early date of the regulatory aspects of their protocol from their institution, Institutional Review Board (IRB), manufacturer of the drug, and/or the appropriate government agencies. Investigators may obtain their own Notice of Claimed Investigational Exemption for a New Drug (IND) to study an investigational drug. Even if no regulatory problems are anticipated, it would still be prudent for the investigator to confirm this impression with the appropriate individuals.

PATENT CONSIDERATIONS

If the proposed study involves an investigational drug, then there may be some patent issues to consider and/or discuss with relevant individuals. In sponsored studies, a clear understanding of the patent status of the investigational drug should be obtained before any information is disclosed to outside individuals. By the time the protocol is being developed, these discussions should have been completed. It is important to realize that patent protection may be obtained for a novel use (indication) of a presently unpatented old drug or chemical ("use" patent). Patent protection may also be obtained for novel pharmaceutical formulations or novel routes of synthesis of new or existing drugs in addition to "use" patents and a patent on the drug per se. A patent on the drug per se is the best type of patent to obtain.

Disclosure of a patentable invention before an appropriate patent application has been filed can have a profound impact on patent protection. In most countries, a nonconfidential disclosure (e.g., in discussion at a scientific meeting) becomes an immediate bar to patentability unless a patent application has been filed prior to the disclosure. In the United States and Canada, however, one may file a patent application up to 1 year after such a disclosure.

Investigators of unsponsored studies should check with their institutional patent officers before publishing data on drugs used in a novel way. In order to clarify whether there are issues that must be considered and resolved in regard to patent protection, it is preferable for investigators of unsponsored studies to consult with their patent office prior to initiating a study.

LEGAL CONSIDERATIONS

The following comments do not purport to provide legal advice relating to clinical studies but raise points that may be discussed further with your attorneys or other individuals who are familiar with the specific details in particular situations and the local laws governing them.

1. The informed consent cannot contain any exculpatory language that would waive or appear to waive any of the patient's legal rights or releases or appear to release the investigator, the sponsor, the institution, or its agents from liability for negligence.
2. Personal injury may result during treatment in the clinical study; however, the occurrence of injury does not indicate that any liability attaches.
3. The investigator's legal obligations towards the patient include obtaining a voluntary informed consent from the patient or the patient's guardian, adhering to a proper and adequate study design and protocol that is approved by an IRB, and providing due care in conducting the study.
4. Indemnification agreements may be entered into between sponsors and institutions, institutions and investigators, and sponsors and investigators.
5. Guidelines for compensation for drug-induced injuries have recently been proposed in the United Kingdom by the Association of the British Pharmaceutical Industry (1983) with an accompanying commentary by Professors Diamond and Laurence (1983).

24 Ethical Considerations

Selected Areas Where There Are Ethical Concerns • Official Groups Concerned with Medical Ethics • Study Designs that Attempt to Avoid Ethical Problems

SELECTED AREAS WHERE THERE ARE ETHICAL CONCERNS

Ethical and moral values often vary to a marked degree in different countries and often vary between different cultures within the same country. Although Institutional Review Board (IRB) and government regulatory bodies are "official" arbiters of ethical issues, every investigator should prepare his protocol with a cognizance of the ethical issues it raises. This sensitivity to ethical concerns is especially relevant when the protocol is intended for another country, social class, or group than that of the person who is developing the protocol. A number of ethical considerations raised in conducting clinical studies in developing countries were discussed by de Maar et al. (1983). These authors also discussed various other aspects of preparing protocols and conducting studies in less developed regions. Ethical considerations are definitely raised in studies performed on infants, children, pregnant or lactating women, prisoners, mentally retarded or psychotic individuals, or other persons who are unable to fully protect their own rights.

Ethical questions concern not only which populations of patients are permissible to study and which study designs are ethical to conduct but also when it is no longer ethically acceptable to continue a study to the scheduled completion (e.g., because of obvious changes in the medical outcomes from what was expected). The means used in terminating a study may raise additional ethical concerns, which are discussed in Chapter 37. These and other ethical questions have been widely discussed in the last few years (Rouzioux, 1979; Levine and Lebacqz, 1979; Schafer, 1982).

OFFICIAL GROUPS CONCERNED WITH MEDICAL ETHICS

A collection of papers concerning medical research on the human fetus as well as the Declaration of Helsinki and The Nuremberg Code of Ethics in Medical Research are presented in the report by the National Commission for the Protection of Human Subjects of Biomedical and Behavioral Research (1976). The Declaration of Helsinki contains recommendations guiding doctors in clinical research that have been adopted by the World Medical Association. The successor to the National Commission for the Protection of Human Subjects of Biomedical and Behavioral Research is the Presidents Commission for the Study of Ethical Problems in Medicine and Biomedical and Behavioral Research. Their first biennial report

(Abram, 1981), provides information on policies followed by all individual U.S. Government Agencies that are involved in research on humans. This report also contains the numerous recommendations from this Commission.

STUDY DESIGNS THAT ATTEMPT TO AVOID ETHICAL PROBLEMS

There are limited alternatives to consider when it is not ethically acceptable to maintain patients on placebo medication in a chronic study. The use of an active drug may be used as a control, but this approach has significant drawbacks, which were discussed in Chapter 4.

A different study design that incorporates both study drug and placebo in a double-blind study but avoids the ethical dilemma of maintaining seriously ill patients on placebo is to incorporate relatively frequent examinations into the protocol with unequivocal criteria for defining clinical improvement and deterioration. In this design, any patient who is observed at the first examination (while on drug) to be worse than at baseline is called a treatment failure and is discontinued from the study. Any patient who has not shown clinical improvement according to defined criteria by the second (or third) examination is likewise called a treatment failure and is discontinued from further study treatment. The advantage of this approach is that patients receiving placebo who deteriorate at first or fail to show improvement by a specific date will be removed from the study and can be given alternative treatment. This study design has been approved by various IRBs as having a sound ethical basis in situations in which routine use of a placebo is not acceptable.

An alternative study design to consider in situations in which an IRB will not accept a placebo control study is a dose–response evaluation. In this situation, a dose that is close to the threshold for activity is evaluated as well as one or two (or more) higher doses that would generate a dose–response relationship. This design has the potential advantages of satisfying IRBs that no placebo is used and of meeting regulatory requirements when use of a placebo would be desirable but not mandatory.

The dose-response study should not be confused with a dose-titration study. In the former design, separate groups of patients receive different doses of the same drug (e.g., Group A receives 10 mg/day, Group B receives 50 mg/day, and Group C receives 100 mg/day), whereas patients on study drug in the latter design may all receive doses from 10 to 100 mg/day depending on their responses, adverse reactions, or other factors. Placebo and/or active drug control groups may be used in either design. A combination of both the dose-response and dose-titration design is possible. In the combination design, patients are titrated within specified dose ranges (e.g., Group A receives 10–40 mg/day, Group B receives 50–90 mg/day, and Group C receives 100–150 mg/day).

Other designs such as the sequential design should also be considered in situations in which the IRB raises various ethical concerns. If strong ethical reservations persist about conducting a given clinical study, then it may be useful to consider a pilot study to obtain data that may indicate whether or not the study design would be acceptable from an ethical perspective.

25 Completing and Reviewing the Initial Draft

Establishing study objectives and choosing a protocol design are usually the initial steps in developing a protocol. In writing a protocol, most of the steps described in Table 14.12 may be performed simultaneously or sequentially. If a sequential order is used, there is no "correct" order to follow for all protocols or for all individuals who could prepare the same protocol. One convenient method of preparing several sections simultaneously is to start rough drafts of each section on separate sheets of paper or by separate dictations. After all sections have been completed, the various parts may easily be brought together and interdigitated to form the first draft.

There are many individual styles used in writing protocols. Two different styles in writing that are discussed in this chapter are the slow and deliberate approach and the fast, "get-it-all-down-quickly" approach. Many individuals find it easier to adopt the latter approach and to improve their protocols through a series of revisions. Each individual who is involved in writing protocols develops his/her own approach.

The first draft of a protocol should be read and rewritten as necessary before copies are submitted to other individuals for review. In reviewing one's own draft, it is helpful to question whether (1) each section is placed in the appropriate order, (2) each paragraph within a section is placed in the appropriate order to carry ideas and statements forward smoothly and without gaps or sudden changes in direction or logic, and (3) each sentence has definite meaning and is required for inclusion in the protocol. Introductory phrases at the start of sentences that do not add meaning to the sentence should be deleted, as well as nonessential words such as "the" or "very" when not required. Check for colloquialisms or clichés that can be replaced by more appropriate terms. Ascertain that all statements are adequately qualified and that one has established the intended limits in latitude and scope that will be placed on the statements' interpretation. For example, it may not be appropriate to state "Include patients, who, in the opinion of the investigator, show little or no evidence of the symptoms of ...," since this statement does not adequately qualify the latitude allowed in the investigator's judgment. Finally, read each sentence by itself, for its connotations as well as denotations, before deciding whether it conveys the intended meaning and should remain in the protocol.

Although the quality of fine literature is often enhanced by the use of a variety of expressions for the same concept, scientific writing is often made confusing when a number of different terms have the same or approximately the same definition. Thus, a concept such as adverse reactions should be written using the same single term throughout the protocol and not sometimes as adverse experiences,

189

adverse events, drug reactions, adverse drug reactions, side effects, or untoward effects. Additionally, if two similar terms are to be used in a protocol with different meanings, then the specific meanings of each term should be made clear. For example, if the term "adverse reactions" is defined as the patient's signs, symptoms, and abnormal laboratory values but does not include other medical events, then another term, such as "adverse experiences," may also be used in a protocol. Each term used must be clearly defined.

Some protocols are written with a substantial amount of repetition between various sections. Other protocols strive to avoid presenting any repetitive information. This aspect of protocol writing is highly individualized, and different authors have different opinions about the amount of repetition that it is appropriate to include in a protocol. If each section of a protocol is able to stand alone, and material may be repeated elsewhere, there is an advantage in generally being able to quickly locate specific information in the protocol. The major disadvantage of repeating information presented elsewhere is in increasing the length of the protocol. Each writer must determine the proper balance between avoiding any repetition and using extensive repetition. A number of the practical considerations described in this section, plus others not described, are listed in Table 25.52.

TABLE 25.52. *General considerations in writing and polishing a protocol[a]*

---

1. Avoid excessively long sentences
2. Use correct and consistent tenses
3. Limit the use of adjectives, adverbs, and other modifiers
4. Use concrete, graphic, and precise words
5. Eliminate unnecessary and hedge words (e.g., very, seemed, etc., presumably)
6. Eliminate clichés and trite phrases
7. Eliminate unnecessary sentences or paragraphs
8. Do not begin numerous sentences or paragraphs with the same word
9. Develop thoughts logically and orderly
10. Describe each significant step in a complete thought or procedure
11. Define ambiguous or potentially ambiguous words or phrases

---

[a]There are exceptions to each of these points, especially when dictated by style.

26   Improving the Protocol

The most obvious technique for improving the quality of a protocol is for the author to review it as critically as possible. It is often useful to conduct this exercise after laying the manuscript aside for several days. A fresh review after a lapse of time usually allows the author to view his/her own work more objectively. It is generally advantageous to mentally check every step required to complete all procedures or aspects of a study and to confirm that all steps have been both accurately and adequately described. All possible problems that can be envisioned should be considered, and a decision made as to which countermeasures to include in the protocol (e.g., if ____situation occurs, then ____). Additionally, in reviewing one's own protocol, it is important to insure that many common pitfalls have been avoided in the preparation of the clinical study. A number of these common pitfalls are listed in Table 26.53.

Another established method for improving the quality of a protocol is to have other professionals and colleagues conduct a review and provide a critique for the author. If the investigator is not the same individual as the author, then the investigator's input is usually obtained, as is that of the statistician who will be analyzing the data. If a roundtable discussion among all investigators, monitors, coordinators, and the sponsor can be held, difficult points can be discussed and, one hopes, resolved. It is the author's assumption that the greater the attention paid to the planning phase, the greater is the likelihood that the study will be conducted as desired.

Protocols have to be approved by Institutional Review Boards (IRBs), and if they are prepared by a sponsor, then the sponsor must also approve the protocol. The various steps followed in evaluating a protocol sometimes lead to useful suggestions for its improvement.

A 15-page form titled *Trial Assessment Procedure Scale* (TAPS) has been prepared by the Pharmacologic and Somatic Treatments Research Branch of the National Institute of Mental Health to assist in the critique of protocols or completed studies. The TAPS procedure was designed to evaluate the quality of a study rather than the data obtained. This form is available by writing to the address listed in the footnote to Table 26.54. One may use all or part of this form to evaluate one's own work, or request that a colleague use this form as the protocol is being developed. The eight general parts of the TAPS forms assess:

1. Research problem
2. Research management
3. Design characteristics
4. Treatment characteristics
5. Subject characteristics

TABLE 26.53. *Common pitfalls in preparing and writing protocols[a]*

A. Study objectives
1. Expressed too generally to allow a specific study design to be constituted
2. Ambiguous or vague
3. Not obtainable with the current study design. Study may be too complex or include too many parts, or there may be inadequate resources to conduct the study
B. Study design
1. Not thoroughly discussed with a statistician, and the design will not adequately address study objectives
2. The design chosen is beyond current state of the art
3. Efficacy tools chosen for the disease being studied have not been adequately validated
4. There is inadequate statistical power for the particular study. The sample size chosen is too small to detect clinically meaningful results
5. Inappropriate use of an active control in a pivotal study
6. Lack of placebo or double blind in a study in which one or both should be incorporated
7. Dose regimen too restrictive in terms of range of doses allowed, alterations of dosing for adverse reactions, or other factors
8. Failure of the investigator or sponsor to consult with statistician before designing the study's randomization
C. Inclusion/exclusion criteria
1. Too stringent to allow adequate numbers of patients to be enrolled
2. Too loose to permit meaningful data to be obtained
D. Screen/baseline/treatment
1. Periods of time for screen and/or baseline and/or treatment are used that are either too long or too short for optimal and appropriate conduct of the study
2. Too few, too many, or an inadequate number of measurements are requested (i.e., the study generates too little or too much data)
3. Patients may be inappropriately entered into the study and begin to receive drug before all screening results are obtained and evaluated
4. Excessive numbers of blood drawings are requested that may cause adverse reactions (headache or dizziness)
5. An excessive period of fasting is required that causes adverse reactions (headache or dizziness). This is especially common in pharmacokinetic studies
E. Drug packaging/dispensing
1. Drug packaging that does not permit all options allowed by protocol to be followed
F. Study blind
1. Study blind easily broken because of "obvious" characteristics (e.g., adverse reactions, changes in laboratory parameters, drug odor) of one (or more) treatment groups (e.g., drowsiness caused by diazepam, colored urine because of phenolphthalein, garlic smell on breath caused by DMSO) that are difficult or impossible to adequately mask
2. Study blind easily broken by observation of drug interactions or other situations by the investigator (e.g., marked improvement in study group or changes in blood levels of concomitant drugs)
3. Study blind chosen for use is not appropriate or optimal for the study
G. Data collection and analysis
1. Poorly designed data collection forms
2. Incorrect statistical methods used to analyze data
H. Overall
1. Ambiguous language used in a protocol that may lead to different results and/or interpretations than desired
2. Too many comparisons requested, which will probably lead to some significant results obtained by chance alone (5 of every 100 independent comparisons will be statistically significant by chance alone, if $\alpha = 0.05$ and there are no true differences between the comparison groups)
3. Presence of conflicting parts of the protocol (i.e., internal consistency is absent)
4. Discretionary judgments by the investigator are allowed, which may seriously affect the quality and/or quantity of data obtained

[a]Numerous pitfalls related to biases are presented in Appendix 1.

TABLE 26.54. *Structure of Trial Assessment Procedure Scale (TAPS)*[a]

1. Research problem	5. Subject characteristics
a. Background and rationale	a. Selection criteria
b. Objectives and/or hypothesis	b. Sample representatives
2. Research management	c. Subject induction
a. External review/monitoring	d. Subject compliance
b. Site selection	6. Data collection
c. Personnel	a. Scope of assessment
d. Trial period	b. Assessment measures
3. Design characteristics	c. Assessment schedule
a. Independent variables	d. Assessment performance
b. Design configuration	7. Data analysis
c. Subject assignment	a. Data preparation
d. Control of treatment-	b. Data presentation
related bias	c. Statistical analysis
e. Control of extraneous variables	d. Data synthesis
4. Treatment characteristics	8. Conclusions and interpretation
a. Description	a. Focus
b. Dosage	b. Logic
c. Duration	c. Application

[a]Taken from DHHS, NIMH, Alcohol, Drug Abuse and Mental Health Administration. Document available from Dr. Jerome Levine, Pharmacologic and Somatic Treatments Research Branch, NIMH, Room 10C-06, 5600 Fishers Lane, Rockville, MD 20857.

6. Data collection
7. Data analysis
8. Conclusions and interpretations

Each of these areas is divided into two to five sections, and each of the individual points is evaluated separately.

Another system for assessing reports of therapeutic studies was proposed by Lionel and Herxheimer (1970). Their checklists can be used by authors who are preparing protocols as an assurance that they have considered each of the important elements that will eventually be utilized and included in a publication.

27 Preparing Data Collection Forms

General Organization of Data Collection Forms • Designing the Data Collection Forms • Measuring and Recording Parameters that Are Not Easily Quantitated • Completing the Data Collection Forms

GENERAL ORGANIZATION OF DATA COLLECTION FORMS

These forms are also referred to as "Case Report Forms" (or other terms) but are referred to as data collection forms (DCFs) in this monograph. One of the first decisions related to the preparation of DCFs that must be addressed is whether or not to organize and group the forms on the basis of separate clinic visits or evaluations (e.g., day A, day B, day C) where all forms for day A are separated from those for day B, etc. An alternative approach is to have the grouping of DCFs based on integrating similar or identical forms (e.g., forms for all physical examinations are placed together, followed by the forms for all laboratory tests, which are placed together, followed in turn by the forms for all efficacy measures, and so forth). In this approach, different copies of the same form (for any parameter) to be filled in on days A, B, and C are all placed together. A third approach to preparing DCFs is to combine both of the approaches described above and to have some forms arranged in a visit-by-visit grouping and other forms integrated by type of examination, test, or form.

The advantages of using a visit-by-visit format in DCFs is that it is easier for investigators to complete the forms, especially if the original DCFs are completed at the time of the patient's visit. One disadvantage of this method is that it is more difficult for either the investigator or a monitor to observe trends in the data. For example, a gradually changing laboratory parameter may be more easily missed in this type of DCF, since the values obtained at each visit are in separate sections of the DCF "book" and are not as easily compared as if all values were on the same or adjoining pages.

An advantage of combining all similar forms together in one section of the DCF book is that monitoring of data and detection of trends are more easily accomplished. For example, if all of the laboratory values obtained at one visit are placed in one column, and one page has several adjacent columns, then reading across the page allows one to quickly scan for any abnormalities or trends in the data. The major problem with this approach is that completing the forms is more difficult, since each form that must be completed at one visit is in a different section of the DCF "book" and must be located.

There are circumstances in which it is advantageous to combine both of the above formats. For example, it may be deemed important to observe specific parameters closely (e.g., laboratory results or seizure counts), but the investigator may prefer to use a visit-by-visit approach for the rest of the study forms. Also, selected data may be more easily kept together (i.e., integrated) in a study of long duration (e.g., daily or weekly drug doses in a study in which the patients come at irregular intervals), and the remaining forms placed in a visit-by-visit section.

DESIGNING THE DATA COLLECTION FORMS

Standardized Information and Forms

Each page of the DCF usually has a standardized section in which spaces are provided for the patient's initials, study number, and specific date relevant to the information on that page. Other standard information that may be printed on each page includes the title of the study, name of the sponsor (if any), page number, title of the information on that page [e.g., electrocardiogram (ECG), Medical History, Laboratory Examination], plus relevant information about the sponsor or drug [e.g., Notice of Claimed Investigational Exemption for a New Drug (IND) number, department organizing the study, code number of the drug]. See Fig. 27.14 for an example. To identify the general contents of any page at a glance when searching through a DCF book, it is useful to print the title of the information contained on that page in much larger (and bolder) type than that used for the rest of the page. It may be relevant to specify on the DCF whether the ECG as well as other tests [electroencephalogram (EEG) or X-rays] will be "read and interpreted" by nonexpert MDs or by MD specialists highly trained in their interpretation.

Investigators of unsponsored drug studies may prefer to utilize some standardized preprinted DCFs. A number of examples related to behavioral and performance tests as well as demographics, diagnosis, and adverse reactions are available from ECDEU (see *ECDEU Assessment Manual for Psychopharmacology*, Guy, 1976).

Developing DCFs requires the use of medical jargon and terminology that will be familiar and suitable for the physicians who will complete the forms. Precoded synonyms or codes for many of these terms will be useful for data entry and analysis. These terms or codes should be prepared prior to the study. Precoding of various responses in the DCFs should be considered as a step to simplify data entry and analysis at the end of the study. Discussing the DCFs with the relevant personnel who will process them after the data have been collected will provide important information on this point.

Closed Versus Open Systems

In preparing DCFs there are many viewpoints, which range from using a "closed system" having almost 100% preprinted multiple-choice responses to questions to having an "open system" with spaces or lines on the DCFs in which responses may

Post Follow-up Evaluation

To Be Completed By Sponsor	
Compound	Project
IND No.	NDA No.
Protocol No.	Study No.
Department	Section

PATIENT'S INITIALS: _ _ _   PATIENT NO. _____
               F M L

INSTRUCTIONS:

This form is to be used to follow any clinically significant findings occuring since the initiation of the treatment period that have not returned to baseline or acceptable values at the time of the final posttreatment visit. Give dates and description of all pertinent events and note action taken, if any.

Abnormal Event(s)   Date of   Date of
                       Onset   Resolution   Check One
1. _____   Has Patient Completed   ___ YES
2. _____   Treatment Period?   ___ NO
3. _____

TESTS PERFORMED

Test	Date	Value	Normal Value Range (Units)	Test	Date	Value	Normal Value Range (Units)

INVESTIGATOR'S COMMENT LOG (Date each entry and indicate actions taken.) _____

_____

_____

_____

_____

FINAL OUTCOME OF EACH ABNORMAL EVENT: _____

_____

_____

                                                                    , M.D.
_____ _____   _____ _____
Edited by   Date   Date   Investigator's Signature

FIG. 27.14. Sample form used for data collected during a post follow-up evaluation (i.e., at a clinic visit outside the normal protocol necessitated by an abnormality present at the post-treatment or last scheduled visit).

be entered. In the former case, data entry and statistical analysis are immeasurably simplified, all investigators will respond in the same or similar manner, and the data obtained may be more easily combined with data from other studies. But there is the chance that meaningful data may not be collected in a totally closed system, and some investigators will undoubtedly balk at this "regimented" approach. In the totally open system, different investigators will probably complete the forms differently, but some of the observations and comments collected on the DCFs may provide valuable insights into the patients and their responses.

It is the author's opinion that a goal in designing DCFs is to have a minimum number of write-in answers or responses. One essential write-in area is for "Investigator's Comments," located either in one central place or on several pages in the DCF. A list of alternative answers should be provided for questions on other DCFs, with instructions to check, cross out, circle, or otherwise indicate the specific response. An additional space or spaces for "other" responses should always be considered. In recording the data from laboratory tests, some individuals prefer indicating the actual number of digits to be used in the answer (e.g., Hematocrit = ____ ____. ____) rather than using a single line (Hematocrit = ____), since this latter method may elicit a different number of digits in some written responses.

In multicenter studies, the units of measurement used at each site must be compared for each test to insure that all laboratories are utilizing the same system of units. This is especially relevant if studies are being run in two or more countries, since only some countries utilize standard international units, and several systems exist for expressing the results of certain laboratory parameters. It may be necessary to include conversion factors in the DCFs or to use conversion factors on selected data after the DCFs have been completed. A category of "NA" (not applicable) or another similar term should be used by investigators to avoid having certain boxes or lines left blank on the DCFs. Blank spaces are undesirable, since they may indicate that the question posed (1) has had no response by the patient, (2) has not been assessed by the investigator, (3) was not found to be relevant at that site, (4) was forgotten to be entered in the DCF, or any of several other possibilities.

Amount of Data to Collect

In determining how much data to collect in a clinical study, there are two extreme positions that may be taken. The first scenario is one in which investigators collect too little data and collect it in a haphazard manner on various pieces of paper they have quickly assembled without conducting a thorough review of the forms required for recording data. This leads to the situation in which results of some tests may be adequately documented but where relevant data generated in other tests are inadequate for appropriate statistical analysis. The "worst-case scenario" with this problem occurs when the study objectives are inadequately addressed because of insufficient data collection.

The opposite extreme occurs when significantly more data are collected than are required to meet the study objectives. The vast amount of data generated may threaten the actual conduct of the study as well as its analysis. The conduct of a study could be affected if excessive time was required by study personnel to spend with patients to generate the data. The investigator, research coordinator, and other personnel may grumble at the redundant work, the patients may feel hassled by excessive demands and testing, the individuals who monitor and enter the data into computers feel burdened, and the statisticians and clinicians who analyze and interpret the data may only utilize part of the data collected in an attempt to avoid being "swamped" by irrelevant information.

To avoid both of these extreme situations (which the author believes are rather common occurrences), the individual responsible for designing and assembling the DCFs must analyze the overall approach to data collection as well as each data form used, adding important measurements and questions and culling extraneous ones. The touchstones for determining the amount of data to collect are (1) how necessary the data are to meet the objectives of the protocol, (2) how the data will fit with data collected from other studies if they may be combined at some point into a regulatory submission, and (3) how the data will be treated in the reports that are generated.

Binders and Paper to Be Used

After the DCFs have been prepared, evaluated, revised, and printed (or photocopied), they should be placed into loose-leaf or other binders or attached together by a different method. A method that allows for replacement forms to be used or for additional sheets to be inserted into the binder has obvious advantages over a rigidly bound set of forms. In addition, if a copy of an ECG, laboratory printout, or official interpretation of a test (or the original) is to be inserted into the record, it is preferable to have an easy means for accomplishing this.

An easy method of separating the different sections of the DCFs is to place divider sheets with side tabs between relevant forms. The side tabs can be printed, or typed labels may be inserted into plastic side tabs attached to heavy stock paper sheets. If both an integrated and visit-by-visit organization of DCFs are used, then the side tabs for each of the two parts may be printed in different colors for ease of identification. Side tabs can be labeled with the name or abbreviation of the test for integrated forms and with the day (week, month), visit number, or date for visit-by-visit forms. There are numerous other approaches that can be used in determining the titles to use on section tabs.

Some sponsors and investigators prefer to prepare DCFs with noncarbon reproducing-type paper. Other individuals prefer single sheets of paper (usually white) that may later be photocopied to obtain additional copies. Noncarbon reproducing paper is often made in different colors. Instructions are often presented in the study that one color page of each form is retained by the investigator and two or more different colors of the same page are sent to the sponsor. If binders are chosen to hold the DCFs together, then the outside color may be utilized as either a means to help identify the specific study if multiple studies are being conducted by the same investigator (e.g., red binders for study A, blue binders for study B) or to identify different groups of patients within the same study (e.g., green binders for group A and yellow binders for group B).

Specialized Data Collection Forms

It is often useful in designing DCFs to include a separate checklist that lists each procedure, test, or examination that will be performed or conducted at that visit. One of these forms may be prepared for each clinic visit or dosing period. It may also be relevant to prepare a checklist for all tests or procedures that are scheduled for a specific (or general) time period of a study. These checklists provide assurance to the investigator and/or others conducting the study that they have not omitted any tests, procedures, or other details that should have been attended to at that particular time or visit. A listing of many of the different parameters or forms to be included in DCFs is shown in Table 27.55. The checklist that is prepared for a study may indicate the page number of the DCF for each item listed as well as

TABLE 27.55. *Sections of data collection forms[a]*

1. Medical history and demographics
   General
   Specific for the disease being evaluated or treated
2. Physical examination
   Complete or abbreviated physical examination
   Complete or abbreviated neurological examination (or other specific parts of the physical examination)
   Vital signs, weight, and height
   Examinations focusing on the disease being evaluated
3. Other examinations
   ECG (specify lead II, 12-lead, or Holter monitor)
   EEG (specify number of channels, and whether photic stimulation, sleep, and/or hyperventilation tests are required)
   Ophthalmological (specify tests)
   X-ray or other examinations
4. Laboratory examinations:
   Hematology
   Blood chemistry
   Urinalysis
   Urine collection
   Study drug samples
   Other samples or specialized studies
5. Adverse reactions
6. Efficacy measurements
7. Study drug medication record (amount of drug prescribed, dispensed, and dose changes)
8. Concomitant drugs
9. Pill count and compliance checks
10. Patient's global evaluation
11. Physician's global evaluation[b]
12. Investigator's comment log[c]
13. Patient discontinuation record[d]

[a]A box or line may be placed next to each item for check-off after the item has been handled or performed.
[b]A numerical code may be used to denote the clinical judgment (e.g., 1, improved; 2, no change; 3, worse).
[c]This form usually consists of blank lines or an open space for comments.
[d]This usually includes a section related to information required in cases of premature patient discontinuation.

including a space or a box next to each item to be marked after that item is completed. The overall time and events schedule (study flow chart) is a convenient reference for study personnel and may be placed in the front of each patient's DCF as well as in other suitable locations. This schedule could be used as a checklist, especially in a long study in which not all patients begin the study at the same time.

If patients are not able to be discharged from the study at their final posttreatment evaluation because of adverse reactions, abnormal laboratory measurements, or other factors, additional visits and possibly additional tests must be scheduled. To collect these data in an efficient manner, it must be determined how data will be entered into the patient's records. One means is to construct a separate form to be filled in (e.g., Fig. 27.14). Another means is to have investigators utilize a form designated as the "Investigator's Comment Log," which is often included in DCFs.

In noting the time of day at which specific events are scheduled and actually performed, there are a number of different systems that may be used. Time measurements may be noted in terms of actual clock time (4:10 P.M.) or the elapsed time after a given point (2.50 hr after drug administration) or both. Either a 24-hr "military" clock or a conventional 12-hr A.M. and P.M. clock may be used to specify the actual clock time. The 24-hr clock is usually preferable for data entry and analysis because it is more suitable for statistical treatment (subtracting or combining times), and it avoids potential problems created by any omission of the A.M. and P.M. notation. The time at which an event is scheduled to occur may be printed on the form used to collect the data. A brief summary of some possible notations relating to time are shown in Table 27.56.

MEASURING AND RECORDING PARAMETERS THAT ARE NOT EASILY QUANTITATED

In examining safety and/or efficacy data after a study is complete, numerous options may be used in compiling, categorizing, and analyzing information. This

TABLE 27.56. *Selected methods to measure and record time in DCFs*

		Tests performed at: Study day (week) 4			
		Tuesday	7	2	80
		Day of week	Month	Day	Year
	Scheduled time				
Hours postdrug	Clock time (use a 24-hr clock)[a]	Actual time test was performed (use a 24-hr clock)[a]			Δ[c] (min)
0[b]	8:00	8:05			5
1	9:00	9:10			10
2	10:00	10:06			6
8	16:00	15:58			−2

[a]A 12-hr clock plus A.M. or P.M. may be used.
[b]Drug is given at "0" time.
[c]Δ, Difference between actual and scheduled times. This value may also be expressed in hours using decimals.

book has stressed the principle that it is important to develop systems for collecting and processing data (insofar as possible) before the clinical study begins.

Even data that may not appear to be easily quantitated should be dealt with in a systematic manner in DCFs and analysis. The example that will be described relates to red blood cell (RBC) morphology in a study in which this parameter is not being systematically investigated. If specific instructions or a DCF are not provided for RBC morphology, then it is most likely that the data will be collected in the form of scattered comments in the DCFs. To analyze these comments most effectively and to collect optimal data, it is initially useful to develop the categories that could be incorporated into the DCFs to classify and quantitate the various comments. The four major categories of RBC morphology are:

1. Poikilocytosis (abnormal shape)
2. Anisocytosis (abnormal size)
3. Color abnormalities (abnormal amount or distribution of hemoglobin)
4. Inclusion bodies (abnormalities inside the cell)

These categories are not mutually exclusive; for example, an RBC may exhibit two or more abnormalities. After the categories are chosen, the terms that will be included under each category may be listed. Definitions of each term may be developed. The most common terms that would be included in the four categories above are listed in Table 27.57.

The next step is to designate a code or codes for grading the intensity of each abnormality. One sample code for categories 1, 2, and 3, shown below, is similar to the code used to grade various aspects of urinalysis (see Table 17.18).

$0 =$ None or negative
$0.5 =$ Trace
  $1 =$ Slight, mild, $1 +$
  $2 =$ Moderate, $2 +$
  $3 =$ Marked, $3 +$
  $4 =$ Severe, loaded, $4 +$

The last of the four categories of RBC morphology (inclusion bodies) may be coded as "present" or "not present." If many abnormalities are noted in this category, however, then a more elaborate code may be developed.

Both the quality and quantity of data obtained in a study will undoubtedly affect how the categories and codes are used and reported. If there are few reports of any abnormalities, then a summary sentence or even paragraph may suffice to treat the results. But if numerous abnormalities are reported, then a more sophisticated handling of the data will have to be developed.

COMPLETING THE DATA COLLECTION FORMS

If the study is sponsored, the investigator(s) and research coordinators should both have an opportunity to evaluate the DCFs before they are printed or photo-copied. In unsponsored studies, a colleague should perform this task. The individ-

TABLE 27.57. *List of terms included in four categories of abnormal RBC morphology*

1. Poikilocytosis	
Common terms (old terminology)	New terminology
Burr cell, berry cell, crenated cell	Echinocyte
Acanthoid cell, spur cell	Acanthocyte
Mouth cell, cup form, mushroom cap, uniconcave disk	Stomatocyte
Spherocyte, microspherocyte	Spherocyte
Schistocyte, helmet cell, fragmented cell	Schizocyte
Ovalocyte, oval cells	Elliptocyte
Sickle cell	Drepanocyte
Target cell, bull's eye cell, Mexican hat cell	Leptocyte
Teardrop cell, tennis racket cell, poikilocyte	Dacryocyte

2. Anisocytosis
   Microcytosis
   Macrocytosis
3. Color abnormalities
   Hypochromic, pale color, thin cell, wafer cell
   Hyperchromic, dark color
   Heterochromasia, polychromasia (blue to orange coloration)
   Abnormal distribution of color
4. Inclusion bodies
   Basophilic stippling (noted in many clinical situations, the rest are seen in more
      specific clinical states)
   Howell–Jolly bodies
   Azuraphilic granulations
   Pappenheimer bodies
   Cabot rings
   Heinz bodies

uals who will be responsible for data entry and data analysis should also have an opportunity to evaluate these forms to insure that the data collected are in the proper format for entry and analysis and may be integrated with data obtained from other studies.

When all of the various forms are brought together and put in order, it is useful to place individual forms in the order that the tests will be performed during the study. Similar types of forms should be grouped together (when possible), such as those relating to patient history, physical examinations, laboratory tests, and specialized procedures or tests. This approach may be followed regardless of whether an integrated or visit-by-visit approach is used to organize the forms.

There are several alternative methods used to collect and enter data onto the DCFs.

One Set of Data Collection Forms Per Patient

All data are entered onto the DCF directly or transcribed from laboratory or other forms. Forms may be bound or removable, as in a three-ring binder.

Two Sets of Data Collection Forms Per Patient

One set is used as a rough copy to fill in during the patient's visit, and the other set is a clean copy that is filled out later. One set may be denoted as a "workbook," and this rough copy should be retained, at least until the monitor has edited the data, in case of any transcription errors. The clean set may contain "no-carbon-required" paper to provide additional copies. Using two sets of DCFs may lead to more errors than a single set and is not generally recommended.

Flow Charts Used with Data Collection Forms

A flow chart may be prepared and used to collect data as it is generated, at the bedside or under conditions in which it is not practical or convenient to use the complete set of DCFs. The data written on the flow chart are later copied onto the DCFs.

Partial Sets of Data Collection Forms for Different Functions or Individuals

The DCFs for each patient may be divided into sections to provide one section to each individual, such as the physician, assistant, nurse, or coordinator who will complete that part. These separate parts are fitted together after they are completed.

It is usually preferable for one individual to enter all data onto the DCFs at one site. If this is not possible, then the smallest number of individuals possible should have this responsibility. In many studies, different individuals have responsibility for specific pages to complete (e.g., the investigator completes the physical examination, and the research coordinator completes the laboratory forms).

It is important for the investigator to sign each patient's DCF. This can take the form of signing (and dating) each page or only the first and/or last page, of the DCF. Other options include having the investigator initial (and possibly date) each page and sign the last page or only sign the last page.

28 Instructions for Patients, Investigators, and Study Personnel

After patients have been accepted for entry into a study, it is often helpful to have a summary of important information prepared for them that they may refer to at any time during the study. This may be achieved by preparing and giving patients an instruction sheet. The form should contain the names and telephone numbers for both day and night of the investigator and research coordinator plus salient points about dosing, appointments, self-rating scales (if applicable), contraindications, and any other related information (see Table 28.58).

An alternative to preparing an instruction sheet is to prepare a text for the investigator to read to all patients prior to the start of a specific test or part of the study. This insures that each patient has heard a standard set of instructions (information).

There are several additional types of instructions that may be prepared for use with a protocol. Many of these are listed in Table 28.59. The purpose of instructions is to standardize the conduct of the study and to help prevent problems in communication between the people involved. Instructions may be placed in an appendix

TABLE 28.58. *Types of information that may be supplied to patients[a]*

---

1. Discussion about the purpose of the study
2. Comments on the dosing schedule. A table of all drugs, dosages, and times of dosing may be appropriate
3. Comments on whether to take drug before, with, or after meals
4. Future clinic or laboratory visits—where, when, and other pertinent data. If all facilities are not located in same building, a map may be useful
5. Information on possible adverse reactions of which patient should be cognizant.
6. Information on whom to call with questions related to the study or if adverse reactions or medical problems occur (include telephone numbers for day and night calls)
7. Details on how to complete any self-rating scale, diary, or other patient-completed test included in the protocol
8. Instructions to bring all medicines and relevant records to all (or some) future clinic visits
9. Comment on types of permissible daily activities, including driving a car or operating potentially dangerous tools (machinery)
10. Instructions on when to take drug doses prior to next (each) study visit
11. Instructions on how to store the drug
12. Comments on nondrug treatments that patients may also be receiving
13. Information on collecting biological samples (e.g., urine)
14. Comments on concomitant medications, food, alcohol, caffeine-containing drinks, or other beverages that may be relevant to the study

---

[a]The information to be given to patients may be preprinted and handed to patients or presented verbally (either formally by reading or less formally in a discussion).

TABLE 28.59. *Types of instructions to be used in conjunction with a protocol*

1. Written instructions to be given to patients
2. Written instructions to be read to and discussed with patients by investigators. These instructions are not given to patients
3. Instructions prepared for investigators relating to the conduct of specific tests
4. Instructions prepared for investigators and research coordinators for filling in each page of data collection forms
5. Instructions for obtaining biological samples containing study drugs plus information on storage, handling, and shipping of these samples
6. Instructions prepared for pharmacists relating to their role in the study
7. Instructions prepared for nurses or any of various specialists relating to their role in the study
8. Other instructions pertaining to specific aspects of study

to the protocol or in the data collection forms (DCFs), or they may be prepared separately and not included in the protocol.

Instructions may also be prepared to describe the accepted means of applying the inclusion criteria, arranging patient visits, completing the DCFs, and dealing effectively with other aspects of the study (see Table 28.59). These instructions and other information may be combined into a "manual of procedures," which is often extremely useful in achieving uniformity among different sites of a multicenter study.

29   Continuation Protocols

An important consideration in studies of investigational drugs that have a specified duration is whether patients who have benefited from treatment will be allowed to continue to receive the drug. If so, a continuation protocol is generally provided. Patients who enter continuation protocols may receive drug under this protocol for a fixed, variable, or unspecified duration. The existence of a continuation protocol is often identified in the initial "feeder" protocol.

In developing a continuation protocol, it is important to determine whether it will be specifically tailored to follow one (and only one) protocol and thus exclude patients who have completed all other protocols with the same study drug. An alternative approach is to design a generic continuation protocol that will accept patients from many protocols in which the same study drug was tested.

In either situation, one must consider all of the probable relationships of patients and study drug that may be presented to the investigator and determine which patients will be entered and which will be excluded from the continuation protocol. For example, it should be determined whether patients may enter a continuation protocol if they have completed their original protocol a number of weeks or months prior to the time of entry into the continuation study or if they have received only placebo treatment in the original protocol. If patients have just completed the feeder protocol and are still receiving active drug, it must be determined whether they must be taken off drug prior to entry into the continuation protocol. Patients who were hospitalized with nonstudy drug-related problems who were dropped from the original protocol may wish to enter the continuation protocol. The manner in which any or all of these groups are permitted to enter the continuation protocol must be determined and specified in the admission criteria for the continuation protocol. Specific criteria for defining the minimal improvement on study drug that qualifies a patient for entry into a continuation protocol comprise an additional factor that must be established. If the continuation protocol emanates from a sponsor, then periodic review of the data generated in the continuation protocol should be conducted by the sponsor and the prerogative maintained (by the sponsor) to cancel any continuation protocol if the drug's development is discontinued or for other defined (or undefined) reasons.

There are many potential semantic problems that may arise in describing the duration of patient treatment in continuation protocols. These can be illustrated by an example of two patients who enter a 1-year continuation protocol. The first question is whether "1 year" refers to a patient's total exposure to drug or to 1 year of additional exposure to drug beyond the time of original exposure. Assume that each patient had previously received drug for 3 months but that Patient 1 stopped receiving drug 2 months prior to the beginning of the continuation protocol and Patient 2 has not stopped drug therapy but has entered the continuation protocol still receiving study drug at a maintenance level. After 1 month of dose escalation, Patient 1 is now at his maintenance level. After the study is half complete, an interim analysis of the data is being prepared, and the question is raised about whether Patients 1 and 2 have each received study drug for the same duration.

There are several different ways of combining data from these patients. The assumptions and details of the techniques used for data analysis should be established prior to the study. One issue is whether to define the duration of time that a patient has been on drug from the time of the original exposure or from the time of entry into the continuation protocol. One solution is to group patients who have been exposed to the drug for different overall periods of time (e.g., 3–6 months and 6–9 months of exposure), but several other alternative methods of calculating exposure to drug are possible. Data from Patients 1 and 2 would be combined in some situations (e.g., total duration of exposure to drug, since each would have been exposed to drug for 9 months) but not in others (e.g., duration of exposure to drug at a maintenance level in the continuation protocol, since Patient 1 would have been receiving drug for 5 months and Patient 2 for 6 months).

The initiation of continuation protocols may be further complicated if the original patients entered in the study were previously evaluated in a double-blind study and, at the time of their entry, there were at least some patients remaining in the original study. At least three dilemmas may arise in this situation. First, if the study blind is broken for the original patients at the time of their entry into the continuation protocol, then the integrity of the original study will be compromised. Second, if patients enter the continuation study in a double-blind manner, then some patients may be receiving placebo. This may raise an ethical issue that must be considered. Third, when the double blind for the first study is eventually broken, there will be implications for statistically treating the data in the continuation protocol if some patients' data were collected entirely in a double-blind manner, some patients' in an open-label manner, and some patients' data under both conditions.

Long-term exposure to a drug may be established in open-label humanitarian or "compassionate" protocols. These types of protocols are designed to expose larger numbers of patients (than were previous exposed to the drug) to a study drug during Phase III, often at many different types of sites. Only a single or a few patients may be enrolled by each investigator. The protocols serve the function of decreasing the depth of the study and increasing the breadth by including a broader population base. In essence, these studies provide data that are useful for premarketing surveillance and serve as a methodological transition to the observational survey studies that are often used in Phase IV postmarketing surveillance studies. Patients followed in this type of Phase III study could continue to be followed after the NDA has been approved and would form a pool of patients from whom postmarketing surveillance studies could be generated. Each of these possible scenarios, or others not described, must be worked out in advance of the implementation of this type of Phase III protocol.

30   Comments on Multicenter Studies

Basic Tenents of Multicenter Studies • *Administrative Considerations*

BASIC TENENTS OF MULTICENTER STUDIES

A multicenter study, by definition, utilizes one protocol at more than one site, although the protocol will usually be implemented and conducted in a somewhat different manner and style at each site.

In choosing the sites to include in a multicenter study, one usually makes an attempt to include institutions (or investigators) that are either similar or different. The specific sites may be chosen on the basis of many factors, including geography, type of institution, or types of patients seen (other factors are listed in Table 32.61). A multicenter study of a drug used to treat chronic back pain could be limited to one type of medical practice (e.g., orthopedic clinics) or hospital (e.g., Veterans Administration Hospitals) or be expanded to include pain clinics, private (or hospital-based) practitioners in family medicine and/or internal medicine, rehabilitation centers, and/or other types of medical centers or facilities at which patients with back pain are treated.

The "golden rules" of multicenter studies are (1) that protocol designs be kept relatively simple and be the same at all centers, (2) that careful planning of the initiation, conduct, and analysis of the study be mandatory and that statisticians be involved in this process, and (3) that communication problems be minimized through all possible techniques (see Section III of this book). Both formal and informal systems of communications should be established to include consideration of all aspects and organizational levels of the study.

The situation often arises in which one investigator wishes to perform an additional test in the study. The claim is usually made by the investigator that the rest of the study will not be affected. The sponsor of the multicenter study and the investigator's own Institutional Review Board (IRB) must approve this additional test. There may be strong reasons to either accept or reject this type of protocol amendment. If the proposed amendment to the protocol is accepted by the sponsor, its implementation may be limited to one site or made optional for the other sites as well.

It is important to determine whether the expected number of patients to be enrolled at each site of a multicenter study will be sufficient for the data to stand alone statistically, since data obtained from various sites may only be combined if they are determined to be compatible. Since the compatability of data from different sites cannot be assured in advance for multicenter studies, the possibility of enrolling adequate numbers of patients at each site should be considered. If this is done, then data from any site may be separated from the other sets of data. Each site may then be analyzed separately and still retain reasonable statistical power. On the other hand, one of the primary reasons for conducting a multicenter study relates to the inability of any single site to enroll an adequate number of patients. If there is a choice of conducting three separate "one-site" studies or one "three-site" multicenter study, the former choice is usually preferable.

ADMINISTRATIVE CONSIDERATIONS

Quality assurance of data obtained in multicenter studies may be conducted by establishing a group(s) to review various aspects of the study. In order to insure uniformity or standardization among centers on (1) criteria of patient eligibility, (2) diagnostic classification, (3) assessment of treatment outcome, or (4) other factors, it is often useful to have one individual or group not directly involved in the study review pertinent information on all patients. This individual or group would be assigned the function of reviewing any or all of the above points (e.g., diagnosis) according to a predetermined format and would thus function as an independent central reviewer. If questions arose on specific information reviewed, then it should be clarified whether the reviewer would contact the relevant investigator directly or contact the sponsor or monitor of the study.

Individuals who are reading and interpreting medical data or tests [e.g., electrocardiograms (ECGs), X-rays, pathology samples] may be blind to patient treatment and should perform their tasks independently of study personnel if possible. If more than one individual will be involved in one activity, then interreviewer variability may be assessed.

In addition to study personnel plus clinicians and scientists at the sponsoring institution, a number of administrative committees are sometimes established to help organize and run large multicenter studies. Many types of committees may be established, such as executive, data-monitoring, data analysis, publications, ethics, and outside advisory committees. A number of major clinical studies in recent years have utilized numerous committees, and their publications provide additional details on the procedures used (e.g., Anturane Reinfarction Trial Research Group, 1980; Winship et al., 1975; Lachin et al., 1981; β-Blocker Heart Attack Trial Research Group, 1981, 1982).

If the establishment of one or more monitoring and organizational groups to help run the drug study is contemplated, then it is essential to clearly define the role(s) of each group. A diagram of the organizational structure of one large multicenter study is shown in Fig. 30.15. (There are numerous reports and papers on the conduct and logistics of multicenter studies that may be consulted for additional details, including the following: Cancer Research Campaign Working Party, 1980; Chan et al., 1983; Friedman et al., 1982; Boissel and Klimt, 1979; Stanley et al., 1981.)

Careful planning, conduct, and analysis of a large multicenter study do not insure that the methodologies used, data gathered, or analyses performed will be accepted

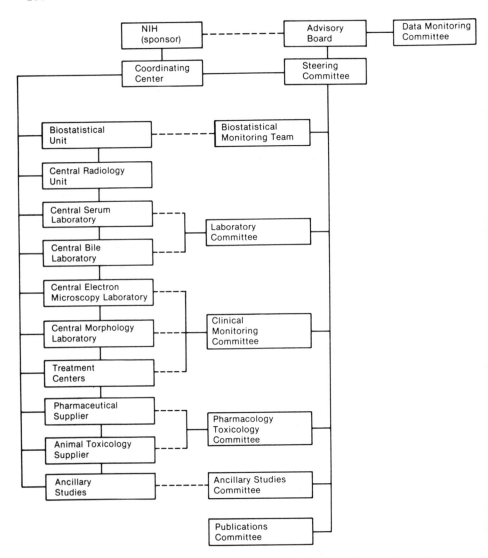

FIG. 30.15. Organizational structure of the National Cooperative Gallstone Study. (Reprinted by permission of Elsevier Science Publishing Co. from Lachin et al., 1981.)

by the medical community or by regulatory agencies. The last two decades have witnessed many of the largest (and most complex) multicenter studies ever conducted, and yet the criticism of several of these studies has been strong, and the studies have been involved in controversy. For example, there has been criticism of the data gathered in the UGDP Trial (Seltzer, 1972; Kilo et al., 1980) and the analyses performed in the Anturane Reinfarction Study (Temple and Pledger, 1980).

There is no simple solution to the dilemma of spending enormous sums of money, energy, time, patient involvement, and other resources on a large multicenter study and yet having the basic approaches or interpretation of the data strongly criticized. If the data are eventually going to be presented to the Food and Drug Administration (FDA) (or other government agency) in support of any claim, then the details of that large multicenter study design should be discussed with the FDA (or other government agency) prior to its implementation.

It may be beneficial to the conduct of a large multicenter study to arrange for an annual or interim meeting of the investigators, monitors, and possibly other study personnel. Meetings of the committees that are overseeing the study may also be held on a periodic basis. If these types of committees are not established but situations arise in which outside input is required, then a group of consultants may be brought together to discuss relevant issues.

Finally, if the results of a multicenter study are published in a monograph, then a succinct article in a widely read journal should also be considered in order to reach a wider audience.

Section III

Planning and Conducting Clinical Studies

31   Introduction

Planning, initiating, conducting, and analyzing the results of a clinical study require knowledge of and use of a large number of procedures. The specific steps followed usually differ among studies in terms of which steps are involved and how they are applied. The purpose of Section III is to present a system that can be utilized to assist individuals in performing these steps in an efficient manner.

There are important differences that are usually present between unsponsored studies initiated in academic institutions, clinics, or private practices and sponsored studies initiated by pharmaceutical corporations, government agencies, or other sponsors. These differences reflect the fact that in unsponsored studies the investigator usually assumes and modifies many of the responsibilities primarily carried out by the sponsor. For example, study monitoring conducted by the sponsor is generally replaced by internal control mechanisms in unsponsored studies; drug packaging by a pharmaceutical corporation in sponsored studies may be performed by a pharmacy for unsponsored studies. Most factors related to study initiation, conduct, and data analysis are addressed by both academicians and sponsors, although the manner in which each addresses the same issue often differs.

The approach of Section III focuses attention on the scientific method and is intended for use by pharmaceutical corporations (or other sponsors) and by clinical investigators involved in both unsponsored or sponsored studies. Some modifications will be required by each group, depending on the perspective of the individual and nature of the clinical study under consideration.

The primary assumption underlying the procedures described is that the major goal of a clinical study is to attain the objectives stated in the protocol. Obviously, this goal has a greater likelihood of being achieved if the study is planned, initiated, and conducted carefully and if the results are systematically evaluated. To achieve

TABLE 31.60. *Conduct of clinical studies*

1. Interview and selection of investigators
2. Clinical study initiation: I. Internal documents and procedures
3. Clinical study initiation: II. Information for the investigator to send to the sponsor
4. Clinical study initiation: III. Information for the sponsor to send to the investigator
5. Prestudy roundtable meeting
6. Conduct of the clinical study
7. Monitoring and troubleshooting a study
8. Clinical study termination
9. Clinical study data entry and analysis

and maintain the highest standards of performance in carrying out these steps, quality assurance methods and an organized approach to the many facets of a study should be incorporated into the overall study, and the various components of the study should be periodically assessed.

The strategy proposed to accomplish the above goals is discussed in terms of the nine categories listed in Table 31.60. A portion of this material was previously reported (Spilker, 1983).

32

Interview and Selection of Investigators

Choosing Investigators to Visit ● General Topics and Information to Discuss ● Specific Topics to Discuss ● Evaluating Patient Availability and Site Facilities ● Evaluating the Investigator

CHOOSING INVESTIGATORS TO VISIT

Some of the points discussed in this chapter will also be considered by academic or other clinical investigators who are initiating studies themselves. These relate to the planning of the study, the choice of collaborators, assistants, or research coordinators as well as to interactions with pharmacists, laboratory personnel, and other individuals who will assist in the study.

Investigators are selected by sponsors on the basis of numerous factors, any one or combination of which may be decisive in the arrival at a decision for a particular study. A list of several factors that are involved in this process is given in Table 32.61. The choice of a particular investigator for a single-site study or of several investigators for a multicenter study may be made at any stage in the development of a protocol. Agreements may be reached before the study design of a particular protocol is established or at any point prior to initiation of the study. In addition, new sites may be added to multicenter studies that are already in progress.

There are many studies in which the choice of a specific investigator(s) was not made prior to the prestudy interview. This chapter is primarily focused on this

TABLE 32.61. *Selected factors involved in investigator selection by a sponsor*

1. Reputation in the investigator's field of expertise, based on publications, references, and numerous other factors
2. Possession of equipment, techniques, or facilities essential or desirable for the study
3. Access to a patient population essential or desirable for the study
4. Geographical location of the study site in terms of ease of accessibility to the sponsor
5. Geographical location of the study site in terms of conducting the study in a desired location or region
6. Type of organization (e.g., VA hospital, nursing home)
7. Anticipated time required to initiate the study
8. Anticipated time required to complete the study
9. Relationship with individuals at the sponsoring institution
10. Budgetary factors (i.e., cost of the study)
11. Previously made agreements
12. Desirability of utilizing a contract organization to locate and enroll investigators

situation and on the process by which an investigator(s) is chosen for a study from among several who have been interviewed.

The initial step in the process of choosing investigators for a study is to develop a list of potential candidates. This is often done by using the factors listed in Table 32.61 as a guide. Any one of these factors may be of major concern in a particular study. If the sponsor prefers to have a contract organization locate and enroll investigators, then many of the processes described in this chapter would be performed by that organization.

Contract groups may be defined as businesses or organizations whose primary activity is the conduct of clinical studies. They may function independently or be an integral part of an established medical school or hospital or associated with one or more schools or hospitals. There are a number of types of contract groups, but essentially they form two basic varieties: these groups either perform clinical studies themselves or serve as middlemen to place the clinical studies at other sites. In the former case, the location of the site used for the clinical study may be at a medical school, hospital, private clinic, or building used primarily for the purpose of clinical studies. The contract groups may specialize in Phase I studies or offer to perform studies from Phase I to Phase IV. A few sites specialize in either Phase II, III, or IV studies. In the situation in which the contract group initiates the study at another site, the amount of planning, protocol writing, monitoring, and data handling, and analysis by the contract group will vary widely, often based on the requirements of the sponsor. Studies may be placed in private clinics, hospitals, or other sites depending on the specific contract organization that is contacted. Sponsors will usually be more aware of the quality and problems of a study and the data that will be provided if they monitor the study even though the contract group may also be monitoring the study. Even if it is not possible to monitor each study site, the sponsor should visit the sites at which the actual study will be performed on at least one occasion.

The sponsor of a clinical study must evaluate a number of areas, such as those discussed below, at an initial meeting with the potential investigator, preferably at the site where the study will be conducted. A list of the more important points to discuss may be prepared prior to the meeting, and a summary of the meeting is generally written after it has taken place. A synopsis of points to be covered is presented in Table 32.62. An important assumption underlying this chapter is that it is valuable to establish an open relationship with all personnel involved as well as a full understanding by each individual of his/her responsibilities in the drug study.

GENERAL TOPICS AND INFORMATION TO DISCUSS

Determine the potential investigator's research experience in general and with new and marketed drugs in particular. Ascertain the major research interests of the potential investigator in clinical and/or nonclinical medicine.

Determine if the investigator has conducted similar drug studies. This may be accomplished through computerized literature searches as well as by direct ques-

TABLE 32.62. *Selected topics to discuss with potential investigators*

---

1. General background, interests, and experience in conducting clinical studies
2. Clinic, office, and/or laboratory organization
3. Patient availability and potential enrollment
4. Protocol to be followed in conducting the drug study
5. Proposed relationship between sponsor and investigator
6. Basis on which a site or sites will be chosen for the clinical study
7. Specific areas to discuss (if indicated)
    Personnel
    Laboratory and pharmacy
    Dispensing of drugs
    Dates for conducting the study
    Data handling and retention
    Budget
    Ethics committee (Investigational Review Board)
    Informed consent and pregnancy waiver
    Biological samples containing study drug
    Publications
    Prestudy roundtable meeting
8. Other responsibilities of the principal investigator

---

tioning. If the investigator has had previous experience, discuss the design, conduct, and entry rate of patients into previous studies plus other relevant aspects (e.g., overall quality and success of the study). Obtain a copy of the published results if available.

Discuss the organization of the investigator's clinic, office, or laboratory, and whether a research coordinator, residents, assistants, laboratory personnel, nurses, or other individuals are to be included or will be available when necessary. If the site performs contract work for numerous sponsors, obtain a copy of the site's rules and regulations. Attempt to visit the site when a study is in progress and evaluate the atmosphere at the study site.

Determine how often the investigator sees the specific type of patient to be included in the study, how many new or return patients the investigator sees each month or year, and how often the investigator obtains blood levels or performs other relevant tests on patients who are followed in the practice (i.e., how patients are treated and followed).

Determine how the investigator reacts to the actual or proposed protocol and how he or she feels about this type of study in terms of its design, efficacy measures, and/or other factors. Discuss why this study is being conducted (i.e., what the study expects to demonstrate or test and/or how this study fits into the overall development of the drug). Discuss specific areas where additional information or input is desired by the sponsor in order to develop a final protocol. It is the author's view that all potential or actual investigators in a sponsored study should be given an opportunity to participate in the protocol's development if at all possible. Determine the investigator's general motivation and enthusiasm for the proposed study. If it has been decided prior to the interview that additional tests can be incorporated by individual investigator(s) into the protocol, then discuss what types of tests are acceptable and determine the investigator's interest in conducting additional tests.

Discuss how the study would be conducted at the investigator's site in terms of the background of the personnel who would be conducting the actual study, the amount of time and in what specific roles the investigator proposes to be involved, and the method(s) with which the investigator will review the work of assistants (or residents, nurses, and/or other personnel). Ascertain whether the investigator desires to have a colleague, partner, or other individual function as a co- or assistant investigator. The advantage of a co- or assistant investigator is that he/she would be familiar with the study and would be able to substitute for the principal investigator if that individual were unable to see patients. The investigator and co- or assistant investigator could each arrange to follow his/her own patients. The co- or assistant investigator(s) would also be empowered to sign data collection forms.

A discussion of the relationship between the sponsor and investigator(s) will include a review of the joint nature of the study to be conducted, since both the investigator and the sponsor will contribute to the overall project. Review the sponsor's contribution to the project, which is often in planning and implementing the study plus monitoring and analyzing data. Discuss the role of the monitor, which is to help insure a high degree of protocol adherence and attention to quality in the study's conduct.

Discuss the basis on which a site or sites will be chosen to participate in the study and whether other sites are being considered. The standards of scientific quality and cooperation and financial arrangements must be discussed with the investigator. Review the importance of the financial bid in site selection. The reputation of other potential investigators in this field may also be discussed. Indicate whether the investigator will have to sign a letter or statement of confidentiality.

Determine if the investigator has ever been audited by the Food and Drug Administration (FDA). If so, what were the conditions and results (i.e., was it a routine audit or was it "for cause")? Advise the investigator that he may be required to permit FDA inspectors to examine medical records with patients' names or previous medical histories.

SPECIFIC TOPICS TO DISCUSS

In addition to each of the areas discussed above, there are also a number of specific topics related to the proposed study that may be discussed with investigators. The specific topics listed in Table 32.62 are briefly presented in this chapter. These subjects are intended to be representative of the types of areas that may be discussed in detail and are not intended to represent a comprehensive list.

Personnel

Define the number and roles of all individuals necessary to conduct the study. Review each of the specific people to be involved in terms of his/her training, experience, and other pertinent matters. Discuss how much time each individual will devote to the study and in which specific roles he/she will be involved.

Determine if it will be necessary to hire additional staff. If new personnel are expected to join the investigator's staff, how certain is their arrival? Will all staff be present for the duration of the study, or will residents and fellows, for example, rotate to other areas and be replaced by others who must be trained? This latter situation may pose serious problems for a study in which the continuity of personnel dealing with patients is important or if it requires a long period to train the professional staff to conduct the clinical study.

Laboratory and Pharmacy

Confirm that both the laboratory and pharmacy are accredited and have adequate facilities and personnel to perform all required functions. If applicable, confirm that they have previously performed similar functions and that successful conduct of all aspects of their role can be counted on with a reasonable degree of assurance. If the pharmacy will be involved in drug packaging or dispensing, speak to the relevant pharmacist and review his/her role in detail.

Dispensing Drugs

Discuss the advantages and disadvantages of having drugs dispensed by a nurse, coordinator, pharmacist, or other individual. Discuss where drugs are kept and who has access to a key. Inspect the facilities of drug storage to confirm that they are adequate and meet reasonable standards for security.

Dates for Conducting the Study

Discuss the proposed or firm dates for conducting the study and, specifically, the expected starting date of the study, the expected rate of enrollment, and the total duration of the study.

Data Handling and Retention

Discuss how raw data will be collected, i.e., using a flow chart, data collection forms, or by other means. Determine who will complete the data collection forms. Indicate that clinical study files on investigational drugs must be retained for 2 years after the New Drug Application (NDA) is approved or for 2 years past the date the Notice of Claimed Investigational Exemption for a New Drug (IND) is cancelled. Discuss who will analyze the data and how it will be shared with all investigators.

Budget

Indicate how the investigator should prepare a budget and whether it will be itemized and whether it will include the cost of the study on a per-patient basis (total cost divided by number of patients) or on the basis of a completed study. Indicate how the sponsor will pay for this study. Clarify whether costs for patients who fail to pass the screen or baseline are included in the budget. Clarify who will pay for patients who enter but do not complete the study. The general basis for compensating patients may be discussed. Even patients who are not compensated for participating in a study may receive some funds for transportation or for other specific items (e.g., meals).

Ethics Committee

Confirm that the investigator is familiar with the process of having a protocol reviewed and approved by his Ethics Committee [Institutional Review Board (IRB)] and that he understands his obligations to them. Review the recent Federal regulations (Food and Drug Administration, 1981*a,b*) and indicate that the sponsor of the study deals with the IRB (if at all) through the investigator and not directly. The IRB must be informed at periodic intervals about progress of the study and advised immediately about any serious adverse reactions that may affect other patients in the study; they must also be informed and approve any significant changes in the protocol. The sponsor should be sent a copy of relevant correspondence between the investigator and the IRB.

Informed Consent and Pregnancy Waiver

An informed consent and pregnancy waiver are to be written at each site by each investigator. Discuss his familiarity with these forms and the regulatory requirements that must be considered in preparing them. The elements that must be included in an informed consent are presented in Table 22.49, and a sample informed consent and pregnancy waiver are illustrated in Figs. 22.11 and 22.12.

Biological Samples Containing Study Drug

Blood, plasma, or other samples that contain the parent drug and/or metabolites are often obtained in drug studies. Usually these samples are sent to the sponsor or to another site for analysis. Instructions on how to obtain and treat these samples must be clearly delineated in the protocol, as must shipping instructions about how to send samples to the sponsor (or to another facility) for analysis (see Table 22.41).

Publications

Discuss any publications that are anticipated and how they will be organized and written. If the study is multicentered, discuss if it will result in a joint publication and at which point each investigator can write individual papers. Review the various criteria for establishing the order of authorship (e.g., seniority, number of patients enrolled, alphabetical order) and decide on one approach if possible. If the study is sponsored, it may be relevant to discuss whether any individuals representing the sponsor will be coauthors.

Prestudy Roundtable Meeting

Indicate that a prestudy roundtable meeting will be conducted with relevant individuals to review and discuss all details and procedures to follow in a study prior to its initiation. This is not generally carried out at the initial prestudy site visit, when the investigator is interviewed, but optimally is conducted within 1 month prior to study initiation. Some of the above points may be discussed at the roundtable meeting rather than at the initial interview (see Chapter 34).

Other Responsibilities of the Principal Investigator

Other responsibilities of the principal investigator should be reviewed. A Final Study Report from the investigator is required by U.S. Federal regulations for the sponsor. This report will summarize the investigator's experiences with each patient in the study plus the investigator's general observations. The investigator may discuss the study in terms of the overall safety and effectiveness of the drug evaluated and compare it with known drugs used for the same clinical condition. An interim report may also be required by the sponsor (and possibly IRB), especially for studies of long duration. Investigators must send certain required information to the sponsor before a study can begin (see Clinical Initiation Form II, Fig. 33.18). This list and the general information published by the Food and Drug Administration (1977*b*, 1978, 1981*a,b*) should be reviewed with each investigator.

EVALUATING PATIENT AVAILABILITY AND SITE FACILITIES

Discuss in detail the number of patients the investigator states can be entered in the study within the proposed time limits, how patients or volunteers are obtained, and how the investigator has derived these projections. Are patients to be recruited from a private practice, clinic, or other source? Discuss whether the investigator can get referrals of patients from other doctors or clinics for this study or whether it would be advisable to advertise for patients. Review "Lasagna's Law" (the incidence of patient availability sharply decreases when a study begins and returns to its original level as soon as a study is completed; Gorringe, 1970), which is illustrated in Fig. 32.16, and discuss its implications for the current study. Discuss the number of dropouts expected and how this estimate has been reached.

A mechanism should be established whenever possible to insure that adequate numbers of patients who meet inclusion and exclusion criteria are available to the investigator prior to commencement of the study. This may be accomplished for studies involving chronic diseases by review of patient charts selected by the investigator prior to the initial visit. If one has arranged for this procedure, then a preprinted form may be prepared to enter selected data pertaining to the inclusion and exclusion criteria. For studies in which the specific patients who could enter the study cannot be identified at this visit, other procedures must be used. These include (1) reviewing records of patients previously treated to obtain an indication of the nature and numbers of patients seen by the investigator, (2) assessing the

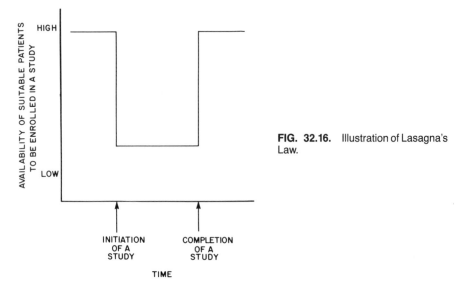

FIG. 32.16. Illustration of Lasagna's Law.

performance of the investigator in previous drug studies by contacting several references, and (3) contacting and assessing the proposed physicians or clinics who will be making patient referrals. The author believes that references from other sponsors should be obtained on all investigators in a sponsored study. Ultimately, the potential of the investigators to enroll patients must be viewed as an educated guess based on all available information.

Visit the facilities to be used in the proposed study. This includes the pharmacy, laboratories, and specialized testing areas as well as all rooms to be used for the study. Evaluate the workload of these groups and determine whether they will be able to participate in the study in a fully acceptable manner. Are the sizes of waiting rooms, offices, and laboratories adequate? Is all of the necessary equipment present and available? Determine that all laboratories to be used by the investigator have appropriate certification. Discuss calibrations, standards, and model numbers if relevant. It is important to meet and spend sufficient time with the personnel who will be involved with the study, such as assistants, coordinators, nurses, administrators, pharmacists, laboratory personnel, or others.

EVALUATING THE INVESTIGATOR

Assess how cooperative the investigator will be with the sponsor through his attitude, approach to the discussion, and willingness to discuss details and return telephone calls, plus any other available clues. The sponsor must judge whether the investigator will disclose confidences. Although it is difficult to estimate accurately the reliability of many investigators, if they are willing to provide information or copies of other protocols and data collection forms to a potential monitor, then they will probably also discuss or provide information on the monitor's protocol to others.

After the meeting has taken place, there may be a variety of materials to send to the investigator, plus items that the investigator may have promised to send or has been asked to send. The completeness and quality of the material sent by the potential investigator and the time of its arrival may be an indication of the investigator's interest in the study and ability to handle relevant details and procedures in the study. It is desirable to discuss the reputation of the potential investigator with other investigators or with other sponsors who have worked with him/her. When selection of investigators must be conducted, the above information plus knowledge of the sponsor's priorities, workload, and the factors listed in Table 32.61 will generally facilitate a decision.

33 Clinical Study Initiation

General Forms to Use as Checklists • Randomization Codes
• Informed Consents

GENERAL FORMS TO USE AS CHECKLISTS

The steps to follow and consider in initiating a clinical study after choosing the investigator(s) are presented in Figs. 33.17, 33.18, and 33.19. These forms may be useful to both sponsors and investigators and can be modified as required for an individual study. They are organized according to whether the documentation and procedures are performed within the sponsoring organization (Fig. 33.17), are sent by the investigator to the sponsor (Fig. 33.18), or are sent by the sponsor to the investigator (Fig. 33.19). Clinical scientists performing unsponsored studies can modify these forms to include only those steps and procedures that they must follow.

These forms are intended to serve as reminders of various steps or procedures that must be followed in organizing and initiating a clinical study. In addition, they are designed to monitor the flow of paperwork as it is routed through various departments and individuals. In formulating the steps in Figs. 33.17 to 33.19, the assumption was made that government approval has been received to investigate the study drug. This approval is called a Notice of Claimed Investigational Exemption for a New Drug (IND) (in the United States) for new drugs or for marketed drugs being evaluated for nonapproved indications. If this step has not been performed, or if the investigator will be conducting the drug study under his/her own IND, then additional documentation must be prepared and submitted to the appropriate regulatory authorities.

RANDOMIZATION CODES

Figure 33.20 illustrates the process by which a randomization code is obtained and utilized. Each randomization code is checked by the individual who requested it unless that person will remain blind to patient randomization. In that situation, another individual will be assigned to check the code(s). Once it is confirmed that the code was generated according to instructions, it may be used to package the drug. Drug packaging may be performed either at the study site (e.g., at the pharmacy), at the sponsor's facilities, or at another location, possibly by an independent contractor. A copy of the randomization code may be sent to the investigator, pharmacist, research coordinator, independent monitoring group, and/or other person to keep during the clinical study. If the study is open label or single blind, then the code will usually not be sealed. If the study is double blind, however,

226

Clinical Study Initiation
Form I: Internal Documents and Procedures

Study Drug: Investigator:
Protocol Number: Site:

Date and Check off each point when completed. NA = not applicable. Add Comments.

Complete 1. **Protocol**

            Draft   With Author _____
                                     With Typists _____
                                     In Review _____
                                     Section (group) _____
                                     Statistics _____
                                     Other Section(s) or Departments _____

            Final   With Typists _____
                                     Department and/or Sponsor Review _____
                                     Approved _____

_____ 2. **Data Collection Forms (DCFs)**
            Draft   In Progress _____
                                     In Review-Section _____
                                     Statistics and/or Data Entry _____
                                     At Art Department _____
            Proofs   In Review _____
                                     At Printers _____
                                     Completed _____
            Finals   Collated _____
                                     Placed in Loose Leaf Binders _____

_____ 3. **Randomization Code(s)**
                                     Requested _____
                                     Received _____

_____ 4. **Drug Supplies**
                                     Bulk Drug Availability _____
                                     Specific Drug(s) for Study Requested _____
                                     Specific Drug(s) for Study Prepared _____
                                     Bottle and Carton Drug Labels
                                     Ordered _____
                                     Bottle and Drug Labels
                                     Prepared _____
                                     Forms Filled Out to Ship Drug(s) _____

_____ 5. **FDA Submittal Forms**
                                     Packet of Forms Routed _____
                                     Approved _____

_____ 6. **Grant Request to Fund Study**
                                     Request Sent to Approve Grant _____
                                     Grant Approved _____

_____ 7. **Initial Grant Payment**
                                     Forms Sent to Have Check Prepared _____
                                     Check Recieved _____

_____ 8. **Book or Forms Prepared to Monitor Study** _____

_____ 9. **Computer Base Set Up to Monitor Study** _____

_____ 10. **Other (ex: Drug(s) needed from other Co.)** _____
                                     _____

FIG. 33.17. Clinical initiation form I: list of procedures that must be addressed within the sponsoring institution for sponsored studies or by the investigator for unsponsored studies.

Clinical Study Initiation
Form II: Information For Investigator To Send To The Sponsor

Study Drug: Investigator:
Protocol Number: Site:

Requested on _____ by letter, phone, visit.   Comments
Date and check off each item when received:

_____   1.   Curricula Vitae* _____

_____   2.   Signed FDA 1572/3 Form* _____

_____   3.   Signature(s) on Protocol Face Sheet* _____

_____   4.   IRB Approval Letter[1]** _____

_____   5.   Informed Consent (Sample)** _____

_____   6.   List of Normal Lab Values[2]** _____

_____   7.   Pregnancy Waiver Form (Sample)** _____

_____   8.   Budget for Study _____

_____   9.   Names of Assistant-or
           Co-investigators _____

_____   10.   Name of Coordinator _____
           (and/or other relevant individuals)

_____   11.   Details of How Checks are to be
           Drawn and Addressed _____

_____   12.   Other _____

_____   _____

_____   _____

* = Required for FDA

** = Required for Files

[1]Plus names and/or occupations of members

[2]The values for the specific population studied (ex: children, women) must be obtained.
The name and address of laboratory, as well as a copy of its certification must also be
received.

FIG. 33.18. Clinical initiation form II: list of information that must be sent by the investigator to the sponsor (for sponsored studies) or be dealt with by the investigator (for unsponsored studies).

then the code must be sent to the relevant individuals in a sealed manner. This may be in the form of a group of individually sealed envelopes, each containing a patient number on the outside and the identity of the treatment inside. Another means by which information in the randomization code may be made available to the investigator in cases of medical emergency is for the third part of a tear-off label on the medication bottle dispensed to have the treatment's identity hidden within the label. This portion of the label would be placed either in the patient's data collection form or in another convenient place when the bottle is dispensed and only opened in case of a medical emergency.

INFORMED CONSENTS

The relatively new Federal regulations covering informed consents (Food and Drug Administration, 1981a) should be reviewed with all investigators. Table 22.49

Clinical Study Initiation
Form III: Information For The Sponsor To Send To The Investigator(s)

Study Drug: Investigator:
Protocol Number: Site:

Date and check off each item when sent. NA = not applicable.

Comments

1. **Letter of Confidentiality**
   1. Sent _____
   2. Signed Copy Received _____

2. **Investigator's Manual (Drug Brochure)** _____

3. **Protocol**
   1. Draft Sent for Comments _____
   2. Final Sent for IRB Approval _____

4. **Drug and Drug Disposition Forms**
   (Add Amount of Drug Sent and Form No.'s) _____
   Additional Drug Sent _____

5. **Data Collection Forms (Add No. Sent)** _____
   Additional DCFs Sent _____

6. **Synopsis of Regulations on**
   Informed Consent _____

7. **Proposed FDA Regulations:**
   Obligations of Clinical Investigators _____

8. **Send on Request Only**
   1. References to Published Literature on
      Study Drug _____
   2. FDA Regulations on Standards
      for IRB's _____
   3. Proposed FDA Regulations of Obligations
      Of Clinical Sponsors and Monitors _____
   4. List of Questions Prepared for and Used
      by FDA Inspectors _____
   5. Samples of Informed Consent or Pregnancy
      Waiver Forms _____

9. **Other Study Material (If Applicable)**
   1. Prescription Blanks _____
   2. Pharmacists Record Book _____
   3. Plasma Labels _____
   4. Plasma Tubes _____
   5. Forms for Mailing Plasma Samples
      (and Procedures to Follow) _____
   6. Boxes for Mailing Plasma Samples _____
   7. Patient Instruction Sheet _____
   8. Other (list): _____
      _____ _____

10. **Letter to Authorize Study** _____
11. **Initial Grant Payment Sent** _____

FIG. 33.19. Clinical initiation form III: list of information that may be sent from the sponsor to the investigator (for sponsored studies) or dealt with by the investigator (for unsponsored studies). The IRB functions as an ethics committee to review protocols and progress of clinical studies.

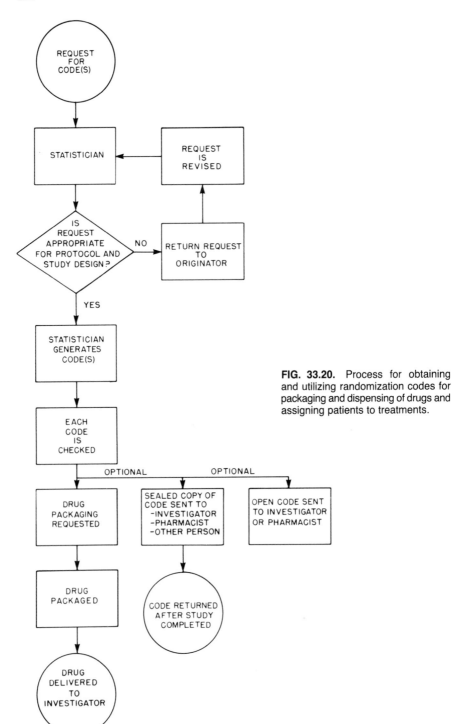

FIG. 33.20. Process for obtaining and utilizing randomization codes for packaging and dispensing of drugs and assigning patients to treatments.

presents the elements of the informed consent that must be included in all such forms according to Federal regulations (Food and Drug Administration, 1981*a*). Figure 22.11 illustrates the information that should be included (when relevant) in the various sections of an informed consent. This topic was discussed in greater detail in Chapter 22.

34 Prestudy Roundtable Meeting

If a multicenter study is being implemented, it is important to bring all investigators together prior to the starting of the study to discuss various aspects of the study and to agree on a uniform approach. Ideally, all research coordinators or assistant investigators will also be present at this meeting, or they will have a separate roundtable discussion. Since problems in communication are usually the source of most major difficulties encountered in multicenter studies, bringing all investigators together to review and discuss important points prior to the start of the study will remove many sources of misunderstanding and help insure a uniform approach.

Even when a relatively uncomplicated clinical study will be conducted by a single investigator with only a single monitor from the sponsoring organization, it is still important to hold this prestudy roundtable discussion. In an unsponsored study, the investigator may hold weekly or periodic meetings with his/her staff to plan and review the study prior to its initiation as well as to assess progress during its conduct.

The outline of a sample agenda for a prestudy roundtable meeting is presented in Table 34.63 and discussed below. This can be modified prior to the meeting to fit the particular nature of the study being discussed. Although the agenda in Table 34.63 is organized for a sponsored study, most of the points covered must also be considered by clinical investigators of unsponsored studies. A more detailed agenda may be preferred.

After the introduction of all people present, the background of the project should be discussed in terms of the investigator's manual (also referred to as an investi-

TABLE 34.63. *Sample agenda for prestudy roundtable meeting[a]*

1. Introduction of all people present
2. Background of the drug project
3. Protocol to be followed
   Introduction
   Materials and methods
   Conduct of the study
   Data analysis and publication(s)
4. Administrative responsibilities of the principal investigator and other personnel involved in the study
5. Financial matters
6. Additional topics

[a]A more detailed agenda may be prepared.

gator's brochure or by other terms) and either prior clinical experience (for investigational drugs) or published literature (for marketed drugs). This should include a general comparison of the study drug with others in the same therapeutic or chemical class. Review the protocol's development (if relevant) and other background material.

As an introduction to the present study, review how it fits into the overall plans for the drug's development and discuss the objectives of the present study. It should be clarified prior to the meeting whether the roundtable is to be used as a working session to polish the protocol and data collection forms or rather as a forum for discussion of a protocol (and data collection forms) that have been formally approved and fixed. It is preferable to allow for input at this session, especially if there has not been a prior opportunity for input or if various issues remain unresolved. Any agreed-on modifications would be incorporated into the draft protocol prior to formal approval (Stage B in Fig. 22.13).

Indicate relevant details about packaging, labeling, storing, and dispensing of the study drug(s). Review all steps of drug movement from shipping by the sponsor to receipt at the institution through dispensing to patients until the unused drug is collected from patients, stored, logged in, and returned to the sponsor. Review the forms to be completed by the investigator to document receipt of drugs and return of unused drugs. Indicate whether all dosing bottles must be saved or whether the patients' returned drugs may be combined, and describe the method of returning unused drugs to the sponsor.

If a study is being initiated in a foreign country, then discuss relevant questions as to import and export customs/regulations, language of the data collection forms, whether a different monitoring system will be used, regulatory requirements, patent considerations, legal concerns, and other related matters. Determine if there are potential problems relating to cultural differences, availability of equipment, ability to perform necessary laboratory tests, and means of converting data from one system of units to another. Decide if the study must meet Food and Drug Administration (FDA) standards. If so, then it must be designed, initiated, conducted, and analyzed accordingly. The various options for transmittal of data to the proper site must be considered (e.g., mail, telecommunications).

If the study is single or double blinded, describe the type of blind to be used and how it will be maintained. Discuss which of the monitors will remain blind and if any of the personnel at the site will be unblinded. Indicate how and when the blind will be broken, both for medical emergencies and at the end of a study. If the study involves a marketed drug, discuss how the placebo has been prepared (i.e., is it identical to the drug in taste, floating characteristics, and other factors in addition to size, shape, and color?).

Discuss any of the following points that are relevant for the conduct of the study: admission criteria, operational definitions to be used in the study, informed consent and pregnancy waiver forms, assignment of subject numbers and medications, and enrollment of backup or alternate subjects. Review any instruction (or other) forms to be handed out to each patient. Other points to consider for discussion are the randomization or stratification procedures to assign patients to different treatment groups, the criteria that will be used to determine whether to change doses or to move to another step in the protocol, and the frequency of monitoring visits plus availability of data to monitors. Also, question the investigators to determine if they anticipate any deviations from the protocol.

Discuss the time and events schedule for each day, week, and/or month. When will vital signs or other tests be performed, i.e., will certain tests be done before or after blood sampling, and how much leeway in time will be permitted in performing each test from the specified times indicated in the protocol? Review how data will be collected and kept until it is entered on the data collection forms and when the data entered on data collection forms will be available to the sponsor. If data are to be originally entered onto forms prepared by the investigator, such as "flow sheets" prior to being transcribed onto data collection forms, then the flow sheets should be reviewed and retained until all reports on the study have been completed. In some situations, data may be initially recorded on one copy of data collection forms and rewritten on a second (final) copy.

Discuss the recording of adverse reactions on data collection forms. Establish and review a brief dictionary of the most common adverse reactions expected. This procedure will help insure that similar symptoms will be described using the same term (e.g., fatigue, drowsiness, tired, sleepy, and sedated may all be described with one term by all investigators for all such adverse reactions). This will prevent a collection of many adverse reaction terms being listed in the data forms that are essentially identical. Discuss the categories chosen to relate the association between adverse reactions and the drug (such as definite, probable, possible, none, unknown). Review the categories chosen to define the intensity of the adverse reaction (mild, moderate, severe), its duration, and the steps taken by the investigator or sponsor to deal with adverse reactions. Stress the importance of the investigator notifying the sponsor of all serious adverse experiences within 24 hr.

Review the policy for premature patient discontinuation and determine which tests or examinations must be performed at the time of discontinuation. The policy for replacing discontinued patients should be reviewed. Discuss the conditions under which patients will not formally be discharged from the study in order to insure that the patients' health has had no adverse carryover effect from drug treatment. Define a "completed" patient and under what conditions (if any) patients may enter a continuation study protocol. Each of these points is discussed in Section II in more detail.

In addition to individual patient discontinuation, a complete study may be discontinued. This would occur for reasons primarily related to the sponsor and drug itself or for reasons related to the site. The conditions should be discussed under which the study, or a particular site in the study, will be discontinued for reasons relating to the investigator's performance or changes at the site.

Review how medical emergencies will be handled. Stress that the investigator must notify the sponsor and the Institutional Review Board (IRB) immediately of any serious adverse reactions. The sponsor will contact the FDA according to

Federal regulations. If the investigator is conducting an unsponsored study, he/she should be familiar with the FDA Adverse Experience Form (FDA 1639), which he/she must submit to the FDA for serious adverse reactions.

Discuss the source of syringes, needles, labels, tubes, and other items to be used for collecting and processing blood or other samples plus the procedures for obtaining, handling, and shipping of samples. Discuss the timing of biological sample collection relative to vital signs or other assessments scheduled at the "same" time. Review the availability of staff needed to conduct specialized tests such as ophthalmological examinations and indicate how patients will be taken to or arrive at the proper facilities for these examinations. Discuss whether special equipment will be required to perform any test(s) at the site, and if it is not present, how this equipment will be obtained and used.

The principal investigator has some administrative responsibilities, which include writing a Final Study Report (an interim report may also be required). Establish a time limit for this report to be received by the sponsor (and/or IRB). The investigator must review each page of the data collection forms and sign or initial the data collection forms in an agreed-on manner. At the roundtable, each unique page of the data collection forms should be reviewed. Indicate how data, notes, and unscheduled tests and examinations are to be entered and how errors on the forms are to be corrected.

Discuss relevant IRB interactions and FDA regulations, including what reports are required by each and whether the sponsor or investigator has primary responsibility. Discuss who will replace or fill in for the investigator if he/she becomes ill or goes on a trip.

Discuss with the principal investigator(s) which items are or are not included in the budget and how bills should be submitted to the sponsor. Review the number of fractional payments to be made and the time points in the study at which each payment will be made. A commonly used arrangement is to pay investigators half of the agreed-on budget at the start of the study (often defined as the entry of the first patient) and the other half at the end of the study, after the Final Study Report has been received. Another common plan is to pay one-third at the outset, one-third when half of the patients are completed, and one-third at the conclusion of the study. Various other alternatives are also used.

It is important to schedule a sufficient amount of time for this meeting so that it is productive and may achieve optimal effectiveness. Although no firm guidelines may be given about how much time is required, it is the author's experience that a half day is necessary for most studies of average complexity and that multicentered studies often require a full day if numerous issues must be resolved. Major national studies with multimillion dollar budgets will probably require both more time and more than just a single meeting to accomplish all of the tasks necessary to successfully launch and maintain such a large-scale project.

35 Conducting the Clinical Study

Strategies • Unanticipated Situations • Patient Recruitment • Patients Lost to Follow-up

STRATEGIES

At the time that a study is being initiated, it is important to plan the strategy of how its monitoring can most effectively be conducted. In this chapter (and Chapter 36) some techniques are described that can be used to achieve the appropriate balance between "tight" and "loose" monitoring. A number of the more common aspects related to conduct of the study are presented in Fig. 35.21.

UNANTICIPATED SITUATIONS

Many unanticipated situations arise during the course of most studies, and it is desirable to have a standard approach available that can be used to deal effectively with the more common situations. This enables the study to proceed (or to be discontinued) with the fewest problems. Some of the unanticipated situations that frequently arise during drug studies include severe adverse reactions or death(s) after the drug, changes in personnel, unapproved modifications introduced into the protocol ("unofficially"), or other protocol violations, and slower than anticipated patient enrollment. In order to minimize the impact of these and other problem situations on the overall conduct of the study, it is advisable for sponsors to choose investigators carefully and to monitor the study closely for early signs of what may later become significant problems. It is advisable for investigators to conduct a "dry run" (prior to starting the actual study) with a fictional or trial patient. This patient will be processed and taken through all steps of the protocol to work out procedures, time requirements, scheduling of tests and visits, and data handling. At the end of the "dry run," the investigator will attempt to devise (or revise) a series of steps to efficiently conduct the study, supply food to patients (if necessary), allow for recreation (if pertinent), and identify and solve potential or real problems that have arisen.

PATIENT RECRUITMENT

Although patients are often recruited for studies from the medical practice of the investigator, there are numerous occasions when this is either not possible or is not the sole source of patient recruitment. A series of articles dealing with recruitment of patients from various other sources was published in the December,

Conducting the Clinical Study

Study Drug: Investigator:
Protocol Number: Site:

Check and Date. Add Number, if relevant, or comments.

1. **Initiation**
    All Forms Received from Investigator _____
    All Forms Approved by Sponsor _____
    All Forms Sent to FDA _____
    Investigator Told to Proceed _____

2. **Monitoring**
    Identify Monitor(s) & Role _____
    Plan Monitoring Strategy (see text) _____
    Plan Frequency of Telephone and Personal Contact_____

3. **Supplies Sent to Investigator(s)**
    Additional Study Drugs _____
    Additional Data Collection Forms (DCFs) _____
    Other:_____

4. **Plasma Samples, DCFs Received From Investigator(s)**
    Plasma or Other Biological Samples _____
    DCFs _____
    Adverse Reaction Report(s) _____
    Other:_____

5. **Financial**
    Additional Funds Requested by Investigator _____
    Forms Sent to Request Funds _____
    Funds Sent to Investigator _____

6. **Unanticipated Situations**
    Protocol Changes, Addenda or Extensions
    (Sponsor & IRB to Approve) _____
    Severe Adverse Reactions or Deaths. Reports from
    (1) Invest. to Sponsor and IRB _____
    (2) Sponsor to Files, FDA and other Invest. _____
    Other:_____ _____
    _____ _____
    _____ _____

FIG. 35.21. List of procedures that may be utilized by the sponsor and/or investigator during the course of a clinical study.

1982 issue of *Circulation* (Agras and Bradford, 1982). These articles discuss the advantages and disadvantages of using the sources of patient recruitment listed in Table 35.64. Another discussion of recruitment in a large multicenter study presented data from the National Cooperative Gallstone Study (Croke, 1979).

It is an accepted generalization that in most clinical situations patient recruitment becomes progressively easier as the admission criteria of the study ease. This was confirmed when Croke (1979) observed that the ability of 10 centers to recruit

TABLE 35.64. *Sources of patient recruitment[a]*

---

1. Government employees (e.g., military)
2. Private industry (e.g., clinics in large industries)
3. Medical referrals from professional colleagues (i.e., from direct contact)
4. Referrals from clinical laboratories
5. Mass media strategies (via newspaper or radio advertisements)
6. Mass mailings
7. Community screening (e.g., health fairs)
8. Participants in other clinical studies
9. Blood banks (blood donors)
10. Local advertisements (notices on bulletin boards)
11. Other sources

---

[a]Other than through the investigator's own practice or through unsolicited visits by patients to the investigator.

TABLE 35.65. *Selected factors that influence patient recruitment[a]*

---

1. Source of patient referral: medical sources, other clinical studies, clinical laboratories, blood banks
2. Number of patients contacted via letter, telephone, or direct approach using mass mailing, mass media, friends, advertisements, or other methods
3. Specific place where mass screening occurs: at work place, educational facility, social group, community location, or elsewhere
4. Socioeconomic composition of the patient pool
5. Resources of time, personnel, and money available to devote to this effort
6. Location of the study site relative to patients' home or work[b]
7. Degree of concern that patients have for their disease
8. Nature of the appeal to patients to enroll in the study[c]
9. Specific requirements and demands of the study (e.g., in terms of difficult or disagreeable tests)
10. Amount of remuneration or other benefits (e.g., meals, transportation) given to patients

---

[a]Most inclusion and exclusion criteria are not considered in this table, but these criteria have a major impact on patient recruitment.
[b]Use of outreach programs and flexible schedules for clinic visits may improve recruitment.
[c]Presenting benefits in a positive approach and concentrating on personal motives of the patients may improve recruitment.

volunteers was increased by loosening the criteria of admission into the study. This change had a far greater impact on the enrollment rate of patients than did any of the other methods used to increase patient enrollment at the different sites. Other discussions of patient recruitment are found in the following references: Agras and Marshall (1979), Prout (1979), Schoenberger (1979), and Benedict (1979). A list of some factors that influence patient recruitment is presented in Table 35.65.

In many studies, problems are encountered as a result of a low rate of patient entry. It is generally useful to develop (prior to the study) a series of alternative techniques to attempt to increase enrollment if the rate of patient enrollment becomes a problem. A list of some of these techniques is presented in Table 35.66. If these techniques are not successful, then it may be necessary to decrease the number of patients in the study. The new number chosen should be reached in

TABLE 35.66. *Selected techniques to increase patient recruitment*

---

1. Loosen the inclusion/exclusion criteria[a]
2. Loosen the demands of the protocol (e.g., eliminate some or all disagreeable tests)
3. Speak informally to additional colleagues directly or by telephone to request referrals
4. Speak at formal or informal professional meetings and request referrals
5. Write letters to colleagues and request referrals
6. Put notices in places where colleagues and/or patients may notice
7. Print leaflets and distribute directly to potential patients
8. Advertise in local or regional sources (newspapers, TV, radio)
9. Contact patients directly at health fairs or by radio and TV appearances (for large multicenter studies with widespread relevance)
10. Add additional sites to the study[a]
11. Increase or initiate payment or other benefits to patients (e.g., include payment for transportation and/or meals)
12. Increase the time of the study's duration[a]
13. Hire additional personnel to help recruit patients
14. Conduct additional chart reviews and/or reviews of pharmacy records (e.g., in a nursing home)
15. Add a continuation protocol so that patients may continue to receive a study drug if they have demonstrated clinical improvement in the study[a]
16. Determine which techniques are working best at sites with high recruitment rates and utilize those techniques at sites with lower recruitment rates

---

[a]This should be evaluated with a statistician and may require Institutional Review Board (IRB) approval.

collaboration with a statistician. Although a lowering of the required sample size is usually accompanied by a decrease in the power of the statistical tests used, it is sometimes possible to decrease the sample size without compromising these values. For example, consideration of a secondary hypothesis may be dropped, or different statistical tests may be found to be more appropriate tools to analyze the data.

There may be a temptation in some Phase II and III studies to encourage patients to enroll in the study by offering overly generous benefits. It is the author's view that neither money nor other nonmedical inducements should be given to patients so that their primary motivation to enroll in a study is for any monetary "reward" that may be offered. This view must be modified for Phase I clinical studies and for bioavailability and selected other studies, where financial benefit is accepted as the primary motivating factor for many volunteers rather than the desire to help medical research. Patients with most chronic diseases usually enroll in a study out of a strong desire to receive an effective treatment for their medical disease. This desire is also shared by many other patients who participate in clinical studies.

Another potential problem with recruitment occurs when recruitment is "too successful" and there are more patients who wish to enter the study than can be handled with available resources. If the patient supply is expected to remain high, then the number of patients entering the study every day (week or month) may be budgeted. If, however, the patient supply is only temporarily high (e.g., students are expected to return home from school), then an attempt can be made to increase or adjust the resources to handle the temporarily increased patient load. There are limits to how many additional patients may be included into virtually all studies within a given time period. The quality of a study will undoubtedly suffer if an excessive number of patients are either rushed through a study or dealt with more superficially than is appropriate.

When patient recruitment has utilized referrals from other physicians, there are a number of additional considerations. Investigators should provide relevant study data and information plus other feedback to colleagues who have referred patients for the investigator's study. This can be done on one or more occasions, depending on the length and nature of the study, and usually takes the form of a letter or possibly a telephone call. This practice should be followed as a matter of professional courtesy as well as a part of the ethical responsibility of temporarily caring for another physician's patient. If the study has a clinically significant effect on the disease for which the patient was being treated by the referring physician, then a detailed account of all clinically relevant events and data should be communicated to the original physician.

PATIENTS LOST TO FOLLOW-UP

In studies that have a long duration (i.e., in terms of months or years), it is sometimes difficult or impossible to locate patients who do not attend scheduled clinics. In most cases, the location of these patients or their medical status is not especially important to determine, but there are studies in which their vital status may be critical to the outcome of the study (e.g., if death is used as an end point). In those particular studies, there are several methods for locating these patients. These methods include contacting a patient's friends, relatives, employers, as well as using social security numbers, national death registries, and even private detectives (see Table 22.44). If these steps might be envisioned as potentially necessary, then relevant information about the patient's outside contacts should be sought at the start of a study. It would also be relevant to indicate to the patients in the informed consent that a search might be conducted at a later date to determine their location, vital status, and medical condition.

36

Monitoring and Troubleshooting a Study

Basic Monitoring Strategy • Monitoring at the Investigator's Site • Monitoring Activities at the Sponsoring Institution

BASIC MONITORING STRATEGY

There are many aspects to the successful monitoring of a clinical study. One of the most important points is to plan a basic strategy at the time of initiation of a clinical study. This strategy will contain a number of different elements. Although the monitoring function suggests that one is referring to a sponsored study, in fact all unsponsored studies involve monitoring through periodic review and internal checks of performance and results. Although the monitoring function may focus on selected aspects of the study, there are four basic areas that must be periodically assessed. These involve confirmation that (1) the facilities remain adequate, (2) the study is proceeding according to protocol, (3) the investigator and other study personnel are fulfilling their various obligations, and (4) the data on the data collection forms are accurate and complete.

One of the rarely perceived functions of monitoring is to help maintain and improve the morale and enthusiasm of the staff. The means of achieving this goal vary among studies and individual monitors, but some attention should be devoted to this consideration by all monitors. These and other functions are listed in Table 36.67. Investigators of unsponsored studies are also concerned with internal monitoring. Thus, the comments below are applicable to both sponsors and clinical investigators (of sponsored and unsponsored studies), even though various aspects will require modification.

Monitoring visits or internal assessments should be conducted on a regular basis. Discuss how frequently and with whom they will occur and also how telephone and/or mail communications will be integrated into the monitoring strategy and how they will be implemented. Consider sending investigators letters that document significant decisions or changes in the study whether the decision was reached during a telephone conversation, at a site visit, or in a different manner. Discuss the role of the monitor(s) with the investigator and any assistants or coordinators participating in the study. Monitors may be associated with the investigator, sponsor, or contract organization setting up the study for a sponsor, or they may function independently and not be directly associated with either sponsor or investigator. This last method is sometimes used in large multicenter studies, where an independent monitoring group is established.

TABLE 36.67. *Selected functions of a clinical study monitor*

A. Related to protocol
   1. Evaluate recruitment rate and number of patients entered into the study
   2. Evaluate eligibility of patients enrolled
   3. Evaluate randomization of patients to treatment groups
   4. Evaluate conduct of the study according to good clinical practices
   5. Evaluate adequacy and accuracy of data obtained
   6. Evaluate timely and accurate entry of data onto data collection forms
   7. Evaluate transmittal of information on all important adverse reactions and other relevant matters to appropriate individuals at sponsoring institution or on monitoring committee
B. Administrative
   1. Insure adequacy of site with regard to good clinical practices
   2. Insure adequacy of professional treatment of patients
   3. Transfer biological samples and data collection forms as directed
   4. Arrange for payment of investigator
   5. Arrange for the availability of adequate drug(s), supplies, data collection forms, and other items
   6. Confirm that proper contacts between the sponsor and Institutional Review Board (IRB) are maintained
   7. Handle *ad hoc* problems and maintain communication with all relevant individuals
   8. Encourage a positive interest and involvement in the study by all study personnel (i.e., attempt to keep morale high)
   9. Assist in study termination procedures
  10. Assist in data handling, data analysis, and publications

---

Confirm that the procedures to be followed for communication are explicit and discuss the purposes for telephone and direct visits. In planning the frequency of visits or internal assessments, consider the personality and reliability of the investigator and/or the staff plus the nature and relative importance of the drug study and also the resources of the sponsor. An independent consultant or group of consultants may be contacted at any stage of a study to assist with problems encountered, interpretation of data, or other matters. In addition, medical consultants at the investigator's site may be contacted prior to the start of the study to evaluate patients if problems are anticipated that would require their expert help in diagnosis or treatment. Clarify that the sponsor must have access to all records generated in this study to insure accuracy of data transcription.

Contact the investigator and/or study coordinator prior to each visit so that he/she is aware of its purpose as well as an estimate of time requirements. This allows the investigator time to prepare for discussions that may focus on specific topics known in advance. Discuss the amounts of drug and supplies that are at the site and whether additional drug or supplies are needed. An agenda may be prepared if indicated. Reconfirm each trip approximately 1 to 3 days prior to its scheduled time to insure that the meeting will be held as scheduled and that the monitoring trip is likely to be productive. In an unsponsored study, the principal investigator should establish procedures and guidelines for the conduct of periodic internal assessments of all aspects of the study. This process of internal monitoring includes observations of physicians, other study personnel, and patients, and assessment of data recording and entry.

MONITORING AT THE INVESTIGATOR'S SITE

An important role of a clinical monitor is to review (edit) the data collection forms at each visit. It is usually more efficient for the monitor to review these records prior to meeting with the investigator and/or research coordinator. The records should be reviewed for:

1. Problems of omission (e.g., missing or incomplete data, dates, or other information). Confirm that a properly signed and witnessed informed consent and pregnancy waiver (when appropriate) are in each patient's chart. The monitor should also confirm that the investigator's notes adequately explain missed visits or tests, patient dropouts, and any relevant abnormalities that are noted by the monitor.
2. Problems of commission (e.g., errors that must be changed on the data collection forms by the investigator or coordinator).
3. Areas to explain or clarify (e.g., abnormal or inconsistent data).
4. Legibility. If a monitor cannot read the form, other people probably cannot either.
5. Use of black ink, since blue ink does not usually microfilm well.
6. Corrections that have been properly entered according to established procedures.

One method to help monitors from reediting a page on a subsequent site visit is to initial each page reviewed, either in a corner of the page or on a blank line titled "edited by" (if one was included on the data collection form). The procedure of initialing a page may be used only after the entire page is completed and has been signed or initialed by the investigator, if that is part of the protocol. Pages should not be altered after they are signed by the investigator without the monitor being informed.

The progress of efficacy and/or safety parameters in some drug studies is followed by collecting selected data on an ongoing basis in a "monitor's book." This book often consists of one or more forms per patient kept in a loose-leaf or other similar binder. The monitor's book should be filled out at each visit and/or updated via telephone contacts. The information collected should concentrate on the most important efficacy and safety parameters. Computers may also be utilized to follow the conduct and results of drug studies. This process will require careful organization and planning prior to study initiation. In a few drug studies to date, data have been transmitted directly from the investigator's site to the sponsor by computer and telephone connections. This process of information transmittal will probably become more widespread in the future.

In addition to the editing function, a monitor should review the data and look for trends, problems, or relevant areas to discuss with the investigator and/or research coordinator. The monitor can perform this role most effectively in double-blind studies if he/she also remains blind to patient assignment. At some sponsoring institutions, it is a standard procedure to have monitors remain blind to patient randomization. Some specific examples of this function include an evaluation of whether the attribution of adverse reactions to the study drug (i.e., possible, definite, unknown, etc.) was the same at subsequent visits to the sites at which the adverse reaction was reported. When terms such as "double vision," "dizziness," and other potentially ambiguous phrases are reported, the specific characteristics observed should be indicated. Also, the monitor should evaluate whether laboratory results are showing gradual changes or trends even if all values are still within the normal range. If a laboratory test is reported to be markedly abnormal in the data collection form, it may be worthwhile to compare the value with the original laboratory slip (report) to insure that there was not a transcription error. Calling the laboratory to discuss the value may also be worthwhile. Determine whether a repeat laboratory test was performed. Consider having duplicate samples sent to two different laboratories. The monitor should confirm that the investigator is notifying the sponsor of all serious adverse reactions within 24 hr.

Checks for protocol adherence include evaluation of the number of missed visits and patient noncompliance as measured by pill counts, plasma level fluctuations, or other methods. Some of the simpler mathematical calculations on the data collection forms should be checked to insure that the numbers are being handled properly and that the numbers are added or subtracted correctly. The data collection forms should be corrected, if possible, during the same site visit. Otherwise, the questioned pages of the data collection forms should be reviewed at the following visit to insure that necessary changes have been made.

The monitor can list specific questions or problems concerning data entry on a preprinted blank form for discussion at that visit with the coordinator and/or investigator. It is often convenient to use one of these forms per patient. In meeting with the investigator and/or coordinator, the monitor should review these forms as well as the specific topics mentioned on the telephone or in a letter that was sent to the investigator prior to the visit. Review questions and problems that concern the investigator and coordinator and discuss how these can be solved. Ascertain that the investigator is maintaining required contact with the Institutional Review Board (IRB).

The monitor should periodically visit the pharmacy (if relevant) and review their dispensing records for the study. A separate "pharmacist's book" can be prepared that will contain information on drug dispensing and returned medication if it will assist in the conduct of the study (see Fig. 18.9 for an example). Insure that returned drug supplies are being properly documented and handled. Discuss questions and relevant procedures with the pharmacist. Examine the biological samples that are being collected. Confirm that the relevant samples have been collected and are properly labeled and stored. Labels may be preprinted with the study number, patient number, sample number, and other relevant data. Adhesive may be required to affix labels to tubes or other containers, and waterproof pens may be sent to investigators if any writing is required on the label.

If a Food and Drug Administration (FDA) audit is being conducted when a monitor arrives at a site, or an audit is initiated while the monitor is working at the site, a policy governing the monitor's behavior must be established by the sponsor. The monitor should obtain the results of any audits conducted at sites with which he/she is in contact.

MONITORING ACTIVITIES AT THE SPONSORING INSTITUTION

During the course of the study, the monitor should confirm the arrival of all drugs, data collection forms, and supplies at each site. This process should include confirmation that the correct number of cartons was received in each shipment. A letter of transmittal should be sent separately from the items shipped to alert the investigator of the pending shipment. Complete any forms required by the sponsor after each visit and document all important decisions and changes related to the protocol or study.

The monitor may be contacted if it becomes necessary to break the study blind for a medical emergency and the randomization code for the patient is not readily available to the investigator. A copy of the randomization code should be accessible for such emergencies. Copies are often maintained both at the sponsor's office and at the home of one of the monitors. Provisions must be made for situations in which the monitor is out of town, "unavailable," or is blind to patient randomization. A standard series of procedures (e.g., obtaining blood and urine specimens and samples of medication for chemical analysis) may be developed for situations in which patients are discontinued for medical reasons.

The monitor may assign unused drugs for backup patients at the study site to patients if problems have occurred and additional drug is required. This should be done with care and preferably after consultation with a statistician. Many unusual and "unique" situations seem to arise in almost all studies, which challenge the imagination and creativity of the monitor in arriving at a satisfactory solution.

37 Clinical Study Termination

Procedures for Terminating a Study • Extending a Study • End-of-Study Questionnaire or Interview

PROCEDURES FOR TERMINATING A STUDY

The process of terminating a study may take less than a day or possibly require more than a year, depending on the complexity and nature of the study as well as the efficiency with which it is dismantled. The major aspects that must be considered in dismantling a study are indicated in Fig. 37.22. This figure is intended as a guide, for both sponsored and unsponsored studies, to indicate many of the steps that must be dealt with to comply with government regulations, Institutional Review Board (IRB) agreements, requirements of the sponsor, and good clinical practice (see Food and Drug Administration, 1977b, 1978, 1981b for details). Prior to following the steps in Fig. 37.22, the investigator must prepare the patients for the study's discontinuation, inform them in some manner about the results, arrange for continuation of their medical care, and collect the final data to be incorporated into the data collection forms. The order and emphasis placed on each step will differ to some degree between studies that are terminated normally and those that are prematurely discontinued. The investigator must also plan for the storage of study documents and forms according to Federal guidelines and regulations. These documents may have great value if questions arise at a later date regarding a patient's toxicity, about details in this particular study, or as an aid in the development of a new study.

In double-blind studies, a decision must be made as to when the investigator will be provided with the drug code. In general, this should occur only after the study is completed and all data collection forms have been signed by the investigator and received by the sponsor. The degree to which the double blind was truly effective could be evaluated by asking the investigator to guess which treatment each patient received. The reason(s) for the investigator's decision in categorizing each patient should also be recorded (i.e., was the decision based on adverse reactions, specific laboratory changes, improvement or deterioration in the underlying disease, or other factors?). Patients in either single- or double-blind studies can be asked to guess which treatment they received as well as the reason(s) for their decision. These surveys may provide useful information for designing more effective controls in future studies.

Clinical studies may be terminated prematurely for positive or negative reasons. A positive reason would be that a beneficial effect was detected in the data that raised ethical concerns about continuing patients in the study who were not receiving this treatment. Negative reasons for premature study discontinuation would

Clinical Study Termination

Study Drug: Investigator:
Protocol Number: Site:

Date and check when completed.   Comments

DCFs

_____ Returned to sponsor[1]   _____

_____ Copy retained at site   _____

Biological Samples

_____ All samples sent (brought) to sponsor (or other facility)   _____

Pharmacy (or person who dispenses drugs)

_____ Records reviewed & copies sent to sponsor   _____

_____ Forms completed, signed and returned to sponsor   _____

_____ Drug returned to sponsor   _____

Principal Investigator

_____ Signed or initialed all DCFs   _____

_____ Final Study Report received by sponsor   _____

_____ Final statement sent to the IRB   _____

_____ Drug forms signed   _____

Financial

_____ Determine number of completed and "partial" patients   _____

_____ Final budget request received from investigator _____

_____ Memo to request funds[2]   _____

_____ Money sent to investigator   _____

Data

_____ Analyses of data[1]   _____

_____ Publishing of data discussed   _____

_____ Article(s) and/or abstract(s) prepared   _____

_____ Article(s) and/or abstract(s) reviewed   _____

[1]See next Figure
[2]After the Final Study Report and all data have been received.

FIG. 37.22. List of procedures to consider during the termination period of a clinical study.

include unacceptable adverse reactions or laboratory abnormalities. This has been described more fully in Section II.

For studies that are discontinued prior to their scheduled ending point, there may be special considerations to evaluate. Should all patients be discontinued or only certain groups, and how should discontinued patients be treated? For studies in which only some patients are discontinued, all patients must be informed of the negative (or positive) data, and a new informed consent obtained. It may be useful to collect additional data not requested in the original protocol at the time of discontinuation. The decision on which specific data to collect will depend on the reasons for the discontinuation and the circumstances related to the conduct of the study (e.g., resources, time availability). The means by which patients will be discontinued must be established. If the scope of the study or the implications of the reason the study was discontinued warrant public notification, then an announcement to the press must be considered.

EXTENDING A STUDY

In addition to the process of terminating a study, situations may arise in which the duration of the study should be extended. Depending on the nature of the study, this may require an amendment to the protocol. The most common reason a study is extended is that fewer patients enrolled than was expected. To extend a study under these conditions, it is usually necessary only to increase the allowable recruitment time and not to modify the protocol. In this situation, the original goal remains intact, i.e., to achieve the originally targeted sample size. A second reason for extending a study is when a larger placebo effect is observed than expected, and the original sample size is found to be too small to achieve the desired power. In this situation, increasing the duration of the study to obtain a greater sample size than originally planned will be necessary to provide adequate power (i.e., the same power as originally intended). A third possibility is that fewer events being measured were observed than had been predicted. In this situation, it might be necessary to modify the protocol and to follow patients for a longer period of time in order to observe the event(s) that are being monitored (e.g., death) or measured (e.g., a specific increase, decrease, or change in a physiological parameter). If patient deaths are being used as an endpoint, then prolonging the study would be expected to increase the total number of events (deaths) observed.

END-OF-STUDY QUESTIONNAIRE OR INTERVIEW

It is often useful to incorporate an end-of-study questionnaire into the clinical study. This questionnaire may explore the adherence to, and quality of, the blind by asking patients to guess which treatment they believed they were receiving, how sure they were of their choice, and the reasons why they made that choice. Table 37.68 lists factors to consider in designing a poststudy questionnaire. Investigators can also be questioned with these or similar questions prior to breaking a blind. This may allow better study designs to be developed for use in future clinical studies. Examples of the data obtained with this type of questionnaire are presented in papers by Karlowski et al. (1975) and Howard et al. (1982). It has been clearly shown by Karlowski et al. (1975) that when patients break a study's blind, it may have a significant impact on the data obtained.

TABLE 37.68. *Factors to consider in designing a poststudy questionnaire*

1. Determine whether all patients or only a sample will be given the questionnaire
2. If a sample is chosen for this test, determine how they will be chosen
3. Determine if a telephone interview, direct interview, written questionnaire, or combination of approaches will be used
4. Appoint or choose the individual(s) who will conduct this phase of the study
5. Determine if a pilot project will be conducted with the questionnaire
6. Decide whether the data from the questionnaire will be analyzed to evaluate the study blind
7. Design a standard series of questions to evaluate the study blind, for example:
   Patients' guess as to their treatment
   Patients' "certainty" as to their guess
   Did patients "test" their medication (e.g., taste, smell)?
   Other questions (e.g., about compliance)
8. Additional questions may be posed to evaluate different factors in the study
9. If a similar questionnaire is to be given to each investigator, evaluate his/her guesses as to each patient's treatment and the reasons for these guesses (were the guesses based on adverse reactions, altered blood levels, clinical improvement, clinical deterioration, or other factors?)

If questions relating to the study blind are posed at the conclusion of a pilot study, then the information obtained may permit a better study design to be created for future studies. For example, if certain clues help an investigator break the study blind, such as changes in blood levels of concomitant drugs or abnormal laboratory values, then this information may be kept from the investigator in a subsequent study by utilizing a technique such as the "two-physician method" discussed in Chapter 3.

A different type of poststudy questionnaire was used by Hassar and Weintraub (1976). They evaluated whether patients in their study understood the risks involved in the study they had completed. The patients' memory of the informed consent that they had signed on entry into the study was also tested. The authors found that patients committed three types of errors in memory. First, many patients did not recall one of the major risks inherent in the study despite the fact that it was verbally reported to each patient on three occasions and each patient had read it twice. Second, patients made errors about the contents of certain discussions held with investigators, and, third, patients constructued entirely fallacious information. The authors suggested means for obtaining an informed consent, which are presented in Chapter 22 of this book.

Prior to incorporating a poststudy questionnaire into a study, it should be reviewed and evaluated for clarity and content. In addition, both colleagues and patients should complete these questionnaires to determine that the instructions for their use are easy to understand and that the form is easy to fill out.

38   Clinical Study Data Entry and Analysis

One approach to the processing and analysis of data is to divide the data into three parts, as shown in Fig. 38.23. This approach focuses on (1) handling of data collection forms by the monitor(s), (2) entering that data into a suitable computer by data processors, and (3) analyzing the data in conjunction with statisticians. These stages are essentially identical for both sponsored and unsponsored clinical studies, although modifications of the steps in Fig. 38.23 will be required for each study.

Data editing is part of the quality control system that is an important aspect of all studies. The data-editing process refers to the procedures by which the coded and/or uncoded data on the data collection forms are reviewed for its presence, completeness, legibility, accuracy, and consistency with prior and subsequent data. This is performed both during the study by monitors and subsequent to the study by monitors and/or specially trained data editors. Unusual or inappropriate values or codes in data entry should be brought to the attention of the data editor and evaluated at the proper stage of data evaluation. For many studies, data are entered twice into the computer, and a program is used to compare every datum in the two files to check for nonidentical information. Any discrepancies between the two files are printed by the computer, and an individual must determine which of the two values is correct. After all the data are correctly entered, a further quality assurance process is utilized wherein a sample of the data entered is compared with the original data collection forms to determine an error rate.

Prior to data analysis, the manner should be determined by which the data will be presented and evaluated. This involves the processes of setting up prototype tables and also determining the criteria and level of significance that will be utilized to define efficacy. The criterion setting should take place during the planning phase of the study and be completed by the time the protocol is approved. The prototype tables may be prepared during or subsequent to the study. A series of prototype tables and figures to present safety data from a hypothetical multicentered double-blind evaluation of a study drug versus placebo is given in Appendix 2 and represents one of several approaches that could be used to present safety data. The major areas covered are study characteristics, physical examinations, electrocardiogram (ECG), laboratory examinations, and adverse reactions.

In addition to the tables presented in Appendix 2, it might be useful to include in an appendix to a Final Statistical Report (1) all raw data, (2) all data summarized by patient, and (3) all data summarized by center in those tables in which the data from all 10 centers are combined (e.g., Tables A.8, A.10, A.11). Data on efficacy would require their own series of prototype tables and figures. Site-to-site differ-

Clinical Study Data Entry and Analyses

Study Drug: _____ Investigator: _____

Protocol Number: _____ Site: _____

Date and check when completed. Comments

DCFs

___ Final Edit at Site or at Sponsoring Inst. _____

Completed _____

___ DCFs Received by Sponsor _____

Completed _____

___ DCFs Logged In _____

___ DCFs Sent to Investigator for Changes _____

___ DCFs Copied and Distributed _____

___ DCFs Sent to Computer Section _____

___ DCFs Received at Computer Entry _____

Computer Entry

___ Personnel Assigned _____

___ Data Entry Planned with Medical Input _____

___ Program Written to Enter Data _____

___ Data Edited _____

___ Data Entered (Single or Double Entry) _____

___ Data Quality Assured _____

___ Data Released for Statistical Analysis _____

Statistical Analyses

___ Personnel Assigned _____

___ Data Analysis Planned with Medical Input _____

___ Draft Report Prepared _____

___ Draft Report Received and Reviewed _____

___ Final Report Released _____

FIG. 38.23. List of procedures to consider during the data entry and analysis period of a clinical study.

ences in the data must be evaluated, and the data obtained at the different sites must be statistically comparable before the data may be combined. If data from different studies are collected with the same data collection forms, analyzed in the same way, and presented in the same format, then the eventual combining of data from different studies will be e: pedited.

The question of whether to perform subgroup analyses not originally intended in the study is a controversial topic. After the data are examined, they may suggest comparisons or observations that were not expected or were not originally sought. The most appropriate use of these analyses is to design further clinical studies in which the new results found with this technique may be systematically examined.

After these procedures are completed and the data are analyzed, a Final Medical Report is usually written by the sponsor. This Final Medical Report prepared by the sponsor differs from the Final Study Report prepared by the investigator participating in a sponsored study. The latter is a brief synopsis of the investigator's experiences with the drug and is often presented as a summary of experiences with each patient and a comparison of the study drug's overall safety and efficacy with known drugs of a similar class. The former report is generally prepared in a format suitable for submission to a governmental regulatory agency. The analogous report prepared by the investigator of an unsponsored study is usually a paper intended for publication. In both sponsored and unsponsored studies, the investigator must adhere to and complete all requirements stipulated by the Institutional Review Board (IRB).

Following good standards of protocol development and study conduct optimizes the chances of achieving a meaningful study whose interpretations will be accepted. It is thus important not to allow the blind to be easily broken, introduce biases, peek at the data without proper allowances, or follow other procedures that would compromise the integrity of the study. Patients who are discontinued for any reason after randomization to treatment should be analyzed in the treatment group to prevent bias, since patient dropouts that are not related to drug-induced adverse reactions may still be study or treatment related. For example, patients may have dropped out of a study if they improved on drug and no longer require treatment, did not improve on treatment and sought other medical help, or were unhappy with the requirements of the study for some reason. Thus, patients should not be eliminated from consideration and analysis once they have been randomized to treatment or, possibly, once they have begun to receive drug treatment.

In conclusion, this book has documented that a clinical drug study is usually a complex event requiring careful planning and attention to many details. Each study differs from others to a greater or lesser degree and requires modifications in the steps followed to initiate and conduct the study. In addition, there are many unanticipated events that occur in virtually all clinical studies that make their conduct difficult to maintain at a uniformly high standard. The information presented, plus the tables and figures, are intended to serve as tools to assist individuals in achieving a high standard of quality and efficiency in planning and conducting these studies. By meeting such standards, the probability is greater that the clinical study will successfully attain its objectives.

Appendix 1

Sources of Bias[1]

(1) In reading-up on the field

  (a) *The biases of rhetoric.* Any of several techniques used to convince the reader without appealing to reason, e.g., Good: A classification of fallacious arguments and interpretations. *Technometrics,* 4:125–132, 1962.

  (b) *The all's well literature bias.* Scientific or professional societies may publish reports or editorials that omit or play down controversies or disparate results, e.g., the debate on "control" and the complications of diabetes, well shown in editorials in *N. Engl. J. Med.,* 294:1004, 1976 and 296:1228–1229, 1977.

  (c) *One-sided reference bias.* Authors may restrict their references to only those works that support their position; a literature review with a single starting point risks confinement to a single side of the issue, e.g., Platt and Pickering on the inheritance of hypertension: Hamilton, Pickering *et al.*: *Clin. Sci.,* 24:91–108, 1963; Platt: *Lancet,* 1:899–904, 1963.

  (d) *Positive results bias.* Authors are more likely to submit, and editors accept, positive than null results, e.g., multiple personal experiences.

  (e) *Hot stuff bias.* When a topic is hot, neither investigators nor editors may be able to resist the temptation to publish additional results, no matter how preliminary or shaky, e.g., recent publications concerning medication compliance.

(2) In specifying and selecting the study sample

  (a) *Popularity bias.* The admission of patients to some practices, institutions or procedures (surgery, autopsy) is influenced by the interest stirred up by the presenting condition and its possible causes, e.g., White: *Br. Med. J.,* 2:1284–1288, 1953.

  (b) *Centripetal bias.* The reputations of certain clinicians and institutions cause individuals with specific disorders or exposures to gravitate toward them, e.g., the striking rate of posterior fossa cerebral aneurysms reported from the University of Western Ontario.

  (c) *Referral filter bias.* As a group of ill are referred from primary to secondary to tertiary care, the concentration of rare causes, multiple diagnoses, and "hopeless cases" may increase, e.g., secondary hypertension at the Cleveland Clinic: Gifford: *Milbank Mem. Fund. Q.,* 47:170–186, 1969.

  (d) *Diagnostic access bias.* Individuals differ in their geographic, temporal and economic access to the diagnostic procedures that label them as having a given disease, e.g., Andersen, Andersen: Patterns of use of health services. In: *Handbook of Medical Sociology.* Freeman *et al.* (ed). Prentice-Hall, Englewood Cliffs, 1972.

  (e) *Diagnostic suspicion bias.* A knowledge of the subject's prior exposure to a putative cause (ethnicity, taking a certain drug, having a second disorder, being exposed in an epidemic) may influence both the intensity and the outcome of the diagnostic process; e.g., the possibility that rubber workers were victims of this bias was studied by Fox, White: *Lancet,* 1:1009–1010, 1976.

  (f) *Unmasking (detection signal) bias.* An innocent exposure may become suspect if,

[1]Modified from Sackett (1979) with permission.

rather than causing a disease, it causes a sign or symptom that precipitates a search for the disease, e.g., the current controversy over postmenopausal estrogens and cancer of the endometrium.

(g) *Mimicry bias.* An innocent exposure may become suspect if, rather than causing a disease, it causes a (benign) disorder that resembles the disease, e.g., Morrison *et al.: Lancet,* 1:1142–1143, 1977.

(h) *Previous opinion bias.* The tactics and results of a previous diagnostic process on a patient, if known, may affect the tactics and results of a subsequent diagnostic process on the same patient, e.g., multiple personal experiences with referred hypertensive patients.

(i) *Wrong sample size bias.* Samples that are too small can prove nothing; samples that are too large can prove anything.

(j) *Admission rate (Berkson) bias.* If hospitalization rates differ for different exposure disease groups, the relation between exposure and disease will become distorted in hospital-based studies. Berkson: *Biometrics Bull.,* 2:47–53, 1946; Roberts, Spitzer, Delmore, Sackett: *J. Chron. Dis.,* 31:119–128.

(k) *Prevalence–incidence (Neyman) bias.* A late look at those exposed (or affected) early will miss fatal and other short episodes plus mild or 'silent' cases and cases in which evidence of exposure disappears with disease onset. Neyman: *Science,* 122:401, 1955.

(l) *Diagnostic vogue bias.* The same illness may receive different diagnostic labels at different points in space or time, e.g., British "bronchitis" versus North American "emphysema": Fletcher *et al.: Am. Rev. Respir. Dis.,* 90:1–13, 1964.

(m) *Diagnostic purity bias.* When "pure" diagnostic groups exclude comorbidity, they may become nonrepresentative.

(n) *Procedure selection bias.* Certain clinical procedures may be preferentially offered to those who are poor risks, e.g., selection of patients for "medical" versus "surgical" therapy: Feinstein: *Clin. Biostatistics,* 76, C.V. Mosby, St. Louis, 1977.

(o) *Missing clinical data bias.* Missing clinical data may be missing because they are normal, negative, never measured, or measured but never recorded.

(p) *Noncontemporaneous control bias.* Secular changes in definitions, exposures, diagnoses, diseases, and treatments may render noncontemporaneous controls noncomparable, e.g., Feinstein: *Clin. Biostatistics,* 94–104, C.V. Mosby, St. Louis, 1977.

(q) *Starting time bias.* The failure to identify a common starting time for exposure or illness may lead to systematic misclassification, e.g., Feinstein: *Clin. Biostatistics,* 89–104, C.V. Mosby, St. Louis, 1977.

(r) *Unacceptable disease bias.* When disorders are socially unacceptable (V.D., suicide, insanity), they tend to be underreported.

(s) *Migrator bias.* Migrants may differ systematically from those who stay home, e.g., Krueger, Moriyama: *Am. J. Publ. Hlth.,* 57:496–503, 1967.

(t) *Membership bias.* Membership in a group (the employed, joggers, etc.) may imply a degree of health that differs systematically from that of the general population, e.g., exercise and recurrent myocardial infarction. Rechnitzer *et al.: Circulation,* 45:853–857, 1972.

(u) *Nonrespondent bias.* Nonrespondents (or "late comers") from a specified sample may exhibit exposures or outcomes that differ from those of respondents (or "early comers"), e.g., cigarette smokers: Seltzer *et al.: Am. J. Epidemiol.,* 100:453–547, 1974.

(v) *Volunteer bias.* Volunteers or "early comers" from a specified sample may exhibit exposures or outcomes (they tend to be healthier) that differ from those of nonvolunteers or "late comers," e.g., volunteers for screening: Shapiro *et al.: JAMA,* 215:1777–1785, 1971.

(3) In executing the experimental maneuver (or exposure)
  (a) *Contamination bias.* In an experiment, when members of the control group inadvertently receive the experimental maneuver, the difference in outcomes between experimental and control patients may be systematically reduced, e.g., recent drug trials involving aspirin.
  (b) *Withdrawal bias.* Patients who are withdrawn from an experiment may differ systematically from those who remain, e.g., in a neurosurgical trial of surgical versus medical therapy of cerebrovascular disease, patients who died or "stroked-out" during surgery were withdrawn as "unavailable for follow-up" and excluded from early analyses.
  (d) *Compliance bias.* In experiments requiring patient adherence to therapy, issues of efficacy become confounded with those of compliance; e.g., it is the high-risk coronary patients who quit exercise programs: Oldridge *et al.*: *Can. Med. Assoc. J.*, 118:361–364, 1978.
  (e) *Therapeutic personality bias.* When treatment is not "blind," the therapist's convictions about efficacy may systematically influence both outcomes (positive personality) and their measurement (desire for positive results).
  (f) *Bogus control bias.* When patients who are allocated to an experimental maneuver die or sicken before or during its administration and are omitted or reallocated to the control group, the experimental maneuver will appear spuriously superior.

(4) In measuring exposures and outcomes
  (a) *Insensitive measure bias.* When outcome measures are incapable of detecting clinically significant changes or differences, type II errors occur.
  (b) *Underlying cause bias (rumination bias).* Patients may ruminate about possible causes for their illnesses and thus exhibit different recall of prior exposures than controls, e.g., Sartwell: *Ann. Intern. Med.*, 81:381–386, 1974 (see also the *Recall bias: 4-k*).
  (c) *End-digit preference bias.* In converting analog to digital data, observers may record some terminal digits with an unusual frequency, e.g., a notorious problem in the measurement of blood pressure: Rose *et al.*: *Lancet*, 1:296–300, 1964.
  (d) *Apprehension bias.* Certain measures (pulse, blood pressure) may alter systematically from their usual levels when the subject is apprehensive, e.g., blood pressure during medical interviews: McKegney, Williams: *Am. J. Psychiatry*, 123:1539–1545, 1967.
  (e) *Unacceptability bias.* Measurements that hurt, embarrass, or invade privacy may be systematically refused or evaded.
  (f) *Obsequiousness bias.* Subjects may systematically alter questionnaire responses in the direction they perceive desired by the investigator.
  (g) *Expectation bias.* Observers may systematically err in measuring and recording observations so that they concur with prior expectations; e.g., house officers tend to report "normal" fetal heart rates: Day *et al.*: *Br. Med. J.*, 4:422–424, 1968.
  (h) *Substitution game.* The substitution of a risk factor that has not been established as causal for its associated outcome. Yerushalmy: In: *Controversy in Internal Medicine*. Ingelfinger *et al.* (eds), 659–688, W.B. Saunders, Philadelphia, 1966.
  (i) *Family information bias.* The flow of family information about exposure and illness is stimulated by, and directed to, a new case in its midst, e.g., different family histories of arthritis from affected and unaffected sibs: Schull, Cobb: *J. Chron. Dis.*, 22:217–222, 1969.
  (j) *Exposure suspicion bias.* A knowledge of the subject's disease status may influence both the intensity and outcome of a search for exposure to the putative cause, e.g., Sartwell: *Ann. Intern. Med.*, 81:381–386, 1974.

(k) *Recall bias.* Questions about specific exposures may be asked several times of cases but only once of controls (see also the *Underlying cause bias: 4-b*).

(l) *Attention bias.* Study subjects may systematically alter their behavior when they know they are being observed, e.g., Hawthorne revisited.

(m) *Instrument bias.* Defects in the calibration or maintenance of measurement instruments may lead to systematic deviations from true values.

(5) In analyzing the data

(a) *Post-hoc significance bias.* When decision levels or "tails" for α and β are selected *after* the data have been examined, conclusions may be biased.

(b) *Data dredging bias (looking for the pony).* When data are reviewed for all possible associations without prior hypothesis, the results are suitable for hypothesis-forming activities only.

(c) *Scale degradation bias.* The degradation and collapsing of measurement scales tend to obscure differences between groups under comparison.

(d) *Tidying-up bias.* The exclusion of outlyers or other untidy results cannot be justified on statistical grounds and may lead to bias, e.g., Murphy: *The Logic of Medicine,* 250, Johns Hopkins University Press, Baltimore, 1976.

(e) *Repeated peeks bias.* Repeated peeks at accumulating data in a randomized trial are not dependent and may lead to inappropriate termination.

(6) In interpreting the analysis

(a) *Mistaken identity bias.* In compliance trials, strategies directed toward improving the patient's compliance may, instead or in addition, cause the treating clinician to prescribe more vigorously; the effect on achievement of the treatment goal may be misinterpreted, e.g., Sackett: In: *Compliance with Therapeutic Regimens.* Sackett D. L., Haynes, R. B. (eds), 169–189, Johns Hopkins University Press, Baltimore, 1976.

(b) *Cognitive dissonance bias.* The belief in a given mechanism may increase rather than decrease in the face of contradictory evidence, e.g., Sackett: In: *Controversies in Therapeutics.* Lasagna, L. (ed). Is there a patient compliance problem? If so, what should we do about it? pp. 552–558, W.B. Saunders, Philadelphia, 1980.

(c) *Magnitude bias.* In interpreting a finding, the selection of a scale of measurement may markedly affect the interpretation, e.g., $1,000,000 may also be 0.0003% of the national budget: Murphy: *The Logic of Medicine,* 249, Johns Hopkins University Press, Baltimore, 1976.

(d) *Significance bias.* The confusion of statistical significance, on the one hand, with biologic or clinical or health care significance, on the other hand, can lead to fruitless studies and useless conclusions, e.g., Feinstein: *Clin. Biostatistics,* 258, C.V. Mosby, St. Louis, 1977.

(e) *Correlation bias.* Equating correlation with causation leads to errors of both kinds, e.g., Hill: *Principles of Medical Statistics,* 9th ed, 309–320, Oxford University Press, New York, 1971.

(f) *Under-exhaustion bias.* The failure to exhaust the hypothesis space may lead to authoritarian rather than authoritative interpretation, e.g., Murphy: *The Logic of Medicine,* 258, Johns Hopkins University Press, Baltimore, 1976.

Prototype Tables and Figures for the Safety Section of a Final Medical Report

PROTOTYPE TABLES ILLUSTRATING SELECTED DATA ON DRUG SAFETY
Tables A.1 to A.3: Study characteristics section of a final medical report
Tables A.4 and A.5: Physical examinations
Tables A.6 and A.7: Electrocardiograms
Tables A.8 to A.11: Vital signs and body weight
Tables A.12 to A.20: Clinical laboratory results
Tables A.21 to A.31: Adverse reactions

PROTOTYPE FIGURES ILLUSTRATING SELECTED DATA ON DRUG SAFETY
Figure A.24: Vital signs
Figure A.25: Laboratory results

COMMENTS

These tables were constructed for a hypothetical double-blind placebo-controlled parallel design multicentered study (10 sites) of 22 weeks' duration (including a 5-week baseline) plus 4 weeks for taper and posttreatment evaluation. For the purposes of constructing these tables, a three-item scale was used for severity of adverse reactions (mild, moderate, severe), and a four-item scale was used for the relationship of the test drug (either study drug or placebo) to the adverse reaction (definite, not related, possible, or unknown). The action taken was one of the categories described in the text. Several tables include sample data.

The section on study characteristics does not present the basic tables of patient demographics or analyses of why some patients did not meet entry criteria.

TABLE A.1. *Reasons why patients did not complete protocol*

A. Patients who received study drug

Reason	Number of patients receiving	
	Study Drug	Placebo
Died		
Moved out of area		
Adverse reactions		
Concomitant illness		
Deterioration of disease		
Protocol violation by patient		
Protocol violation by staff		
Improvement of disease		
Laboratory abnormality		
"Personal" reasons unrelated to study		
Reason(s) not stated		
Other (list)		
Total		

B. Patients who did not receive study drug

Reason	Number of patients
Each reason is listed	
Total	

TABLE A.2. *Summary of concomitant drugs for patients in the protocol[a]*

Concomitant drugs	Number of patients on concomitant drugs plus	
	Study drug	Placebo
Individual drugs used[b]		
X		
Y		
Most common drug combinations[c]		
C + D		
E + F		
Other combinations of drugs used		
G + H		
I + J		
G + J		

[a]All patients entered in the study are described for both individual drugs and combinations. Concomitant drugs were used to treat primary disease. If only a few patients are in the study, list concomitant drugs by patient.

[b]Patients are counted more than once if they are taking more than one drug. X, Y, and C to J each represent a different drug.

[c]Patients are counted only once.

TABLE A.3. *Dose administered by treatment week—combined centers[a]*

Week[b]	Study drug			Placebo		
	Mean	Median	Range	Mean	Median	Range
6						
7						
8						
9						
10						
11						
12						
13						
14						
15						
16						
17						
18						
19						
20						
21						
22						
23						
24						
25						
26						

[a]Values are expressed in mg/kg per day. Separate tables for each of the 10 centers could be constructed.
[b]Weeks 1 to 5 are baseline, 6 to 11 are dose ascension, 12 to 22 treatment, and 23 to 26 taper and posttreatment.

TABLE A.4. *Physical examinations—overall incidence of baseline versus treatment abnormalities[a]*

	Number of patients					
	Normal baseline			Abnormal baseline		
	Norm. tr.	Abn. tr.	Total	Norm. tr.	Abn. tr.	Total
Study drug (*N* =)						
Placebo (*N* =)						
Total						

	Number of reports					
	Norm. bl.	Abn. bl.		Norm. tr.	Abn. tr.	Total
Study drug (*N* =)						
Placebo (*N* =)						
Total						

[a]Data from any specialized physical examinations (e.g., neurological) would be presented separately.
Tr., treatment period; bl., baseline period; Norm., normal; Abn., abnormal.

TABLE A.5. *Clinically significant abnormalities noted on physical examination during treatment[a]*

Body system	Treatment group (S, Plac.)	Patient no.	Site no.	Specific abnormality	Observed at (weeks)	Related to severity (M, Mo, S)	Related to study drug (Y, N, P, U)	Action taken
Head and neck	S	302	3	Gingeval Hyperplasia	4	Mo	N	None
				Gingeval Hyperplasia	6	Mo	P	↑ Surveillance
				Skin Rash	8	S	Y	D/C drug
	Plac.	417	4	Lymphadenopathy	6	M	U	↑ Surveillance
Respiratory	Plac.	821	8	Wheezing	10	M	U	None
				Wheezing	14	M	P	↑ Surveillance
				Wheezing	20	Mo	N	D/C other drug

[a]An evaluation should be conducted to determine which abnormalities were present during baseline.
S, study drug; Plac., placebo; M, mild; Mo, moderate; S, severe; Y, definite; N, not related; P, possible; U, unknown.

TABLE A.6. *Electrocardiogram within- and between-treatment comparison for screen versus termination*

| Screen | Number of patients at termination | | | | | |
| | Study Drug ($N = y$) | | | Placebo ($N = x$) | | |
	Normal	Abnormal	NA	Normal	Abnormal	NA
Normal	a					
Abnormal	b					
NA	c					
Total	d					

NA, not assessed.

TABLE A.7. *Patients with abnormal electrocardiograms on treatment but not at screen*

Treatment group (S, Plac.)	Patient no.	Site no.	Abnormality noted	Clinical significance (Y, N)	Related to study drug (Y, N, P, U)	Comment
Plac.	331	3	RVH	Y	N	Not on study drug
S	415	4	LAH	Y	P	Consult doubted a relationship
S	711	7	RBBB	N	N	Noted in past
S	712	7	LVH	N	N	Artifact of electrode placement

S, study drug; Plac., placebo; Y, definite; N, not related; P, possible; U, unknown.

APPENDIX 2

TABLE A.8. *Summary of blood pressure data—combined centers*[a]

	Study week[b]	Study drug				Placebo			
		N	Mean	± SE	Range[c]	N	Mean	± SE	Range
Systolic blood pressure (mm Hg)	0								
	2								
	4								
	6								
	7								
	8								
	9								
	10								
	11								
	12								
	13								
	15								
	18								
	21								
	24								
	25								
	26								
Diastolic blood pressure (mm Hg)	0								
	2								
	4								
	6								
	7								
	8								
	9								
	10								
	11								
	12								
	13								
	15								
	18								
	21								
	24								
	25								
	26								

[a]A similar table would be constructed for pulse rate, respiration rate, temperature, or body weight. Body weights are to be presented separately for patients 2 to 11.99 years and 12 to 18 years (ages are determined at start of baseline). Separate tables for each of the 10 centers could be constructed.
[b]Weeks 0 to 5, baseline; 6 to 22, drug treatment; 23 to 26, taper and posttreatment.
[c]Range, minimum and maximum values.

TABLE A.9. *Patients with clinically significant abnormal blood pressure values during treatment[a]*

Treatment group (S, Plac.)	Patient No.	Site No.	Blood pressure value (mm Hg)	Observed at (weeks)	Related to study drug (Y, N, P, U)	Action taken	Outcome
S	321	3	150/80	8	U	None	Improved
			140/75	22	P	↑ Surv.	Improved
	482	4	170/80	24	N	None	Improved
Plac.	214	2	100/20	10	N	None	Improved
	220	2					
	244	2					

[a]A similar table would be constructed for each vital sign plus each body weight group.
S, study drug; Plac., placebo; Y, definite; N, not related; P, possible; U, unknown; ↑ Surv., increase surveillance.

TABLE A.10. *Blood pressure[a]: within-treatment-group-changes, combined centers*

| | | Study drug | | | | | Placebo | | | |
| | | | | Change score ANOVA | | | | | Change score ANOVA | |
Study week[e]	N	Treatment (mean ± SE)	Baseline (mean ± SE)	Est. diff.[b]	p^c	N	Treatment (mean ± SE)	Baseline (mean ± SE)	Est. diff.[b]	p^c
Systolic blood pressure										
6										
7										
8										
9										
10										
11										
12										
13										
15										
18										
21										
24										
Diastolic blood pressure										
6										
7										
8										
9										
10										
11										
12										
13										
15										
18										
21										
24										

[a]A similar table would be prepared for each vital sign and body weight group. Separate tables for each of the 10 centers could be constructed.
[b]Treatment week 7 or 8, etc. minus baseline.
[c]Two-sided test.
[d]Baseline (mean ± SE) is the baseline measurement at week 5 or last baseline visit.
[e]In other studies this column could represent hours postdose or other time measurements.
N, number of patients evaluated each week in the study drug (or placebo) group; ANOVA, analysis of variance.

TABLE A.11. *Blood pressure: between-treatment-group changes, combined centers*[a]

| | Study week | Treatment − Baseline[b] | | | | Between-treatment analysis[c] | |
| | | Study drug | | Placebo | | | |
		N	Mean ± SE	N	Mean ± SE	Mean diff. ± SE	p[d]
Systolic blood pressure	6						
	7						
	8						
	9						
	10						
	11						
	12						
	13						
	15						
	18						
	21						
	24						
Diastolic blood pressure	6						
	7						
	8						
	9						
	10						
	11						
	12						
	13						
	15						
	18						
	21						
	24						

[a]A similar table would be constructed for each vital sign and body weight group. Separate tables for each of the 10 centers could be constructed.

[b]T − B. These data could also be presented as baseline − treatment (B − T).

[c]Between-treatment (mean treatment − baseline for study drug) minus (mean treatment − baseline for placebo).

[d]Two-sided test.

TABLE A.12. *Overall percent incidence of clinically significant abnormal elevations[a] in hematology and urinalysis measurements: within-treatment-group changes, combined centers[b]*

Test	Baseline			Treatment			Within-treatment change scores analysis[e]		
	N	% Pts.[c]	% Reps.[d]	N	% Pts.[c]	% Reps.[d]	N	p(% Pts.)	p(% Reps.)
Study drug									
Hematology									
Hemoglobin									
Hematocrit									
Total WBC count									
Neutrophils									
Lymphocytes									
Monocytes									
Eosinophils									
Basophils									
Total RBC count									
MCV									
MCH									
MCHC									
Fibrinogen									
Reticulocytes									
Prothrombin time									
Partial thromboplastin time									
Urinalysis:									
Specific gravity									

Placebo
Hematology
  Hemoglobin
  Hematocrit
  Total WBC count
  Neutrophils
  Lymphocytes
  Monocytes
  Eosinophils
  Basophils
  Total RBC count
  MCV
  MCH
  MCHC
  Fibrinogen
  Reticulocytes
  Prothrombin time
  Partial thromboplastin time
Urinalysis
  Specific gravity

[a] Same table for "decreases" in laboratory values would be prepared. Separate tables for each of the separate centers could be constructed.
[b] Baseline, values at week 5 or last baseline visit (other definitions of baseline values may be established).
Treatment, any clinically significant value while on study drug is included (other definition of treatment values may be established).
[c] % Pts., the overall percent of all patients on study drug (or placebo) who experienced a clinically significant abnormal elevation in a specific parameter during baseline or treatment.
[d] % Reps., the overall percent of all reports on study drug (or placebo) in which a clinically significant abnormal elevation was indicated for a specific parameter during baseline or treatment.
[e] Change score, treatment − baseline.

TABLE A.13. *Hematology and urinalysis measurements: within-treatment-group changes, combined centers*

Test	Baseline[a]			Termination[b]			Within-treatment change scores analysis[c]		
	N	Mean ± SE	Range	N	Mean ± SE	Range	N	Mean ± SE	p
Study drug									
Hematology									
Hemoglobin (g/dl)									
Hematocrit (%)									
Total WBC count (%/cmm)									
Neutrophils (%)									
Lymphocytes (%)									
Monocytes (%)									
Eosinophils (%)									
Basophils (%)									
Total RBC count (millions/mm³)									
MCV (fl)									
MCH (pg)									
MCHC (g/dl)									
Fibrinogen (mg/dl)									
Reticulocytes (%)									
Prothrombin time (sec)									
Partial thromboplastin time (sec)									
Urinalysis									
Specific gravity									

Placebo
Hematology
  Hemoglobin (g/dl)
  Hematocrit (%)
  Total WBC count (%/cmm)
  Neutrophils (%)
  Lymphocytes (%)
  Monocytes (%)
  Eosinophils (%)
  Basophils (%)
  Total RBC count (millions/mm^3)
  MCV (fl)
  MCH (pg)
  MCHC (g/dl)
  Fibrinogen (mg/dl)
  Reticulocytes (%)
  Prothrombin time (sec)
  Partial thromboplastin time (sec)
Urinalysis
  Specific gravity

---

[a]Baseline, values obtained at week 5 or last baseline visit (other definitions of baseline values may be established, e.g., average of all or specific values).
[b]Termination, values obtained at last visit on study drug (other definitions of termination values may be established). Separate tables for each of the 10 centers could be constructed.
[c]Change scores, termination − baseline.

TABLE A.14. *Hematology and urinalysis measurements: between-test-group changes, combined centers[a]*

| Test | Treatment − baseline[b] | | | | Between-treatment analysis[c] | | |
| | Study drug | | Placebo | | Mean difference | ± SE | p[d] |
	N	Mean ± SE	N	Mean ± SE			
Hematology							
Hemoglobin							
Hematocrit							
Total WBC count							
Neutrophils							
Lymphocytes							
Monocytes							
Eosinophils							
Basophils							
Total RBC count							
MCV							
MCH							
MCHC							
Fibrinogen							
Reticulocytes							
Prothrombin time							
Partial thromboplastin time							
Platelet count[e]							
Urinalysis							
Specific gravity							

[a]Separate tables for each of the 10 centers could be constructed.

[b]Alternative approaches to presenting the treatment data are to (1) only list treatment data for study drug and placebo, ignoring the baseline, (2) use baseline minus treatment, especially if this will yield positive numbers, (3) adjust all treatment data for baseline using the least-square means technique, (4) use the format in Table A.15.

[c]Between treatment, (mean treatment − baseline for study drug) minus (mean treatment − baseline for placebo).

[d]Two-tailed test.

[e]The terms thrombocytosis and thrombocytopenia are not used in these tables, since they refer to an interpretation of the data, which may be discussed in the text of the report.

TABLE A.15. *Hematology and urinalysis measurements within- and between-test-group changes, combined centers[c]*

Test	Treatment	Study period	N	Mean	SE	SD	Min. value	Max. value	Normal range	Within-group p^a	Between-group p^b
Hemoglobin	Study drug	Screen									
		Posttreatment									
	Placebo	Screen									
		Posttreatment									
Other											

[a]Two-tailed test comparing the study drug screen and posttreatment values (i.e., within-group) with respect to change scores (i.e., posttreatment values minus screen value).

[b]Two-tailed test comparing the study drug and placebo treatment groups (i.e., between groups) with respect to change scores, i.e., (study drug posttreatment minus screen value) minus (placebo posttreatment minus screen value).

[c]This test presents data shown in Tables A.13 and A.14 in a different format. Separate tables for each of the 10 centers could be constructed.

TABLE A.16. *Patients with clinically significant abnormalities in hematological parameters[a]*

Abnormality	Treatment group (S, Plac.)	Patient no.	Site no.	Observed at (weeks)	Related to study drug (Y, N, P, U)	Action taken	Outcome
Decreased hematocrit	S	204	2	8	N	None	No change
				12	U	↑ Surv.	No change
				16	P	→ Dose	Improved
	Plac.	215	2	8	Y	→ Dose	Improved
	Plac.	331	3	12	P	None	No change
				16	P	None	No change
				24	Y	↑ Surv.	No change
Decreased hemoglobin	S	111	1	10	N	None	Improved

[a]Same table would be prepared for RBC morphology, blood chemistry, and urinalysis.
S, study drug; Plac., placebo; Y, definite; N, not related; P, possible; U, unknown; ↑ Surv., increase surveillance; ↓ Dose, decrease dose.

TABLE A.17. Overall incidence of all reported abnormalities in red blood cell morphology[a]

	Anisocytosis													Poikilocytosis													
	Study drug treatment					Placebo treatment					Study drug treatment					Placebo treatment				
	Mild	Mod.	Marked	Sev.	N	Mild	Mod.	Marked	Sev.	N	Mild	Mod.	Marked	Sev.	N	Mild	Mod.	Marked	Sev.	N
Anisocytosis																				
Normal																				
Mild																				
Moderate																				
Marked																				
Severe																				
Poikilocytosis																				
Normal																				
Mild																				
Moderate																				
Marked																				
Severe																				

[a]Patients are entered only once in each category, under the maximal intensity observed for anisocytosis and similarly for poikilocytosis.
Mod., moderate; Sev., severe; N, number of patients.

TABLE A.18. *Overall percent incidence of clinically significant abnormal increases in blood chemistry measurements: within-treatment-group changes, combined centers[a]*

Test	Baseline			Treatment			Within-treatment change scores analysis[d]		
	N	% Pts.[b]	% Reps.[c]	N	% Pts.	% Reps.	N	p(% Pts.)	p(% Reps.)
Study drug									
Calcium									
Total protein									
Albumin									
Phosphorus									
Glucose									
Bilirubin									
BUN									
Alk. phosphatase									
Uric acid									
LDH									
Cholesterol									
SGOT									
Sodium									
Potassium									
Chloride									
CO_2									
Creatinine									
Serum iron									
TIBC									

Placebo
Calcium
Total protein
Albumin
Phosphorus
Glucose
Bilirubin
BUN
Alk. phosphatase
Uric acid
LDH
Cholesterol
SGOT
Sodium
Potassium
Chloride
CO_2
Creatinine
Serum iron
TIBC

[a] Same table for "Decreases" would be prepared. The clinical significance of an abnormal parameter was judged by the investigator. Separate tables for each of the 10 centers could be constructed.

[b] % Pts., the overall percent of all patients on study drug (or placebo) who experienced a clinically significant abnormal elevation in a specific parameter during baseline or treatment.

[c] % Reps., the overall percent of all reports on study drug (or placebo) in which a clinically significant abnormal elevation was indicated for a specific parameter during baseline or treatment.

[d] Change score, treatment − baseline.

Baseline, values at week 5 or last baseline visit (other definitions of baseline values may be established).

Treatment, any clinically significant value while on study drug is included (other definitions of treatment values may be established).

TABLE A.19. *Blood chemistry measurements: within-treatment-group changes, combined centers[a]*

Test	Baseline			Termination			Within-treatment change scores analysis[c]		
	N	Mean ± SE	Range	N	Mean ± SE	Range	N	Mean ± SE	p[d]
Study drug									
Calcium (mg/dl)[b]									
Total protein (g/dl)									
Albumin (g/dl)									
Phosphorus (mg/dl)									
Glucose (mg/dl)									
Bilirubin (mg/dl)									
BUN (mg/dl)									
Alk. phosphatase (IU/liter)									
Uric acid (mg/dl)									
LDH/(IU/liter)									
Cholesterol (mg/dl)									
SGOT (IU/liter)									
Sodium (mEq/liter)									
Potassium (mEq/liter)									
Chloride (mEq/liter)									
CO_2 (mEq/liter)									
Creatinine (mg/dl)									
Serum iron (μg/dl)									
TIBC (μg/dL)									

Placebo
  Calcium (mg/dl)
  Total protein (g/dl)
  Albumin (g/dl)
  Phosphorus (mg/dl)
  Glucose (mg/dl)
  Bilirubin (mg/dl)
  BUN (mg/dl)
  Alk. phosphatase (IU/liter)
  Uric acid (mg/dl)
  LDH (IU/liter)
  Cholesterol (mg/dl)
  SGOT (IU/liter)
  Sodium (mEq/liter)
  Potassium (mEq/liter)
  Chloride (mEq/liter)
  CO_2 (mEq/liter)
  Creatinine (mg/dl)
  Serum iron (µg/dl)
  TIBC (µg/dl)

[a]Baseline, values obtained at week 5 or last baseline visit (other definitions of baseline values may be established). Termination, values obtained at last visit on study drug (other definitions of termination values may be established). Separate tables for each of the 10 centers could be constructed.

[b]mg/dl = mg/100 ml = mg%.

[c]Change scores, termination − baseline.

[d]Two-tailed test.

TABLE A.20. *Blood chemistry measurements: between-treatment-group changes, combined centers*[a]

| Test | Treatment − baseline[b] | | | | Between-treatment analysis[c] | | |
| | Study drug | | Placebo | | | | |
	N	Mean ± SE	N	Mean ± SE	Mean difference	± SE	p[d]
Calcium							
Total protein							
Albumin							
Phosphorus							
Glucose							
Bilirubin							
BUN							
Alk. phosphatase							
Uric acid							
LDH							
Cholesterol							
SGOT							
Sodium							
Potassium							
Chloride							
CO_2							
Creatinine							
Serum iron							
TIBC							

[a]Separate tables for each of the 10 centers could be constructed.

[b]Alternative approaches to presenting the treatment data are listed in footnote *b* of Table A.14.

[c]Between-treatment = (mean treatment − baseline for study drug) minus (mean treatment − baseline for placebo).

[d]Two-tailed test.

TABLE A.21. Overall incidence of total adverse reactions (A.R.) by treatment group and phase for each center

| | Study drug | | | | | | Placebo | | | | | |
| | Baseline | | Treatment period | | | | Baseline | | Treatment period | | | |
Center	No. pts. with A.R.	Total No. pts.	No. pts. with A.R.	Total No. pts.	No. rep.[a] of A.R.	Total No. of ass.[a]	No. pts. with A.R.	Total No. pts.	No. pts. with A.R.	Total No. pts.	No. rep. of A.R.	Total No. ass.
01												
02												
03												
04												
05												
06												
07												
08												
09												
10												
Total patients	X	X	X	X			X	X	X	X		
Total reports or assessments					X	X					X	X

[a] Ass., assessments (number of times that an A.R. was potentially able to be observed; rep., reports (actual number of occurrences of an A.R.).

TABLE A.22. Overall incidence of specific adverse reactions by treatment (study drug vs. placebo), combined centers[a]

Adverse reactions	Study drug					Placebo				
	Baseline	Treatment period				Baseline	Treatment period			
	% of patients ($N = X$)	% of patients ($N = Y$)	No. of reports	% of reports[b]		% of patients ($N = C$)	% of patients ($N = D$)	No. of reports	% of reports[b]	
Behavioral										
Neurological										
Autonomic										
Cardiovascular										
Other										
Total no. of reports			$C/D = E\%$					$U/V = W\%$		
Total no. of assessments	$A/B = C\%$					$R/S = T\%$				

[a]Separate tables for each of the 10 centers could be constructed.
[b]This column is the total number of reports obtained for each adverse reaction in the treatment period of the placebo (or study drug) group divided by the total number of assessments for that symptom in the group studied (i.e., placebo or study drug) during that treatment period ($\times 100$).

TABLE A.23. *Percent incidence of adverse reactions for study drug versus placebo[a]*

A. Percent of patients

Adverse reaction	Study drug (S) $(t - b)^b$	Placebo (P) $(t - b)^b$	Study drug − placebo $S(t - b) − P(t - b)$ (percentage units difference)
Effect M	+ 7	+ 17	+ 10
Effect N			+ B
Effect O			+ C
Other			
			$\cdots\cdots c$
Effect P	+ 4	− 11	− 15
Effect Q			− 5
Effect R			− F
Other			

B. Percent of reports

Effect N			
Effect O			
Effect J			
Effect Q			
Other			
			$\cdots\cdots c$
Effect V			
Effect X			
Effect Y			
Other			

[a]For all adverse reactions for which $S(t - b) − P(t - b)$ is 10 or more percentage units different. This factor of 10 can be raised (or lowered) as deemed appropriate.

[b]t, treatment; b, baseline.

[c]This dashed line divides those adverse reactions for which patients (reports) were more prevalent in the study drug group (above the lines) from those for which the percent of patients (reports) was greater in the placebo group (below the lines).

TABLE A.24. *Incidence of adverse reactions by assessment period, combined centers*[a]

| | Percent of patients | | | | | | | | | | | | |
| | 2 (Baseline) ($N = a$) | 4 (Baseline) ($N = b$) | Study drug treatment: study week | | | | | | | | | 27 (Posttreatment) ($N = m$) |
Adverse reaction			6 ($N = c$)	8 ($N = d$)	10 ($N = e$)	12 ($N = f$)	15 ($N = g$)	18 ($N = h$)	21 ($N = j$)	24 ($N = k$)	
Behavioral											
___											
___											
Neurological											
___											
___											
___											
Autonomic											
___											
___											
Cardiovascular											
___											
___											
Other											
___											
___											
Total no. of reports for each symptom	A	B	C	D	E	F	G	H	J	K	M
Total no. of assessments for each symptom											

[a]This table would have a second page for "Placebo Treatment." All of these data could be plotted with a different adverse reaction on each graph. Separate tables for each of the 10 centers could be constructed.

TABLE A.25. *Overall intensity of adverse reactions, combined centers*[a]

	Study drug													Placebo												
	Baseline period % of patients (N = a)			Treatment period							Baseline period % of patients (N = c)			Treatment period							
				% of patients (N = b)			% of reports							% of patients (N = d)			% of reports			
Adverse reaction	Mild	Mod.	Sev.	Mild	Mod.	Sev.	Mild	Mod.	Sev.	N	Mild	Mod.	Sev.	Mild	Mod.	Sev.	Mild	Mod.	Sev.	N
Behavioral																				
___																				
___																				
Neurological																				
___																				
___																				
Autonomic																				
___																				
___																				
Cardiovascular																				
___																				
___																				
Other																				
___																				
___																				
Total (% reports)																				
Total (% patients)																				

[a] Separate tables for each of the 10 centers could be constructed.
N = number of assessments.

TABLE A.26. *Relationship between adverse reactions and treatment, combined centers*[a]

Adverse reaction	Study drug (N = A)													Placebo (N = B)												
	% of patients				% of reports							% of patients					% of reports			
	Yes	Poss.	No	Unk.	N	Yes	Poss.	No	Unk.	N	Yes	Poss.	No	Unk.	N	Yes	Poss.	No	Unk.	N
Behavioral																				
Neurological																				
Autonomic																				
Cardiovascular																				
Other																				
Total (%)																				

[a]Treatment period only. Only the most definite relationship will be considered (i.e., "yes" before "possible," "possible" before "unknown," "unknown" before "not related").

Poss., possible; Unk., unknown; No, not related; Yes, definite; N, number of assessments. Separate tables for each of the 10 centers could be prepared.

TABLE A.27. *Frequency of patients with adverse reactions judged drug related during the treatment phase, by center and treatment*[a]

Center	Study drug	Placebo	Together
01	X/B (C)	A/Y (D)	$X + A/B + Y$ (E)
02			
03			
04			
05			
06			
07			
08			
09			
10			
Combined			

[a]According to the physician investigator who evaluated the adverse reactions.
Numbers in parentheses represent percents.

TABLE A.28. *Action taken as a result of adverse reactions, combined centers,[a] study drug (N = A)*

Adverse reaction	None		↑ Surveillance		Contraactive Rx		Change dose		D/C study drug		Total	
	No. pts.	No. reps.	No. pts.	No. reps.	No. pts.	No. reps.	No. pts.	No. reps.	No. pts.	No. reps.	No. pts.	No.reps.
Behavioral												
Neurological												
Autonomic												
Cardiovascular												
Other												

[a]Same table would be prepared for placebo. Separate tables for each of the 10 centers could be prepared.

TABLE A.29. *Patients whose treatment was discontinued because of an adverse reaction*

Treatment group (S, Plac.)	Patient no.	Age	Sex	Site no.	Drug week	Dose (mg/day)	Adverse reaction	Intensity (M, Mo, S)	Related to study drug (Y, N, P, U)
S	420			4					
	682			6					
	943			9					
Plac.	174			1					
	560			5					
	592			5					

S, study drug; Plac., placebo; M, mild; Mo, moderate; S, severe; Y, definite; N, not related; P, possible; U, unknown.

TABLE A.30. *Patients with severe adverse reactions whose treatment was not discontinued*

Treatment group (S, Plac.)	Patient no.	Age	Sex	Site no.	Drug week	Dose (mg/day)	Adverse reaction	Intensity (M, Mo, S)	Related to study drug (Y, N, P, U)	Action taken
S	440									
	681									
Plac.	112									
	145									
	268									
	294									
	412									
	654									

S, study drug; Plac., placebo; M, mild; Mo, moderate; S, severe; Y, definite; N, not related; P, possible; U, unknown.

TABLE A.31. *Frequency of patients with a given number of reports of adverse reactions, combined centers[a]*

No. of reports	Study drug ($N = a$)		Placebo ($N = b$)	
	No. of patients	% of patients	No. of patients	% of patients
0				
1				
2				
3				
4				
5				
6–8				
8–10				
10–12				
12–15				
15–18				
18–21				
Other				

[a]Separate tables for each of the 10 centers could be prepared.

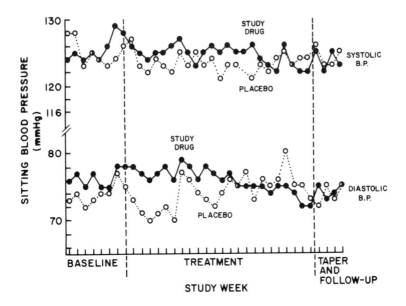

FIG. A.24. Mean blood pressure by treatment group, combined centers. This is a prototype illustration of one of the vital signs. Similar figures would be prepared to illustrate supine blood pressure, pulse rate, respiration, and temperature. Similar figures could also be prepared to illustrate changes in other parameters such as body weight.

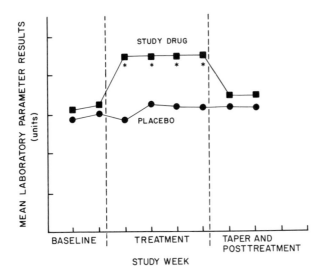

FIG. A.25. Prototype of mean laboratory parameter results by treatment group, combined centers. $*p < 0.05$, change from baseline.

References

Abram, M. B., Chairman, Presidents Commission for the study of Ethical Problems in Medicine and Biomedical and Behavioral Research (1981): Protecting human subjects (First biennial report on the adequacy and uniformity of Federal rules and policies, and their implementation, for the protection of human subjects in biomedical and behavioral research), No. 040-000-00452-1. United States Government Printing Office, Washington, D.C.

Abrams, W. B. (1976): The development of clinical protocols. In: *Factors Influencing Clinical Research Success*, edited by M. J. Finkel, pp. 7–23. Futura, Mt. Kisco, New York.

Agras, W. S., and Bradford, R. H. (1982): Recruitment for clinical trials: The lipid research clinic's coronary primary prevention trial experience. *Circulation*, 66(Suppl. IV):1–78.

Agras, W. S., and Marshall, G. (1979): Recruitment for the coronary primary prevention trial. *Clin. Pharmacol. Ther.*, 25:688–690.

Allen, P. A., and Waters, W. E. (1982): Development of an ethical committee and its effect on research design. *Lancet*, 1:1233–1236.

Amene, P. C. (1983): Activation of pulmonary tuberculosis following intralesional corticosteroids. *Arch. Dermatol.*, 119:361–362.

American Academy of Pediatrics Committee on Drugs (1977): Guidelines for the ethical conduct of studies to evaluate drugs in pediatric populations. *Pediatrics*, 60:91–101.

American Medical Association (1983): From the NIH. 1. Sensitivity to pain greater in a clinical than in a laboratory setting. *J.A.M.A.*, 250:718.

American Psychiatric Association (1980): *Diagnostic and Statistical Manual of Mental Disorders*, third ed. American Psychiatric Association, Washington, D.C.

Anturane Reinfarction Trial Research Group (1980): Sulfinpyrazone in the prevention of sudden death after myocardial infarction. *N. Engl. J. Med.*, 302:250–256.

Association of the British Pharmaceutical Industry (1983): Compensation and drug trials; guidelines: Clinical trials–compensation for medicine induced injury. *Br. Med. J.*, 287:675.

Banker, G. S., and Rhodes, C. T. (1979): *Modern Pharmaceutics*. Marcel Dekker, New York.

Benedict, G. W. (1979): LRC coronary prevention trial: Baltimore. *Clin. Pharmacol. Ther.*, 25:685–687.

Berry, H., Bloom, B., Mace, B. E. W., Hamilton, E. B. D., et al. (1980): Expectation and patient preference—does it matter? *J. R. Soc. Med.*, 73:34–38.

β-Blocker Heart Attack Study Group (1981): The β-blocker heart attack trial. *J.A.M.A.*, 246:2073–2074.

The Beta-Blocker Heart Attack Trial Research Group (1981): Beta blocker heart attack trial: Design features. *Control. Clin. Trials*, 2:275–285.

β-Blocker Heart Attack Trial Research Group (1982): A randomized trial of propranolol in patients with acute myocardial infarction. I. Mortality results. *J.A.M.A.*, 247:1707–1714.

Blackwell, B. (1972a): For the first time in man. *Clin. Pharmacol. Ther.*, 13:812–823.

Blackwell, B. (1972b): The drug defaulter. *Clin. Pharmacol. Ther.*, 13:841–848.

Blanc, S., Leuenberger, P., Berger, J.-P., Brooke, E. M., and Schelling, J.-L. (1979): Judgments of trained observers on adverse drug reactions. *Clin. Pharmacol. Ther.*, 25:493–498.

Boissel, J. P., and Klimt, C. R. (Eds.) (1979): *Multicenter Controlled Trials—Principles and Problems*. INSERM, Paris.

Brown, J. H. U. (1979): Functions of an institutional review board and the protection of human subjects. *Fed. Proc.*, 38:2049–2050.

Buckalew, L. W., and Coffield, K. E. (1982): An investigation of drug expectancy as a function of capsule color and size and preparation form. *J. Clin. Psychopharm.*, 2:245–248.

Buros, O. K. (Ed.) (1972): *The Seventh Mental Measurements Yearbook*. The Gryphon Press, Highland Park, New Jersey.

Cancer Research Campaign Working Party (1980): Trials and tribulations: Thoughts on the organization of multicentre clinical trials. *Br. Med. J.*, 281:918–920.

Cato, A. (1982): Design of clinical trials. *Drug Inform. J.*, 16:44–50.

Chan, Y. K., Archibald, D. D., and Peduzzi, P. N. (1983): Management of a multicenter clinical trial. *Trends Pharmacol. Sci.*, 4:21–24.

Chaput de Saintonge, D. M. (1977): Aide-mémoire for preparing clinical trial protocols. *Br. Med. J.*, 1:1323–1324.

Conners, C. K. (1976): Rating scales for use in drug studies with children. In: *ECDEU Assessment Manual for Psychopharmacology*, DHEW Publ. No. (ADM) 76-338, edited by W. Guy, pp. 303–312. U.S. Government Printing Office, Washington, D.C.

Conney, A. H., Pantuck, E. J., Hsiao, K.-C., Kuntzman, R., et al. (1977): Regulation of drug metabolism in man by environmental chemicals and diet. *Fed. Proc.*, 36:1647–1652.

Croke, G. (1979): Recruitment for the national cooperative gallstone study. *Clin. Pharmacol. Ther.*, 25:691–694.

Davis, K. V., Sprague, R., and Werry, J. (1969): Stereotyped behavior and activity level in severe retardates: The effects of drugs. *Am. J. Ment. Def.*, 73:721–727.

de Maar, E. W. J., Chaudhury, R. R., Kofi Ekue, J. M., Granata, F., and Walker, A. N. (1983): Management of clinical trials in developing countries. *J. Int. Med. Res.*, 11:1–5.

Diamond, A. L., and Laurence, D. R. (1983): Commentary. *Br. Med. J.*, 287:676–677.

Dittert, L. W., and DiSanto, A. R. (1973): The bioavailability of drug products. *J. Am. Pharm. Assoc.*, NS13:421–432.

Epstein, L. C., and Lasagna, L. (1969): Obtaining informed consent. *Arch. Intern. Med.*, 123:682–688.

Evans, E. F., Proctor, J. D., Fratkin, M. J., Velandia, J., and Wasserman, A. J. (1975): Blood flow in muscle groups and drug absorption. *Clin. Pharmacol. Ther.*, 17:44–47.

Evans, J. T. (1979): Internal monitoring: Patient and study management at the clinic. *Clin. Pharmacol. Ther.*, 25:712–716.

Feinstein, A. R. (1967): *Clinical Judgment*. Williams & Wilkins, Baltimore.

Folb, P. I. (1980): *The Safety of Medicines—Evaluation and Prediction*. Springer-Verlag, New York.

Food and Drug Administration (1974): General guidelines for the evaluation of drugs to be approved for use during pregnancy and for treatment of infants and children: A report of the Committee on Drugs, American Academy of Pediatrics to the Food and Drug Administration, U.S. DHEW. American Academy of Pediatrics, Evanston, Illinois.

Food and Drug Administration (1977a): FDA Bureau of Drugs Clinical Guidelines. General considerations for the clinical evaluation of drugs in infants and children, FDA 77-3041. Superintendent of Documents, U.S. Government Printing Office, Washington, D.C. (Over 24 separate guidelines are available for evaluation of different types of drugs in adults and children.)

Food and Drug Administration (1977b): Clinical Investigations: Proposed Establishment of Regulations on Obligations of Sponsors and Monitors. *Federal Register*, 42(187, Tuesday, September 27, 1977, Part IV):49612–49630.

Food and Drug Administration (1978): Obligations of Clinical Investigators of Regulated Articles: Proposed Establishment of Regulations. *Federal Register*, 43(153, Tuesday, August 8, 1978, Part V): 35210–35236.

Food and Drug Administration (1981a): Protection of Human Subjects; Informed Consent. *Federal Register*, 46(17, Tuesday, January 27, 1981):8942–8958.

Food and Drug Administration (1981b): Protection of Human Subjects; Standards for Institutional Review Boards for Clinical Investigations. *Federal Register*, 46(17, Tuesday, January 27, 1981):8958–8979.

Foulds, G. A. (1958): Clinical research in psychiatry. *J. Ment. Sci.*, 104:259–265.

Friedman, L. M., Furburg, C. D., and De Mets, D. L. (1981): *Fundamentals of Clinical Trials*. J. Wright, PSG, Boston.

Goldman, J., and Katz, M. D. (1982): Inconsistency and institutional review boards. *J.A.M.A.*, 248:197–202.

Goldsmith, M. A., Slavik, M., and Carter, S. K. (1975): Quantitative prediction of drug toxicity in humans from toxicology in small and large animals. *Cancer Res.*, 35:1354–1364.

Gorringe, J. A. L. (1970): Initial preparation for clinical trials. In: *The Principles and Practice of Clinical Trials*, edited by E. L. Harris and J. D. Fitzgerald, pp. 41–46. E. & S. Livingstone, Edinburgh, London.

Gray, B. H., Cooke, R. A., and Tannenbaum, A. S. (1978): Research involving human subjects. *Science*, 201:1094–1101.

Guy, W. (1976): *ECDEU Assessment Manual for Psychopharmacology* (revised), U.S. DHEW Publ. No. (ADM) 76-338, U.S. Government Printing Office, Washington, D.C.

Harris, E. L., and Fitzgerald, J. D. (eds.) (1970): *The Principles and Practice of Clinical Trials*. E. & S. Livingstone, Edinburgh, London.

Hassar, M., and Weintraub, M. (1976): "Uninformed" consent and the wealthy volunteer: An analysis of patient volunteers in a clinical trial of a new anti-inflammatory drug. *Clin. Pharmacol. Ther.*, 20:379–386.

Henkin, R. I., Schechter, P. J., Friedewald, W. T., Demets, D. L., and Raff, M. (1976): A double blind study of the effects of zinc sulfate on taste and smell dysfunction. *Am. J. Med. Sci.*, 272:285–299.

Hill, A. B. (1971): *Principles of Medical Statistics*, 9th ed. Oxford University Press, New York.

Howard, J., Whittemore, A. S., Hoover, J. J., Panos, M., and the Aspirin Myocardial Infarction Study Research Group (1982): How blind was the patient blind in AMIS? *Clin. Pharmacol. Ther.*, 32:543–553.

Hussar, D. A. (1980): Patient compliance. In: *Remington's Pharmaceutical Sciences*, 16th ed., edited by A. Osol, pp. 1703–1713. Mack, Easton, Pennsylvania.

Hutchinson, T. A., Leventhal, J. M., Kramer, M. S., Karch, F. E., et al. (1979): An algorithm for the operational assessment of adverse drug reactions. II. Demonstration of reproducibility and validity. *J.A.M.A.*, 242:633–638.

Jacobs, K. W., and Nordan, F. M. (1979): Classification of placebo drugs: Effect of color. *Percept. Mot. Skills*, 49:367–372.

Joubert, P., Rivera-Calimlim, L., and Lasagna, L. (1975): The normal volunteer in clinical investigation: How rigid should selection criteria be? *Clin. Pharmacol. Ther.*, 17:253–257.

Karch, F. E., and Lasagna, L. (1975): Adverse drug reactions. A critical review. *J.A.M.A.*, 234:1236–1241.

Karlowski, T. R., Chalmers, T. C., Frenkel, L. D., Kapikian, A. Z., et al. (1975): Ascorbic acid for the common cold. A prophylactic and therapeutic trial. *J.A.M.A.*, 231:1038–1042.

Kilo, C., Miller, J. P., and Williamson, J. R. (1980): The Achilles heel of the University Group Diabetes Program. *J.A.M.A.*, 243:450–457.

Klimt, C. R., and Canner, P. L. (1979): Terminating a long-term clinical trial. *Clin. Pharmacol. Ther.*, 25:641–646.

Knapp, T. R. (1983): A methodological critique of the 'ideal weight' concept. *J.A.M.A.*, 250:506–510.

Kramer, M. S., Leventhal, J. M., Hutchinson, T. A., and Feinstein, A. R. (1979): An algorithm for the operational assessment of adverse drug reactions. I. Background, description, and instructions for use. *J.A.M.A.*, 242:623–632.

Krauth, J. (1982): Objective measurements of the quality of life. In: *Clinical Trials in Early Breast Cancer*, edited by M. Baum, R. Kay, and H. Scheurlen, pp. 402–451. Birkhauser Verlag, Boston.

Lachin, J. M., Marks, J. W., Schoenfield, L. J., NCGS Protocol Committee, and the National Cooperative Gallstone Study Group (1981): Design and methodological considerations in the National Cooperative Gallstone Study: A multicenter clinical trial. *Control. Clin. Trials*, 2:177–229.

Lachman, L., Lieberman, H. A., and Kanig, J. L. (1976): *The Theory and Practice of Industrial Pharmacy* (2nd ed.). Lea & Febiger, Philadelphia.

Lancaster, H. O. (1974): *An Introduction to Medical Statistics*. John Wiley & Sons, New York.

Lasagna, L. (1977): Prisoner subjects and drug testing. *Fed. Proc.*, 36:2349–2351.

Lasagna, L. (1982): Historical controls. The practitioner's clinical trials. *N. Engl. J. Med.*, 307:1339–1340.

Lasagna, L. (1983): Discovering adverse drug reactions. *J.A.M.A.*, 249:2224–2225.

Leventhal, J. M., Hutchinson, T. A., Kramer, M. S., and Feinstein, A. R. (1979): An algorithm for the operational assessment of adverse drug reactions. III. Results of tests among clinicians. *J.A.M.A.*, 242:1991–1994.

Levine, R. J., and Lebacqz, K. (1979): Some ethical considerations in clinical trials. *Clin. Pharmacol. Ther.*, 25:728–741.

Lionel, N. D. W., and Herxheimer, A. (1970): Assessing reports of therapeutic trials. *Br. Med. J.*, 3:637–640.

Melmon, K., Chairman, Joint Commission on Prescription Drug Use, U.S. Senate Committee on Labor and Human Resources. Subcommittee on Health and Scientific Research (1980): Final Report. U.S. Government Printing Office, Washington, D.C.

Melzack, R. (1975): The McGill pain questionnaire: Major properties and scoring methods. *Pain*, 1:277–299.

REFERENCES

Merz, B., Hager, T., and Macek, C. (1983): New methods of drug delivery. *J.A.M.A.*, 250:145–147, 151–153.

Morgenstern, H., and Bursic, E. S. (1982): A method for using epidemiologic data to estimate the potential impact of an intervention on the health status of a target population. *J. Community Health*, 7:292–309.

Naranjo, C. A., Busto, U., Sellers, E. M., Sandor, P., et al. (1981): A method for estimating the probability of adverse drug reactions. *Clin. Pharmacol. Ther.*, 30:239–245.

National Commission for the Protection of Human Subjects of Biomedical and Behavioral Research (1977): Research on the fetus (Appendix). U.S. DHEW Pub. No.(OS)76-128. U.S. Government Printing Office, Washington, D.C.

Osol, A. (1980): *Remington's Pharmaceutical Sciences*, 16th ed. Mack, Easton, Pennsylvania.

Pearson, R. M. (1982): Who is taking their tablets? *Br. Med. J.*, 285:757–758.

Peck, C. L., and King, N. J. (1982): Increasing patient compliance with prescriptions. *J.A.M.A.*, 248:2874–2877.

Penta, J. S., Rozencweig, M., Guarino, A. M., and Muggia, F. M. (1979): Mouse and large-animal toxicology studies of twelve antitumor agents: Relevance to starting dose for phase I clinical trials. *Cancer Chemother. Pharmacol.*, 3:97–101.

Prout, T. E. (1979): Other examples of recruitment problems and solutions. *Clin. Pharmacol. Ther.*, 25:695–698.

Redwood, D. R., Rosing, D. R., Goldstein, R. E., Beiser, G. D., and Epstein, S. E. (1971): Importance of the design of an exercise protocol in the evaluation of patients with angina pectoris. *Circulation*, 43:618–628.

Riley, T. L., Porter, R. J., White, B. G., and Penry, J. K. (1981): The hospital experience and seizure control. *Neurology (N.Y.)*, 31:912–915.

Rodda, B. E. (1974): Sequential analysis in phase I and phase II clinical trials. In: *Importance of Experimental Design and Biostatistics*, edited by F. G. McMahon, pp. 19–27. Futura, Mt. Kisco.

Rodnan, G. P. (ed.) (1973): Primer on the rheumatic diseases. *J.A.M.A.*, 224(Suppl. 5):662–805.

Rossi, A. C., Knapp, D. E., Anello, C., O'Neill, R. T., et al. (1983): Discovery of adverse drug reactions—a comparison of selected phase IV studies with spontaneous reporting methods. *J.A.M.A.*, 249:2226–2228.

Rouzioux, J. M. (1979): The ethical problems of human therapeutic trials. In: *Multicenter Controlled Trials—Principles and Problems*, pp. 253–264. INSERM, Paris.

Rozencweig, M., Von Hoff, D. D., Staquet, M. J., Schein, P. S., et al. (1981): Animal toxicology for early clinical trials with anticancer agents. *Cancer Clin. Trials*, 4:21–28.

Ryan, K. J., Chairman, National Commission for the Protection of Human Subjects of Biomedical and Behavioral Research (1977): Research involving children. U.S. DHEW Pub. No. (OS) 77-0004. U.S. Government Printing Office, Washington, D.C.

Sackett, D. L. (1979): Bias in analytic research. *J. Chronic Dis.*, 32:51–63.

Schafer, A. (1982): The ethics of the randomized clinical trial. *N. Engl. J. Med.*, 307:719–724.

Schechter, P. J., Friedewald, W. T., Bronzert, D. A., Raff, M. S., and Henkin, R. I. (1972): Idiopathic hypogeusia: A description of the syndrome and a single blind study with zinc sulfate. *Int. Rev. Neurobiol. [Suppl.]*, 1:125–140.

Schoenberger, J. A. (1979): Recruitment in the coronary drug project and the aspirin myocardial infarction study. *Clin. Pharmacol. Ther.*, 25:681–684.

Schwartz, M. L., Meyer, M. B., Covino, B. G., Narang, R. M., et al. (1974):Antiarrhythmic effectiveness of intramuscular lidocaine: Influence of different injection sites. *J. Clin. Pharmacol.*, 14:77–83.

Seltzer, H. S. (1972): A summary of criticisms of the findings and conclusions of the University Group Diabetes Program (UGDP). *Diabetes*, 21:976–979.

Shubin, S. (1981): Research behind bars. Prisoners as experimental subjects. *The Sciences*, 21:10–13,29.

Spilker, B. (1983): Practical considerations in planning and conducting clinical trials with investigational or marketed drugs. *Clin. Neuropharmacol.*, 6:325–347.

Spilker, B., Bruni, J., Jones, M., Upton, A., Cato, A., and Cloutier, G. (1983): A double-blind crossover study of cinromide versus placebo in epileptic outpatients with partial seizures. *Epilepsia*, 24:410–421.

Sriwatanakul, K., Kelvie, W., Lasagna, L., Calimlin, J. F., et al. (1983): Studies with different types of visual analog scales for measurement of pain. *Clin. Pharmacol. Ther.*, 34:234–239.

Stanley, K., Stjernsward, J., and Isley, M. (1981): *Recent Results in Cancer Research, Vol. 77: The Conduct of a Cooperative Clinical Trial.* Springer-Verlag, New York.

Strom, B. L., Miettinen, O. S., and Melmon, K. L. (1983): Postmarketing studies of drug efficacy: When must they be randomized? *Clin. Pharmacol. Ther.*, 34:1–7.

Tallarida, R. J., Murray, R. B., and Eiben, C. (1979): A scale for assessing the severity of diseases and adverse drug reactions: Application to drug benefit and risk. *Clin. Pharmacol. Ther.*, 25:381–390.

Taves, D. R. (1974): Minimization: A new method of assigning patients to treatment and control groups. *Clin. Pharmacol. Ther.*, 15:443–453.

Temple, R. (1982): Government viewpoint of clinical trials. *Drug. Inform. J.*, 16:10–17.

Temple, R., and Pledger, G. W. (1980): The FDA's critique of the Anturane reinfarction trial. *N. Engl. J. Med.*, 303:1488–1492.

Thompson, E. I. (1980): Application of restricted sequential design in a clinical protocol. *Cancer Treat. Rep.*, 64:399–403.

von Kerekjarto, M. (1982): Considerations for the impact of medical therapy on quality of life. In: *Clinical Trials in Early Breast Cancer,* edited by M. Baum, R. Kay, and H. Scheurlen, pp. 388–396. Birkhauser Verlag, Boston.

Weintraub, M., Francetić, I., Hasday, J. D., Jacox, R. F., and Atwater, E. C. (1980): Tiopinac in rheumatoid arthritis: A three-phase dose-ranging, efficacy, and aspirin-withdrawal protocol. *Clin. Pharmacol. Ther.*, 27:579–585.

Weintraub, M., Sriwatanakul, K., Sundaresan, P. R., Weis, O. F., and Dorn, M. (1983): Extended-release fenfluramine: Patient acceptance and efficacy of evening dosing. *Clin. Pharmacol. Ther.*, 33:621–627.

Weissman, L. (1981): Multiple dose phase I trials—normal volunteers or patients? One viewpoint. *J. Clin. Pharmacol.*, 21:385–387.

Winship, D. H., Summers, R. W., Singleton, J. W., Best, W. R., et al. (1979): National cooperative Crohn's disease study: Study design and conduct of the study. *Gastroenterology*, 77:829–842.

Working Party on Ethics of Research in Children—British Paediatric Association (1980): Guidelines to aid ethical committees considering research involving children. *Arch. Dis. Child.*, 55:75–77.

Zelen, M. (1979): A new design for randomized clinical trials. *N. Engl. J. Med.*, 300:1242–1245.

Subject Index